Leon P. Bignold
Brian L. D. Coghlan
Hubertus P. A. Jersmann

David Paul von Hansemann: Contributions to Oncology
Context, Comments and Translations

Birkhäuser Verlag
Basel · Boston · Berlin

Authors:

Leon P. Bignold
Division of Tissue Pathology
Institute of Medical and
Veterinary Science
P. O. Box 14
Rundle Mall, SA 5001
Australia

Brian L.D. Coghlan
Centre for European Studies
and General Linguistics
University of Adelaide
Adelaide, SA 5005
Australia

Hubertus P.A. Jersmann
Department of Medicine
University of Adelaide
Adelaide, SA 5005
Australia

Library of Congress Control Number: 2006934676

Bibliographic information published by Die Deutsche Bibliothek
Die Deutsche Bibliothek lists this publication in the Deutsche Nationalbibliografie;
detailed bibliographic data is available in the Internet at <http://dnb.ddb.de>.

ISBN 13: 978-3-7643-7768-7 Birkhäuser Verlag, Basel – Boston – Berlin

The publisher and editor can give no guarantee for the information on drug dosage and administration contained in this publication. The respective user must check its accuracy by consulting other sources of reference in each individual case.
The use of registered names, trademarks etc. in this publication, even if not identified as such, does not imply that they are exempt from the relevant protective laws and regulations or free for general use.
This work is subject to copyright. All rights are reserved, whether the whole or part of the material is concerned, specifically the rights of translation, reprinting, re-use of illustrations, recitation, broadcasting, reproduction on microfilms or in other ways, and storage in data banks. For any kind of use permission of the copyright owner must be obtained.

© 2007 Birkhäuser Verlag, P.O. Box 133, CH-4010 Basel, Switzerland
Part of Springer Science+Business Media
Printed on acid-free paper produced from chlorine-free pulp. TCF ∞
Printed in Germany
Cover illustration: Portrait of David Paul von Hansemann. Courtesy Wolfgang von Hansemann, Bonn
ISBN-10: 3-7643-7768-2   e-ISBN-10: 3-7643-7769-0
ISBN-13: 978-3-7643-7768-7   e-ISBN-13: 978-3-7643-7769-4

9 8 7 6 5 4 3 2 1

Table of Contents

Preface and Overview xi
Acknowledgements xv
Notes on the Works and Translations xvii
Table of Chronology xix

Part I   Background   1

Chapter 1:
Family, education and career 3
Family background 3
Education 5
Rudolph Virchow as a teacher 7
Post-graduate career 9
Notes to chapter 1 10

Chapter 2:
Aspects of philosophy in the culture and science of Germany in the nineteenth century 25
Introduction 25
Influence of the Ancient Greeks 25
German philosophy and literature after the Reformation; *Streitkultur* . . 27
"Romantic biology" and *Naturphilosophie* 28
Characteristics of Virchow's thinking 28
Virchow's "Cellular Pathology" as a philosophy of pathology 29
Darwinism in Germany 30
Altruism, "cellular altruism" and "biologistic sociology" 32
Militarism and *Junkertum* 33
Notes to chapter 2 35

Chapter 3:
Aspects of biomedical science in the nineteenth century 41
Introduction 41
Microscopy 42
Normal histology 43
Virchow's "Cellular Pathology" – an analysis 45
Virchow and the origin and lineage fidelity (an aspect of "specificity")
    of cells 46

Embryology 46
Genetics – general considerations 48
Heredity at the level of the whole individual (ancestral heredity) 48
Heredity material in sexual reproduction 49
Cellular heredity in embryonic development 49
Heredity in cell populations which turn over in adults 50
Applications of the word "differentiation" 51
"Capacity for independent existence"; in normal, pathological and
    experimental studies 53
Notes to chapter 3 54

Chapter 4:
Theories of tumours prior to Hansemann 57
Introduction 57
The concept of "plasias" 57
Virchow's concepts of tumours 59
"Embryonal" theories of cancer 61
"Egg-like" features of cancer cells 62
"Fecundation/fertilisation/fusion" theories 63
The role of mitosis in heredity at the time of Hansemann ... 63
Chromosomes in tumour cells 66
Difficulties of diagnosis of tumours by histopathology in the 1890s:
    the case of the laryngeal cancer of Emperor Friedrich III 70
Notes to chapter 4 71

Chapter 5:
Hansemann's ideas of the nature of cancer: description and analysis .. 75
Introduction 75
The original version of the theory (Hansemann 1890a) 75
Further analysis of the oogenic model 78
Further analysis of de-differentiation and numbers of chromosomes
    in tumour cells 79
Later modifications to the detail of the theories 80
Hansemann on mitoses and chromosomes in general 82
Hansemann on abnormal mitoses and chromosomes in pathological cells ... 83
Hauptplasmen and *Nebenplasmen* 85
The problem of excessive growth of tumour cells 85
The application of anaplasia and de-differentiation to the diagnosis
    of malignant tumours 86
Hansemann's philosophy 87
Notes to chapter 5 90

Table of Contents

Chapter 6:
Critics, reviewers, the forgetting of Hansemann, and what might have been 91
Introduction 91
Ribbert and the theory of "control by connective tissue" 91
Lubarsch 92
Borst 95
O. Israel 96
Other critics: Beneke, Wolff 101
Boveri's ideas were similar to Hansemann's 101
Hauser; Farmer, Moore and Walker; Bashford 104
Other reviewers 1900–1919 105
Whitman – overlooked insights 106
Reviewers in the 1920s and after 107
Subsequent developments in cancer research 110
Why was Hansemann forgotten? – more fruitful fields of research 111
Why was Hansemann forgotten? – scientific faults of his work 112
Why was Hansemann forgotten? – other factors 114
What might have been 116
Notes to chapter 6 117

Part II   Translations   121

Chapter 7:
On the asymmetrical division of cells in epithelial carcinomata and their biological importance (1890a) 123

Chapter 8:
On pathological mitoses (1891a) 145

Chapter 9:
Karyokinesis and "Cellular Pathology" (1891c) 159

Chapter 10:
On the anaplasia of tumour cells and asymmetric mitosis (1892a) 167

Chapter 11:
"Studies on the Specificity, the Altruism and the Anaplasia of cells with Special Reference to Tumours" (1893c) 179
Introduction 182
I   Specificity 185
II Altruism 219
III Anaplasia 234

Chapter 12:
Hansemann's other articles and books on tumours and related topics . 277
Introduction 277
Pathological/anatomical and histological experiences
    after Koch's treatment (1891b) 277
Pathological/anatomical and histological observations
    after Koch's treatment (1891g) 278
Cell division in the human epidermis (1891h) 278
The cancer stroma and Grawitz' theory of dormant cells (1893a) 279
Critical reflections on the aetiology of carcinomas (1894a) 279
On the specificity of the division of cells (1894i) 280
On the so-called interstitial cells of the testis and their significance in
    pathological conditions (1895b) 281
Pathological anatomy and bacteriology (1895d) 281
The diagnosis of malignant tumours: a clinical lecture delivered at the
    University of Berlin (1895i) 282
On cure and curability (1897g) 283
"The Diagnosis of Malignant Tumours" (1897o) (second edition, 1902h) 283
On the term "anaplasia" and its essential nature (1900b) 286
On nuclear division figures of malignant tumours:
    addendum to the short communication of Messrs Farmer, Moore
    and Walker (1904c) 287
Malignant growths and normal reproductive tissues (1904q) 289
On the functional abilities of cancer cells. A discussion – observation on
    Beneke's position paper on physiological and pathological growth
    (1905c) 291
Critical contemplations on the tumour theory (1905f) 292
Talks by Prof von Hansemann and *Geheimrat* von Leyden on
    "The Aetiology of Cancers" at the Berlin Society of Medicine
    8th March 1905 (1905k) 293
What do we know of the origin of malignant tumours? (1905l) 295
On the function of tumour cells (1906c) 296
A few remarks on the anaplasia of tumour cells (1907c) 297
On the nomenclature of epithelial neoplasms (1908d) 298
What is anaplasia? (1909a) 298
"Origin and Pathology. Studies and Thoughts in Comparative Biology"
    (1909f) 299
"Atlas of Malignant Tumours" (1910k) 302
Pathological anatomy and the diagnosis of cancer (1910l) 304
Experimental chemotherapy of animals with tumours (1912a)
    (with v. Wassermann) 304
Discussion (of Experimental chemotherapy of animals with tumours)
    (1912b) 305

Experimental chemotherapy of animals with tumours (1912c)
(with v. Wassermann) 305
On altruistic diseases: A talk delivered to the Society for Doctors'
continuing education in Görlitz, 13th January, 1912 (1912d) 305
"On Conditional Thinking in Medicine and its Importance for Practice"
(1912f) 308
On precancerous conditions (1913e) 313
Demonstration of slides produced by Herr Fibiger concerning
the artificial induction of cancer (1913g) 313
A working hypothesis for research on Leukemia (1914a) 314
On changes in the tissues and tumours after ray treatment:
Demonstration lecture before the Hufeland Society
19th March 1914 (1914b) 314
On the cancer problem (1914d) 314
Cancer therapeutics in theory and practice (1914i) 315
The problem of cancer malignancy (1920a) 315

Appendix A:
Hansemann's early *curriculum vitae*; letters 317

Appendix B
Supplementary index entries to "The Science of Cancerous Disease
from Earliest Times to the Present" (Wolff, 1907) 319

Appendix C
Published obituaries 323

Appendix D
Bibliography of David Paul von Hansemann 331

Literature cited 347

Index 363

Preface and Overview

This book developed from the historical part of a general study of theories of genomic disturbances which might induce normal cells to become tumourous. It was found that in 1890, David Paul Hansemann (1858–1920) described a chromosomal theory of cancer based on a supposed pathogenic role of asymmetrical mitoses – essentially "non-disjunction" of chromosomes – in somatic cells. Hansemann was also recorded as having coined the words "anaplasia" and "dedifferentiation", which have been used for the description of tumours ever since. However, little else could be found in the literature. In view of the resurgence of interest since the 1970s in the genomic abnormalities, including aneuploidy, of tumour cells a review of Hansemann's work was considered overdue.

The work specifically for the book began with a fortuitous meeting between Drs Jersmann and Bignold at the Royal Adelaide Hospital, South Australia. Dr Jersmann translated the titles of all Hansemann's publications which could be found in the Index Medicus 1885-1920, and the complete texts of the first articles on tumours (1890a, 1891a, 1891c, 1892a – chapters 7–10) and also of the last (1920). These works revealed that Hansemann's ideas were rational, logical, well-considered and relevant to what disturbances of the genome might cause the histopathological complexity of tumours. Professor Coghlan was then approached for help with the project and agreed without hesitation to translate the remainder of Hansemann's books and articles, as well as the relevant publications of other German authors. All three of us then worked together on the content and format of this volume.

Hansemann's contributions to oncology began in 1890 with the first comprehensive theory that the conversion of normal cells to tumourous ones involves the acquisition of intracellularly-arising abnormalities in their hereditary material (not Boveri in 1914, as has been commonly asserted). Next, Hansemann emphasised the fact that – for many tumour types – there are *always* some cells which have hyperchromatic nuclei and some which have hypochromatic nuclei. Hansemann noted that these changes of nuclear chromatism are at least partly due in turn to the nuclei having excess or reduced numbers of chromosomes respectively. This was the first assertion of significance for the phenomenon of "aneuploidy" for these types of tumours. While considering the significance of altered numbers of chromosomes in cells, Hansemann noted August Weismann's theory that differentiation of cells in embryos occurs by way of loss of chromosomal material. Hansemann then proposed that asymmetric mitoses in normal cells result in cells which are both tumourous and suffer a "loss of differentiation" (*Entdifferenzierung*). Further, Hansemann recognised that the particular type of differentiation which was lost during the change of a normal cell into a tumourous one could not be the same type of differentiation which the previously-normal cell had acquired during its embryological development. Instead, Hansemannn proposed that the dedifferentiation manifest by tumour cells is similar to the changes of oogenesis in the ovary, i.e. loss of "germinal epithelial" features during progress towards an independent cell (the egg). It was for this oogenesis-like biological process of supposed "de-differentiation" that Hansemann introduced the word "anaplasia". Thus the processes of "anaplasia" and "de-differentiation" were in fact parts of an abstract, theoretical "superstructure" which Hansemann added on to his basic idea, namely that some alteration in the hereditary material of a normal cell converts it into a tumourous one. In this article too, he proposed even more abstract concepts of cell physiology – especially their "specificity" and "altruism".

Within two years of Hansemann's original article, Weismann retracted his theory of "differentiation by loss of chromosomal material". Hansemann accepted this, and therefore had to admit that there was no known chromosomal or genetic basis available to account for "anaplasia" and "de-differentiation". Hansemann (1892a) changed his definition of "anaplasia" accordingly. The result of the change of definition was to increase the already-existing confusion concerning the meaning of the words. However, for the rest of his life, Hansemann continued to insist that some genome-altering process is at work in tumour formation such that commonly associated morphological and physiological/behavioural abnormalities appear together at the same time in a normal cell when it is converted into a tumour cell. When expanding on all these ideas in a book ("Studies on the Specificity, Altruism and Anaplasia of Cells" – 1893c) Hansemann gave greater emphasis to the abstract concepts of "specificity" and "altruism". In fact this book amounted to an attempted "systematisation of cancerous phenomena", which can be interpreted as a "philosophy of cancer".

Hansemann's theoretical concepts were not well-received at the time. Nevertheless he began to describe the application of his theory of "anaplasia" to the practical problem of the diagnosis and nomenclature of tumours. His resulting book ("The Microscopic Diagnosis of Malignant Tumours" 1897o, 2nd edn 1902h) is of great significance for the history of histopathology as a part of the practice of medicine. This volume described how to diagnose malignant tumours using the supposed properties of the theoretical process: – i.e. anaplasia. Hansemann addressed the issue that tumour cells can vary in their degrees of abnormality not only between cases of the same type of tumour, but also in the same individual case of tumour. Previously the latter lesions had been described by Virchow (1888) as "mixed tumours" (different tumour types in the same lesion). Hansemann insisted that they are cases deriving from the same cell type but showing differences in degrees of "anaplasia" and "de-differentiation". Therefore "The Microscopic Diagnosis..." (1897o, 1902h), together with Hansemann's colour "Atlas" (1910k), were the original analyses of the histopathology of tumours in the ways which histopathologists have used throughout the world ever

Preface and Overview

since. Thus Hansemann was not only the original father (*Urvater*) of the idea of the endo-cellularly-altered-genome concept of tumour formation, but also of the current method of describing the microscopic appearances of tumours for diagnostic purposes.

Hansemann made yet further contributions to pathology and medicine. He was an exceptionally clear thinker on a variety of medical matters. Although all these topics cannot be pursued in this book, it may be noted that Hansemann made original contributions to the understanding of the causation of rickets (noted by Porter, 1999), and provided the first descriptions of malacoplakia and of cerebral cryptococcosis. Hansemann is a good example of the rigorously objective, rational and thorough intellectualism of many German scientists in the late nineteenth century. Indeed, he could be adopted as a model for any cancer theorist today because of his demand for *Gesamtheit*: that any acceptable theory of tumours must explain **all** the phenomena – clinical behaviour in the patient as well as the pathological, epidemiological and aetiological characteristics – of tumours.

To give some reasonable account of Hansemann and his ideas, it was decided (and our publisher agreed) that the main part of this book should be our translations and abstracts of Hansemann's works. However, we also have tried to understand many underlying issues concerning Hansemann and his *travail*. These are especially: What was his family, social and educational background? What cell biological knowledge did Hansemann rely on for his ideas? Why did Hansemann add a philosophical superstructure to his chromosomal theory? What were Virchow's possible influences on Hansemann? Why was Hansemann so concerned with "specificity" of cells? Why were the debates at the time so vigorous, sometimes to the point of being personal? Were there any particular reasons why Hansemann was forgotten during the twentieth century? Do Hansemann's ideas have relevance to cancer research today, and did Hansemann ask any important – if forgotten – questions concerning cancer biology?

We have addressed these questions in the six introductory chapters. We hope that they will be a sufficient guide for the easy understanding of the translated and summarised works which form the rest of the book.

As a last note, we are aware that among the translations, there is some repetition of ideas. However, we felt that if any text were deleted from any of the major articles or from "Studies..." (1893c) some readers would be concerned that something of interest to them had been omitted.

We are very grateful to our publisher, and particularly Dr Beatrice Menz, Senior Editor, for agreeing to publish such a large amount of translation in this way.

L. P. Bignold, Adelaide, South Australia, September 2006
B. L. D. Coghlan,
H. P. A. Jersmann

Acknowledgements

We wish to acknowledge first our teachers, who fostered our skills and interests in our disciplines: in particular Professor Donald L. Wilhelm, late Head of the Department of Pathology at the University of New South Wales (L. P. B.), Professor Roy Pascal, late Head of the Department of German at the University of Birmingham (B. L. D. C.) as well as Dr. med. H.-G. Shiel and Dr. med. U. Claussen (H. P. A. J).

At an early stage in the development of the book, Mr Thomas Kruckemeyer, of GLS -German Language Services (Adelaide), very kindly provided the translation of the section "Anaplasia" in Hansemann's (1893c) book as it appears in chapter 11 of this volume.

Ms Mary Peterson assisted with research in Berlin and London and advised on the later drafts of the introductory chapters. She took the photographs of the pathology buildings at the Friedrichshain Hospital and at the Klinikum Rudolph Virchow, as well as of the Hansemann mausoleum, all in Berlin.

Herr Wolfgang von Hansemann, grandson of David Paul, discussed the project with us at length and has allowed us to use the portrait of his grandfather and other family members as well as the photographs of the family.

Ms Elizabeth Goodwin typed many of the translations from dication tapes and assisted with the compilation of the bibliography.

Dr Jürgen Hammerstein (Director of the *Kaiserin-Friedrich-Stiftung*) gave permission to use photographs of that post-graduate medical institute. Ms Elke-Barbara Peschke, Director of the Historic Book Collection of Humboldt-Universität Library, Berlin, provided the photograph of Virchow originally taken about 1890, and the photograph of Hansemann in middle age.

The copies of Hansemann's letters were obtained by courtesy of the Manuscript Department (*Handschriftenabteilung*) of the *Staatsbibliothek* in Berlin; the *Referat Handschriften-Rara* of the *Staats- und Universitätsbibliothek* Bremen; and the *Bayerische Staatsbibliothek*, Munich.

For discussions and other help we thank Professor Dr. med. Thomas Schnalke (Director of the Institute of Medical History at the Virchow Museum, Charité, Berlin), Professor Steffen Hauptmann (Professor of Pathology, Univerity of Halle), Dr Frank Orro (Pathologist at the Friedrichshain Hospital), Dr Lothar Nunnemacher (formerly Librarian at the Klinikum R. Virchow, Berlin), and Dr. med. Barbara Fey (Director of the Berlin Society for Cancer Research).

We must thank especially Ms Jennifer Harbster of the Library of Congress, Washington DC; Mr Jeremy Cullis of the Fisher Library, University of Sydney;

and Ms Tricia Boyd of the Edinburgh University Library for assistance with particular references.

We are also grateful to the staffs of the Library of the American Philosophical Society, Philadelphia PA; and of the Libraries of the Universities of Adelaide; Clark (Delaware); Melbourne and Leipzig; as well as of the British Library, London; the Royal Australasian College of Physicians, Sydney; and the Town Archives, Eupen, Belgium.

Dr Jürgen Real, Emeritus Professor Dr. med. Werner Schoop, Professor Dr. Dieter Lohmeier, Dr. Gert Sieper, Mr Harald Ohlendorf, Dr. John Hatch, Ms Marie-Louise Krone and Ms Carol Guppy gave assistance with references and other material.

We received much support and encouragement from our family members: James Bignold, Monica Bignold, Sybil Coghlan, Adrian Coghlan and Samantha, Stephanie and Mia Jersmann.

Dr Beatrice Menz, our Senior Editor at the publishers, has been unfailingly kind and helpful with suggestions on content and style.

Notes on the Works and Translations

Some German nineteenth century academic works achieved complexities of expression and thought which have been little rivalled at any time in the English-speaking world. In addition, the works of some German authors were notorious for lack of obvious structure, for repetitions, sudden changes in lines of thought, long sentences, complex grammatical constructions and so on. In brief, the styles of writing of Kant and Hegel (see chapter 2) cast a long shadow. As an example in the field of biology, W. M. Wheeler, the translator of Roux's Introduction to the *Archiv für Entwickelungsmechanik der Organismen* (1894) included a note:

> "Besides the difficulties resulting from the great compactness of Professor Roux's style, there are others, not the least of which is the great conciseness of meaning with which all the terms are used, and the often very delicate qualifications of the leading ideas in the various paragraphs and sentences" (see Maienschein, 1986).

Some of these features are prominent in Hansemann's early work. Mainly, the problem is of *Eingesponnenheit* ("spinning into oneself") which applies to spinning thoughts further and further while ensuring that no particle of an idea is left behind. Thus Hansemann's sentences frequently are very long, with many qualifications and continuous flows of ideas. The sequences of ideas, especially in parts of the first article (1890a) and in "Studies..." (1893c) often seem to have no order at all. In addition, and especially when he was unsure of the truth of his suggestions, Hansemann used complex qualifying clauses within clauses to make up long sentences (*Schachtelsätze*). He also exhibited the habit of "*mitdenken*" ("thinking along"), for example, when a verb is mentioned once, it in fact applies to the next clause as well. Some phrases are almost reminiscent of the more esoteric forms of old-style literary commentary. (This style became effectively obsolete after 1918).

However, in the later works, and especially when Hansemann was sure of his ideas, his writing for the greater part was simple and straightforward. In fact, Hansemann often repeated his points in successive sentences, in a way which is almost that of *"Faust auf den Tisch"* – "fist on the table".

The aim of the present translations has been to render nineteenth century German into Victorian-Edwardian English, and evoke the spirit of the age, i.e. the comity of *fin de siècle* Europe. Frequently in Hansemann (1890a) and (1893c), we have found it necessary to break sentences and introduce colons, semi-colons and dashes to achieve readability. Excessive compactness of style has been countered with insertions of words, which are indicated in brackets, and if several words are introduced, "-eds" is included. Except for this, we have tried to preserve the style of the longer sentences which often achieves a cumulative effect (*Steigerung*).

We have tried to avoid presenting more meaning than was evident in the original (*hineininterpretieren*).

On specific points:

- As was normal at the time, summaries in any form were lacking in most of Hansemann's articles. We have provided them.
- *Reiz* can mean either "irritation" or "stimulation", the latter even to the point of "attractiveness" as in *eine reizende Frau* (a really attractive woman). Virchow (1858) quite specifically used the word to mean irritation. In Hansemann's works on oncology, we think that *Reiz* has been used in the sense of an irritation, especially because it is always applied to carcinogenic agents, which are never "attractive".
- *Bindegewebe* has been rendered as "connective tissue" although the meaning is perhaps more accurately "supportive tissue" as indicated by the translator (M. Campbell) of part 1 of Hertwig's "The Cell. Outlines of General Anatomy and Physiology" (1892). *Richtungkörperchen* is not now used in German, but Hansemann used it initially for polar bodies in oogenesis according to Hertwig's description (Hertwig, 1890). Later, *Polkörperchen* ("polar bodies") was preferred.
- *Entdifferenzirung* means "de-differentiation", not "un-differentiation". Thus if one defuses an explosive mine, one uses the term *Entsorgen* – to take the fuse out. (In English, the usages are less strictly observed: thus "undressing" really means "de-dresssing").
- *Konditional* we have translated as "conditional" and *Bedingung* we render as "pre-condition".
- *Offenbar* can mean either "apparently", "evidently", "clearly" or "obviously" and in many instances, Hansemann's precise meaning is unclear.
- We indicate our author as "Hansemann" when referring to his articles before 1902 and as either "Hansemann" or "von Hansemann" when dealing with articles or issues which arose after the family was ennobled "von" in 1902.
- Where emphasis in the original is indicated by increased font and spacing between letters (*Sperrdruck*), we have ignored the style if it applied to an author's name, and generally rendered it in SMALL CAPITALS if originally indicating emphasis.
- *Italics* have been reserved for all foreign language, and italics in inverted commas if the foreign words form a significant phrase, e.g. "*omnis cellula e cellula*". Where emphasis was indicated in original English-language material, generally such text has been transcribed in **Bold**. Otherwise, **Bold** has been mainly reserved for headings in our own text.
- For abbreviations such as "a. a. O", for which Latin abbreviations ("op. cit.") are often used in English publications, everyday English has been used.

Table of Chronology

1790	David Justus Hansemann born in Finkenwerder, near Hamburg.
1793	Family moved to Heiligenfelde in the Electorate of Hanover.
1806	Napoleon defeated Prussia at the Battle of Jena. By the subsequent Treaty of Tilsit, Prussia lost approximately half of its territory. Napoleon created the "Confederation of the Rhine"; Hanover was divided and experienced very mixed fortunes.
1810	University of Berlin founded according to a plan prepared by August Wilhelm von Humboldt. The philosopher Friedrich Schleiermacher was first Rector.
1815	At the Treaty of Versailles Prussia regained the territories lost in 1808, and acquired additional lands, especially in the Catholic Rhineland. Kingdom of Hanover promulgated, within the new "German Confederation" which replaced the old "Holy Roman Empire".
1817	Active German national-liberal and democratic sentiments began, exemplified by the mass meeting of German students on the Wartburg near Eisenach: Luther tercentenary. David Justus began trading in wool on his own account in Aachen.
1819	Carlsbad Decrees proscribed both national-liberal and democratic movements in German Confederation.
1821	Birth of Virchow.
1825	David Justus founded Aachen Fire Insurance Mutual Company.
1826	Birth of Adolph Hansemann.
1827	Discovery of the mammalian egg by von Baer.
1828	Raspail coined the phrase *"omnis cellula e cellula"*.
1829	Birth of Gustav Hansemann.
1834	Customs Union of German States (*Zollverein*) formed, leading to greater opportunities for the German commercial and industrial entrepreneurs.
1835	Practicable achromatic lenses for microscopes invented. First railway in Germany (Nürnberg to Fürth in Bavaria).
1837	Affair of the "Göttingen Seven" marked an attempt to resist illiberalism in German Academia.
1838	Müller published volume on the microscopic appearances of tumours.

1842–1854	Publication of Comte's major works on Logical Positivism, including the concept of "Altruism".
1844	Silesian weavers' revolt against poor living conditions and industrialisation.
1845	David Justus elected to the Rhenish Provincial Assembly.
1847–8	Virchow sent to investigate epidemics in Silesia; reported that the causes were lack of sanitation associated with poor living conditions. Virchow evolved a radical "biologistic" social philosophy. Founded his journal later known as "Virchow's Archives".
1848	Liberal/Democratic Revolution in many European states. Publication of Marx' and Engels' "Communist Manifesto". David Justus appointed Finance Minister in Camphausen Government of 1848. Virchow among the revolutionaries.
1849	Liberal all-German regime ("Frankfurt Parliament"). However, Virchow forced to leave Berlin; became Professor of Pathology at Würzburg. Subsequently illiberalism increased in German society and academia throughout the remainder of the century.
1854	Pasteur described fermentation of sugar by bacteria.
1855	In an essay on "Cellular Pathology" Virchow stated that all disease is due to disturbed physiological activities of cells. Addison described syndrome associated with adrenal cortical insufficiency.
1851	David Justus founded the Discount Bank.
1856	Virchow returned to Berlin as Director of Pathology at the Charité and Professor of Pathology at the University of Berlin.
1857	Control of the Discount Bank passed to Adolph.
1858	Birth of David Paul Hansemann, son of Gustav Hansemann. Virchow's "Cellular Pathology" published, popularising *omnis cellula e cellula*.
1859	Darwin's "Origin of Species" published in England.
1860	Pasteur enunciated the dictum: "*omne vivum e vivo*".
1861	Virchow member of Prussian Assembly, cofounder of the Progress Party (*Fortschrittspartei*) in the Assembly in Berlin.
1862	Bismarck became Minister President in Prussia.
1864	Danish-Prussian War: Prussia gained hegemony over Schleswig-Holstein, the latter subsequently incorporated into Prussia. David Justus Hansemann died. Pope Pius IX issued the "Syllabus of Errors", which was a precursor of the doctrine of papal infallibility (Vatican Council, 1870).
1865	Introduction of haematoxylin as a stain for nuclei.

Table of Chronology

1866	Defeat of Austria in the Austro-Prussian War led to exclusion of Austria from the German Confederation. Establishment of a new "North German Confederation" dominated by Prussia. Klebs, previously an *Assistent* to Virchow, accepted a position in Bern, and began research in bacteriological causation of disease, leading to later acrimonious arguments with Virchow.
1869	Foundation of the German Social Democratic Party.
1870–1	Franco-Prussian War. Annexation of Alsace-Lorraine; declaration of the German Second Reich, excluding Austria. Reparations from France were used extensively to build many new hospitals and associated medical schools throughout Germany.
1870s	Beginning of *Kulturkampf* in which Virchow's party joined with Bismarck, thus severely reducing the influence of Liberalism in Germany.
	Hansemann family moved to Berlin. Adolph became even more successful as a financier and industrialist, with a large house on the Tiergartenstrasse. David Paul attended gymnasia in Berlin. Gustav Hansemann published books on mathematics and philosophy.
1873	Widespread collapse of banks. After this, markedly prosperous period (*Gründerzeit*) for German Reich.
1875	Hertwig described fertilisation of eggs by single sperm. Strassburger described nuclear division occurring in plant cells. Vol. 1 of Herbert Spencer's "System of Synthetic Philosophy" published in German translation.
1876	Microscopes with apochromatic lenses introduced by Zeiss. Koch discovered that anthrax is caused by a specific bacterium.
1878	Discovery of nuclear "filaments" "threads" "loops" (later named "chromosomes").
1879	Accommodation was reached between Bismarck and the Catholic Church; end of *Kulturkampf*. Arnold described abnormal nuclear division in tumour cells.
1880s	Bismarck introduced "welfare state" legislation – often considered a form of "state socialism".
1881	Pasteur invented an anti-anthrax vaccine. Hansemann began medical studies, mainly in Leipzig, but with one semester in Kiel and one in Berlin.
1882	Flemming introduced the word "mitosis". Koch invented culture of bacteria on solid substrates. Virchow opposed to almost all concepts of microbial aetiology of human disease, and did not support Koch when the latter was provided with extensive funds for research at the University of Berlin.

1884	Van Beneden introduced the term "chromosomes" and, along with other authors, described their replication by longitudinal splitting.
1885	Hansemann obtained his medical degree from Leipzig.
1886	Hansemann began as Professional Assistant (*Assistent*) to Virchow in Berlin.
1888	Weismann proposed that "differentiation" in embryonal tissues occurs by loss of chromatin material, while Hertwig and Nägeli believed that differentiation is achieved by sequential variations in the influences of the hereditary units ("gemmules" – Darwin; "plasmas" – Weismann; "ids" – Nägeli). Boveri described reduction of chromosome numbers during divisions of cells in Ascaris gonads. Death of Kaiser Wilhelm I. Accession of Emperor Friedrich III, who died three months later of laryngeal cancer. Virchow had initially suggested that the Kaiser's lesion might be syphilitic. Emperor Wilhelm II ascended the throne.
1890	Hansemann published chromosomal theory of cancer suggesting that tumour cells "lose differentiation" in an "anaplastic"/oogenesis-like way. Koch announced the discovery of the tubercle bacillus. Kaiser Wilhelm II dismissed Bismarck from all his offices of State.
1891	Hansemann publicly disagreed with von Leyden about the value and safety of the tuberculin test for tuberculosis in humans.
1892	Weismann retracted his theory that "differentiation" occurs by chromosomal loss, leaving the Hertwig/Nägeli hypothesis unopposed.
1893	Hansemann published his book "Studies... etc" (1893c) in which many of the known biological features of cancer cells were grouped into the abstract concepts of "Specificity", "Altruism" and "Anaplasia". Radical social sentiments in Gerhart Hauptmann's play "The Weavers" (based on the Silesian weavers' revolt of 1844 – above) deeply offended Emperor Wilhelm II.
1894	Hansemann published an article suggesting that the use of diphtheria convalescent serum may be harmful to patients with this disease.
1895	Hansemann appointed prosector at the Friedrichshain Hospital, Berlin.
1897	Hansemann's "The Microscopic Diagnosis of Malignant Tumours" published. Hansemann appointed Titular Professor (*Extraordinarius*) of Pathology, University of Berlin.

Table of Chronology

1900+	Hansemann published many attempts to clarify the meaning of "anaplasia" in the face of much misunderstanding.
	Fruitful lines of investigation into the aetiology (X-rays, chemical carcinogens, infectious agents) and treatment of cancer (especially with X-rays) were developed. Relatively speaking, interest in the precise nature of the abnormality in cancer cells declined.
1901	Gustav Hansemann (and hence David Paul) ennobled *von*.
1902	Gustav Hansemann died.
	Sutton and Boveri suggested independently that the pairing of chromosomes parallels Mendel's "paired factors".
	Second edition of Hansemann's "The Microscopic Diagnosis … etc".
1905	Experimental genetic researches conducted by Morgan, Sturtevant, Wilson, Bridges and Muller on Mendelian genetics published but given little attention by pathologists in Germany.
	Hansemann and von Leyden expressed completely opposite views in a public debate on the nature of cancer.
1906	Hansemann attempted to clarify his views on the functions of tumour cells.
1912	Hansemann defended his idea of "altruistic" diseases. In doing so, he denied that the anti-diabetic factor is produced by the islets of Langerhans. Hansemann also drew simplistic conclusions from pathological observations concerning the functional capacity of endocrine glands.
	Hansemann stated that transplantable mouse tumours have no relevance to human cancers.
1914	Boveri's book on the origin of malignant tumours was published. It was simplistic and selective in its approach. Its major idea was based on a mitotic mechanism already described by Hansemann.
	Outbreak of W.W. I, Hansemann served on the Eastern Front as Chief Army Pathologist.
1914–19	W.W. I broke previous cultural links between Germany and the rest of the world; also hindered and delayed reception in Germany of the new genetics principles which derived from the work of Morgan's group.
	War and the epidemic of Spanish Influenza also depleted the numbers of German young men and the facilities for their education.
1918	Kaiser abdicated. Widespread popular reaction against the war. Armistice.

1919+	First German republic (Weimar). Government coalition led by Social Democrats (Scheidemann, Ebert). Civil unrest and assassinations of republican and left wing leaders. Hansemann returned to Berlin and resumed academic duties.
1920	Hansemann developed cancer of the throat and died.
1920+	Traditional German cultural and scientific value systems essentially unchanged despite some artistic and social adventurism. Boveri's supposed originality for a chromosomal theory of cancer stated by Borst and Bauer. This error was repeated by many later authors. Additional reasons for forgetting Hansemann were that he was considered "too philosophical". His ideas became harder to understand by younger scientists who were not aware of Hansemann's historical or scientific contexts.
1960+	Interest in chromosomes and DNA in cancer increased because many carcinogens are found to react with DNA and cause strand breaks; xeroderma pigmentosum is found to be due to a hereditary defect of DNA repair; genomic instability confirmed as a major phenomenon in malignant cells.

Part I:

Background

Chapter 1

Family, education and career

Family background

Scientists come from all socio-economic levels and family circumstances, and their careers follow various paths. These outcomes are sometimes in keeping with the abilities and industriousness of the scientists themselves, and sometimes not. The degrees to which these factors affect the quality of the contribution which each researcher makes to science is debatable, and not usually considered in detail in books of this type. However, David Paul Hansemann's family was very prominent in Germany at the time, and his scientific work and career have many unusual features. Hence many details of his background are given here, especially because all of the sources are in German and perhaps less accessible to readers who are unfamiliar with this language.

The Hansemann family name was recorded in the region of the city of Hanover in the middle of the sixteenth century (von Hansemann, 1968). There were, however, apparently few notable members of the family until the nineteenth century (Dabritz, 1954). David Paul's great-grandfather was a Lutheran pastor, who for a time had a parish at Finkenwerder near Hamburg, where David Paul's grandfather (David Justus Hansemann, 1790–1864, Fig. 1) was born. The family moved to the Hanover area in 1795, and later to other parishes in the region. After leaving school, David Justus was employed in the textile industry, and in 1817 he established a commission business in the wool trade in Aachen (buying wool in eastern Germany, and selling it to the newly-established woollen mills in the Rhineland) with capital from his own savings. In 1821 he married Fanny Fremerey (1801–1876) whose father owned a woollen mill in Eupen (now in Belgium). They had four daughters and two sons.

The times after the Congress of Vienna (1815) were favourable to enterprising Prussians. Napoleon I had abolished the residual aspects of feudalism in many German states, and because that system could not be restored, a free labour market was created. The Congress restored to Prussia the territories it had lost during the wars with Napoleon, and gave her considerable additional territory in the Rhineland. The resulting greatly increased opportunities for individual Prussians were enhanced again by the German customs Union (*Zollverein*) in 1834 and later economic reforms (Henderson, 1984; Lee, 1991; Brophy, 1998).

David Justus' prominence in business began in 1824–5 when he founded the Aachen Fire Insurance Co, on the model of the English mutual-shares company. Only the fourth of its type in Germany, the company rapidly expanded to Munich, becoming the Aachen and Munich Fire Insurance Society. In 1835 David

Justus founded the Rhineland Railway based in Cologne, and later established the Aachen branch of the Society for the Encouragement of Industriousness (*Arbeitsamkeit*). This society was a labour-organisation somewhat resembling the Cooperative Movement in England (Dabritz, 1954), and it later contributed a large sum to the foundation of the Technical College (*Technische Hochschule*) in Aachen (Dabritz, 1954; Corr and Richter, ND).

From the 1840s David Justus devoted himself to politics and political writing on the liberal side. At this time, the state governments of the Rhineland and the south-west of Germany were generally politically more liberal than those of Prussia proper and the overarching goal of the leading politicians in the region was constitutional monarchy for Prussia as whole and the smaller states and principalities.

In 1845 David Justus represented Aachen in the Rhenish Provincial Assembly (*Landtag*) which sat in Coblenz. In 1847, he was a member of the unified Prussian provincial assembly which was summoned to Berlin by Friedrich Wilhelm IV (b 1795, d 1861, r 1840-1858). This parliament demanded constitutional monarchy for Prussia and was dismissed by Friedrich Wilhelm, thus precipitating the 1848 Revolution in Prussia. (A similarity to the summoning of the Estates General to Paris in 1789 and the ensuing revolution may be discerned in this). David Justus was Finance Minister in the first revolutionary government led by Camphausen (1812–1896) (Hofmann, 1981), and on the latter's retirement in June 1848, formed a government with Auerwald (1795–1866). This government was dissolved later in 1848, when the conservatives regained control (*Reaktion*) from the revolutionaries (Taddey, 1977). Subsequently, David Justus was a member for several Rhenish provinces of a democratic assembly which was later convened to consider constitutional matters, but he withdrew entirely from politics in 1852 when that assembly was suppressed by the military, and royal autocracy was reinstated as the system of government (Dabritz, 1954).

David Justus Hansemann returned to a banking career, becoming Chief of the Prussian Bank 1848–1851, and founding the Discount Bank 1851. He died in 1864. In 1884, a statue of him (Fig. 2) was erected in the *Hansemann Platz* in Aachen.

David Justus' elder son and fourth child Adolph (1826–1903) was even more successful commercially than his father. At first, he was apprenticed in a textile firm in Leipzig, but after two years returned to the Rhineland. At 17, he entered the cloth factory of his cousin Wilhelm (mother's side) in Eupen. Adolph prospered at the Eupen firm, so that when David Justus entered politics in the 1840s, he left all financial affairs to Adolph. In the 1850s Adolph worked jointly with his father in the development of the Discount Bank, and became managing director and joint owner in 1857. Subsequently Adolph played a significant part in the financing of the Danish War (1864), the Austro-Prussian War (1866), and the Franco-Prussian War (1870–1). Adolph's other activities included raising loans for railways, expansion of the Discount Bank into the

Education

other states of Germany, and then overseas, with branches in London, South America, East Asia, Italy and Romania. He indulged successfully in property speculation during the boom years (*Gründerzeit*) after 1870, and colonial enterprises. He was ennobled (allowing the use of the title *von*) in 1872. His wife Ottilie (née von Kusserow, 1840–1919) was responsible for a large donation for the foundation of a women's college (originally the *Viktoria-Lyzeum*, now *Haus Ottlie von Hansemann*) in Charlottenburg for the University of Berlin in 1908. Their home on the Tiergartenstrasse in Berlin was apparently palatial but has not survived. The street is now lined mainly by new embassy buildings. Adolph's son Ferdinand (1861–1900) and hence David Paul's cousin, was not significantly involved in commerce, but participated indirectly in nationalist politics, especially in the foundation of the German Eastern Marches Society (Dabritz, 1954).

David Justus' other son, Gustav (1829–1902, Fig. 3) married – in 1855 – Mathilde Vorländer (1827–1880), daughter of Dr med. Daniel Vorländer and Maria Anna Fuhrmann. Gustav was less inclined to commerce than his brother, but managed a woolen mill in Eupen (Fig. 4). The children of Gustav and Mathilde were (1) Fanny Marianne (b Eupen 1856–1923), m 1876 Paul Maximilian *Freiherr*[1] von Reibnitz (1838–1900) Vice Admiral ret., Law Knight in the Order of St John; and (2) David Paul (1858–1920), the subject of this book, who was born in Eupen (von Hansemann, 1968).

In the 1870s, Gustav retired from industry and became a mathematician and physicist in Berlin. He published three books (von Hansemann 1863, 1871a, 1871b), of which the last has considerable philosophical content. Gustav's side of the Hansemann family seems to have been financially comfortable, but not as wealthy as Adolph's family. Gustav was ennobled *von* in 1901.

Other descendants of the family were prominent in academic, commercial and diplomatic circles. For example, Daniel Vorländer (1867-1941) was born in Eupen as the fourth child of Gustav Hansemann's sister Sophie. This Vorländer became professor of chemistry at Halle, and discovered the first liquid crystal material (Buchwald, 1996).

David Paul Hansemann's education and medical career are detailed in the next sections. Here we can note that in 1885 David Paul married Elizabeth Amalie Wilhelmine Walter (b in Eisenach 1863, d in Berlin 1935), daughter of the *Post-Geheimrat*[1] Fritz Walter and his wife Theresa (née Frankenstein). David and Elisabeth had one child, a son (for further details see von Hansemann, 1968).

Education

According to his curriculum vitae described in a letter held in the State Library in Berlin (Appendix A) Hansemann did not attend a primary school, but was tutored at home in the style of the high school for students intending commercial careers (*Realschule*)[2] until the age of fifteen. At some unknown time, he decided on a career in natural sciences. When the family had moved to Berlin, David Paul attended a high school of *Gymnasium*-type in Charlottenburg[3]. He later went to the Friedrich-Wilhelm *Gymnasium*[4] in central (*Mitte*) Berlin, from which he matriculated at Easter in 1881. Throughout this period, he would have received substantial education in the Classics (Latin and Ancient Greek languages) according to the German educational philosophy of "(properly) formed-ness" (*Bildung*[5]). It is not known precisely when he decided to become a medical doctor, or whether his maternal grandfather (Dr med. Daniel Vorländer, see above) influenced this decision.

Hansemann's undergraduate career studies occurred within the German university system[6] in general and the university medical school system in particular. David Paul began his medical course in 1881, and apparently spent three semesters in Berlin[7], one in Kiel and three in Leipzig (Appendix A). During the long summer holidays of 1883, at Leipzig, Hansemann completed an elective in pathology, with Cohnheim[8], and in the subsequent semester, carried out a special pathology assignment under Weigert[9]. The excellence of the German medical schools in comparison to those of all other countries in the period 1860–1914 is well recognised (see Bonner, 1963; Jarausch, 1982; Cocks and Jarausch, 1990). We assume that Hansemann would not have felt particularly out of place in his Medical School environment, because of all medical students, 17 % came from families of the "business elite", 15 % from the "Government elite" and 23 % from "High Office" (Jarausch, 1982). We are unaware of his membership of the student voluntary organisations[10], which were such a prominent part of German student life at the time.

The schools attracted students from all parts of the world, and particularly exerted a great influence on American medicine (Bonner, 1963). For example, the original staff of the Johns Hopkins Hospital were trained mainly in Germany (Sigerist, 1942) and the Mayo brothers, when developing the Mayo Clinic in Minnesota, made numerous trips to Germany to study the latest treatments (Clapesattle, 1941). Hun (1893) in his "Guide to American Medical Students in Europe" (1883) notes many details, ranging from the student accommodation available in the various German cities to assessments of the teaching at the various schools. The entries regarding the medical schools at which Hansemann studied include the following.

Leipzig. "The advantages for studying anatomy in Leipzig are probably unsurpassed in the world." ... "The laboratories etc belonging to the university are handsome new buildings ..." ... "One of the most popular courses in Leipzig is that of Prof. Cohnheim on pathological anatomy. He holds a course on demonstrative pathological anatomy ..."

The academic staff at Leipzig included an illustrious group of medical scientists: His[11] (histology), Thiersch (surgery), E. L. Wagner (internal medicine),

Carl Ludwig (experimental physiology) and Weigert[9] (elementary pathological histology; infectious diseases). On a lighter note, Hun records that "Leipzig has a good opera and several good theatres"

Berlin. Hun (1883) records: "There is much rivalry between Berlin and Vienna ... but there will probably have to be an entire change in the method of instruction in Berlin before it will become very attractive to the foreign medical student...."

"Prof. Virchow gives systematic lectures on pathological anatomy, illustrated by specimens, daily in the winter semester, from 1 to 2 PM and in the summer semester from 11 to 12 M. In the first part of the hour, he exhibits any interesting pathological specimens which he may have, whether or not they are connected with the subject of his lecture; and then, while these specimens are passing about from student to student, he proceeds with his regular lecture. On Mondays from 8 to 10 AM in the winter semester, and from 7.30 to 9 AM in the summer semester, autopsies are made before the class by Prof. Virchow in the first part of the semester and by his students under his criticism during the last part of the semester. The examination of the body and viscera is very minute and accurate. On Wednesdays and Fridays at the same hour, Prof. Virchow exhibits macroscopic pathological specimens and lectures upon them, and passes microscopic sections of them about among the students. These exercises, and the autopsy exercise, are exceedingly valuable. On Tuesdays, Thursdays and Saturdays at the same hour, the assistant gives a course in which the students cut and examine under the microscope fresh pathological specimens...."

"Privatdocent Dr Friedlander (sic) gives a good course on pathological histology. Prof Jacobson gives a course on experimental pathological investigations. Dr Schiffer gives a course on experimental pathology and therapeutics."

(For further notes on Virchow as a teacher, see below).

Kiel. This medical school is mentioned in Hun's book (1883) only by a list of courses, and the names of the academic staff. The Professor of Anatomy from 1876 to 1901 was Walter Flemming (see chapter 3), who conducted so much of the research into chromosomes in this period, and presumably had a great influence on von Hansemann. Kiel was a wealthy city, the largest in Schleswig-Holstein.

Because Hansemann was an undergraduate in these departments, and was later accepted as an Assistant to Virchow, it seems likely that his education in pathology was thorough, and that he was academically gifted. However, before further studies, Hansemann did compulsory military service (Appendix 1 and Fig. 5).

Rudolph Virchow as a teacher

After completing his university studies and discharging his military duties (see Appendix 1), Hansemann began his training in pathology with Rudolf Virchow (Fig. 6)[12] (1821–1902) in Berlin in the Institute (Fig. 7) associated with the Charité

Hospital[13]. Virchow was the most influential pathologist in the world at the time, and as well had been responsible for numerous improvements in public health in Germany. He was also a leading Liberal statesman in the Imperial Assembly (*Reichstag*), a prominent member of the Berlin City Administration and a founder of the discipline of physical anthropology, so that justly, his life continues to be celebrated in Germany. Several biographies (Ackerknecht 1953; Schipperges 1994; Andree 2002; Goschler 2002) have been published, and there are valuable entries in Garrison/Morton (1970) and Dhom (2001). A pathological society in New York was named after him. A bibliography of Virchow's medical and anthropological works was published in the year after his death (Schwalbe, 1901). Rather (1990a) has provided commentaries on Virchow's medical articles.

Virchow's career is sketched in note[12] of this chapter; his philosophical inclinations in chapter 2; his ideas on pathological histology in chapter 3; and his ideas on tumours in chapter 4. Virchow's personal and professional attributes are described in the biographies (above) and in English also by Byers (1989). Here is noted some additional material relevant to Virchow's possible interactions with his Professional Assistants (*Assistenten*[6]).

In his early days as an academic, Virchow was undoubtedly a popular teacher and mentor (Ackerknecht, 1953). However, by the time Hansemann joined the Institute, Virchow may have been less tolerant of students (perhaps not an uncommon concomitant of increasing age). Ackerknecht (1953) quotes sources suggesting that Virchow had "rigidity of thought", "cold enthusiasm for truth" and a taste for polemics. Lubarsch (1921), writing in an issue of Virchow's Archives celebrating the centenary of Virchow's birth, suggested that when an elderly professor, Virchow's participation in seminars was irregular, and his contributions often pedantic, or irritable, or both. Oskar Israel (1903)[14], Virchow's long-serving deputy at the Institute, in an obituary (Israel, 1903) made no mention of Virchow's personality, recording only his ability to disagree without personal insult, and his toleration of the ideas of others.

In general, however, Virchow was undoubtedly a courteous and tolerant person throughout his life, and was obviously very careful to express differences of opinion without giving offence. Virchow held a different opinion from many others on the topic of lineage specificity of cells. However, in his article (1884) on metaplasia Virchow's tone is even-handed and polite in discussing all aspects of this phenomenon in normal and tumourous cells. In dealing with Elie Metchnikoff[15] (Metchnikoff, 1921), whose views on the functions of leukocytes were diametrically opposite to his own, Virchow was supportive and courteous during their personal meeting at Messina (Bibel, 1982). Virchow accepted Metchnikoff's work for publication in his (Virchow's) Archives. An indication of Virchow's considerate nature also can be gained from letters to his parents, to his daughters and his wife, which were published by his daughter and have been translated and published in English (Rabl, 1907).

For Hansemann, Virchow seems to have obtained funding for a new third *Assistent* position immediately before Hansemann was appointed (Wirth, 2005). This implies, but does not prove, that Virchow had the position created for Hansemann. Also, Virchow's toleration of the ideas of others was probably the most significant aspect of his temperament. Hansemann's theory of cancer was contrary to Virchow's views on many points (chapter 5). Hansemann expressed something of this in his dedication of his "Studies ..." (1893c). Virchow (1891) mentioned the possible future significance of the study of karyokinesis in medical research, but did not mention Hansemann's work or any aspect of cellular genetics in an article on recent progress in science and medicine (Virchow, 1898). Nor in any article did Virchow refer to Hansemann's then-new system of diagnosis of malignant tumours according to the principle of anaplasia.

As a final point here, it seems an extraordinary coincidence that Hansemann should have had a grandfather who was a leader of the constitutional government in Berlin during the 1848 revolution, and as a mentor, the pathologist who was most famously of similar political sentiments.

Post-graduate career

Hansemann obtained his Dr med. for work on tuberculosis of mucous membranes. It is not clear whether any dissertation was presented for this (see Appendix A; Wirth, 2005). Hansemann joined Virchow's Institute (Fig. 7) in 1886. He was apparently awarded his habilitation doctorate (*Dr habil.*[16]) in 1890, on the basis of his studies of mitoses in tumours, but no mention of any dissertation was made by Hansemann in his own publications, nor are they mentioned in the writings of other authors we have read. There is no record of such a dissertation in the British Library, Wellcome Institute Library or "The European Library" (on-line catalogues). Hansemann was awarded the University title of Lecturer (*Privatdocent*) at the University of Berlin in 1892 or 1893.

In 1895, Hansemann was appointed Prosector at the Friedrichshain Hospital[17] (Fig. 8). His photograph (Fig. 9) may have been taken at this time or later. The portrait of Hansemann's wife (Fig. 10) was painted in that year, and the family photographs (Figs 11 and 12) are from about the same time. Hansemann was awarded the title of Adjunct Professor[6] (*Extraordinarius, Titularprofessor*) in 1897. He gave lectures on Pathology at the main college in Berlin for post-graduate medical study (the *Kaiserin-Friedrich-Stiftung*[18], Fig. 13) from its foundation in 1906. In the same year, he was appointed Director of Pathology at the then-new Rudolph-Virchow Hospital[19] (Fig. 14) in Wedding, Berlin and in 1912 made an honorary full University Professor (*ordentlicher Honorarprofessor*) of Pathology (Lüder, 2000).

Hansemann was secretary of the Committee for Cancer Research, and Editor of Z. f. Krebsforschung. For a period, he was co-editor of Virchow's Archives.

During his career, he had arguments with others, especially Ribbert and Lubarsch as described in chapter 6. These arguments, especially with von Leyden (chapter 12 and Appendix A), may have affected his promotion at the University of Berlin. In the profession and society as a whole, the arguments may have been less important, as indicated by the positions he held (see above) and the recognition he received by virtue of his appointment as *Geheimrat*[1] for medicine in approximately 1912. His involvement in the anti-Ultramontane movement[20] was probably of little significance to his career.

In W.W.I Hansemann (Fig. 15) served as a General in the Pathology services of the Army on the Eastern Front, being awarded an Iron Cross First Class. After the war, he returned to his duties at the University of Berlin, but died, on August 28th, 1920 of laryngeal carcinoma. His body was buried in the family mausoleum in the old St Matthäus Cemetery in the district of Schöneberg, Berlin (Fig. 16).

An obituary of 1937 (Appendix D) suggests that Hansemann wrote a "personal account" while serving during the war, and after the war was a favourite of returned German soldiers at Medical School, and this is also stated by Wirth (2005). However, David Paul's grandson has no knowledge of this manuscript, and we have not been able to establish whether or not the document existed, and thus have not been able to examine its contents.

We have found no evidence of Hansemann having racist or anti-Semitic sentiments. In his book "Origin and Pathology" (1909f) which would have been the probable place to express such views, there is no mention of Jewish people, or of human "races" at all, except in relation to the inherited disorder of excessive hairiness (hirsutism).

Notes to chapter 1

1. *Freiherr* indicates the lowest order of hereditary title similar to that of a baronet in the English system.

   The title of *Geheimrat* derived from Privy Councillor (*Geheimer Rat* – a member of the supreme organ of government under the Prince or equivalent ruler in many German States. In the nineteenth century in Prussia, it was used to indicate a high official (e.g. *Geheimer Finanzrat*) but also awarded as a mark of distinction to persons with no governmental function at all (e.g. that of *Geheimer Commerzienrat*, for an eminent man of commerce). The system was abolished in 1918.

   References: Encyclopaedia Britannica, 11th edn (1911); Schwarz (1943).

2. By the 1870s, most states in Germany had three types of high schools, which, with some regional variations, had curricula as follows.

   (i) *Hauptschule* (sometimes *Realschule*), which gave a basic secondary education in six years.

   (ii) *Realschule* or *Oberrealschule* and sometimes *Realgymnasium* (if it included some study of the classics) offered a nine-year course, for those intending a career in commerce, and also for engineers, technicians and scientists intent on tertiary education in Technical Colleges (*Technische Hochschulen*).

(iii) *Gymnasien*, which first appeared during the Counter Reformation as private institutions of secondary education, and offered a nine-year course, based on *Bildung* (see note[5] below). Their curricula featured "humanistic" subjects embracing the liberal arts and the classical languages, as well as science and mathematics. *Gymnasien* were for the intellectually elite students who were destined for the professions, as well as the higher levels of the State Administration, of the diplomatic service, of the Church and of the Military. The education provided was approximately equivalent to the high school grades and a liberal Arts college in the American system.

References: Reinhardt (1960); McClelland (1980), Hahn (1998).

3. Hansemann (Appendix A) states that he went to a "*Gymnasium* in Charlottenburg" which may have been one of the following: the Joachimsthal Gymnasium in Kaiser Strasse (now 1–12 Federal Avenue), the K. K. (*Kaiserlich und Königlich* – "Imperial and Royal") Augusta Gymnasium off Berliner Strasse, or the "Bismarck Gymnasium", which was closer to Wilmersdorf.

Reference: Berlin street map, in Baedeker's "North Germany" (1910).
http://www.lib.utexas.edu/maps/historical/baedeker_n_germany_1910/berlin_1910.jpg

4. The Friedrich-Wilhelm *Gymnasium* was perhaps the most famous in Berlin, having Bismarck and several noted philosophers among its alumni.

5. The ethos of *Bildung* is possibly derived from Aristotle's "educatedness" (*paideia*) as opposed to "special knowledge" (*epistēmē*) (Boylan, 1983) and Thomasius' (1655–1724) *Gelehrtheit* versus *Gelahrtheit* (see chapter 2), and probably began to develop in Germany during the Reformation. There is no exact English-language equivalent for *Bildung* but it aims at the formation and shaping of high-level intellectual and emotional maturation of the individual by humanistic education, especially through study of the Classics. Perhaps most neatly, Paulsen (1895) stated that the educational aim of *Bildung* in relation to students was

"… to produce, not a narrow person, but a broad person sharpened to a point."

References: Paulsen (1895), Jarausch (1982), Broman (1996).

6. The German Universities had several important features.

(i) They were founded on a state-by-state basis by the individual reigning princes (*Landesväter*) and governments, so that these universities were under governmental control and were in many respects part of the Civil Service of each state, and often exhibited rivalries accordingly. With illiberal trends in Germany in the period 1870–1914 (Jarusch, 1982), the German academic community became more and more beholden to officialdom.

(ii) They were much more numerous than in England or France, and so tended to be relatively small and thus unable to cover many academic subjects in great depth. Many students therefore studied different parts of their degrees at different universities, as Hansemann did.

(iii) Because of the fragmented nature of German political and social life which was exacerbated by the religious divisions and bitterness associated with the Reformation, the Counter-Reformation and the Thirty-Years War (1618–1648), there was no capital city of Germany to form a focus of German national life, and by default, German universities became a major unifying cultural focus for the German-speaking peoples.

(iv) German intellectuals were often University academics (e.g. Kant at Königsberg; Hegel at Jena, Heidelberg, and Berlin; Fichte at Jena and Berlin, and August von Schlegel at Jena and Bonn. By contrast, many English and Scots philosophers, such as Locke, Hume, Bentham, J. S. Mill and Charles Darwin were never university staff members. Similarly in France, Voltaire, Rousseau, and Diderot were not staff members of any University.

(v) The strength of the German university system lay in the academic excellence of the Professors. *Professores Ordinarii* were heads of Departments and wielded more influence over their departmental staff than occurred in other countries. When a new *Ordinarius* took over a Department, the contract staff associated with the previous *Ordinarius* was sometimes dismissed *en masse*. Thus the pressure on Lecturers to obtain Professorial positions was enormous. The peak of the cult of the all-powerful *Ordinarius* coincided with the period of Hansemann's career.

Professores Extraordinarii ("A. o.") were usually of higher standing than an "Associate Professor" in current English and American universities, and were tenured although having a status and salary below those of an *Ordinarius*. As with Hansemann, at the University Hospitals, the Professorial title could be awarded without salary (*Honorarius*), similar to "Clinical Professors" in some British and American institutions. A *Privatdocent* was equivalent to a Lecturer in the British system. An *Assistent* (Professional Assistant) was a combination of tutor, as well as personal and research assistant to the Professor. A *Famulus* was essentially a technical assistant to a Professor, and lower in status than an *Assistent*. Professors were well-salaried, and in addition, received students fees (*Hörgelder*) directly. On the other hand, lecturers, professional assistants and technical assistants (*Privatdocenten, Assistenten* and *Famuli*) were generally poorly paid and on limited-term contracts. Many supplemented their incomes with part-time paid teaching outside the particular university of their primary affiliation.

(vi) The German University system was extensively reformed thanks to Wilhelm von Humboldt in 1808-1810, who, as Minister for Education in Prussia, established the University of Berlin (see below). He strongly supported the "three freedoms" of German University life: freedom of teaching, freedom of research and freedom of movement (for both staff and students). These changes came to be applied to all Universities in the newly-enlarged Prussia after 1815 (see above), and the further enlarged territories of the Second German *Reich* (Empire) after 1871. Universities in the German speaking areas outside the *Reich* (essentially Austria and German-speaking Switzerland) tended to follow suit.

References: Boyesen (1878), Paulsen (1895), Virchow (1894), Spranger (1960), Reinhardt (1960), Flexner (1968), Sweet (1978), McClelland (1980), Parkinson (1988), Solomon and Higgins (1993), Mautner T (1995), Audi (1999), Dematteis and Fosl (2002), Charle (2004), Rüegg (2004).

7   The medical faculty of the University of Berlin was established in 1810, with Rodolphi as Foundation Professor of Pathology. He was succeeded in 1832 by Johannes Müller. The latter became perhaps the most remarkable teacher of science in modern history. Müller's own works included the first studies of the cellular nature of tumours (Müller, 1838) and "Elements of Physiology" (1840). His students included the histologists Schwann, who proposed the Cell Theory for animals (see chapter 3), His (1811–1887), Henle (1809–1885) and Kölliker (1817–1905). Other students made major contributions to other disciplines, including Virchow (see note), Helmholtz (1821–1894), who conceived the law of conservation of energy as well as contributing to optics and acoustics, and Wilhelm Wundt (1832–1920), who founded experimental psychology. Another of Müller's students was Brücke (1819–1892) who in turn was a major influence on Sigmund Freud (1856–1939).

References: Haggard and Smith (1938), Rather et al. (1986), Bringman et al. (1997).

8   Julius Friedrich Cohnheim (1839–1884), b Demmin, Pomerania, graduated in medicine at the University of Berlin 1861; assistant to Virchow 1864–1868; then successively Professor of Pathology at Kiel, Breslau and finally Leipzig (1876–1884). He is best known for discovering that cells in pus are emigrated blood leukocytes, and for the "embryonal rest" theory of the nature of cancer (Wolff, 1907). A popular and successful teacher, his three-volume "Lectures in General Pathology" was widely acclaimed and the 2nd edition was translated into English in 1889.

References: Malkin (1984), Dhom (2001).

9   Carl Weigert (1845–1904), b Münsterberg, Silesia; graduated in medicine; received training in pathology under Waldeyer, Lebert and Cohnheim (1878–1884). In 1885 (having been refused the

Chair at Leipzig after Cohnheim's death), he received the call to Frankfurt am Main, as Professor of Pathology at Senckenberg's Institute. His main interests were bacteria and histological stains. The most frequently used of his stains today is "Weigert's stain" for myelin.

Reference: Wohlrab and Henoch (1988); Dhom (2001).

10 The largest group of student voluntary organisations consisted of "Duelling Corps" which, in 1903, involved 39 % of all students. The *Burschenschaft* (the most military in tone) comprised only one type of these Corps. Other associations were "Colour-Carrying Corps" (22 %), religious groups (13 %), and scholarly, political, sports, social and other associations (all less than 10 % of students each).

Reference: Jarausch (1982).

11 Wilhelm His (1831–1904) is remembered for the "bundle of His" in the electrical conducting system of the heart. Carl Thiersch (1822–1895) studied the histopathology of skin cancers, concluding that skin cancers must come from epidermis; he also founded plastic surgery. Carl Ludwig (1816–1895) is remembered for his contributions to experimental physiology in cardiology, nephrology and anaesthesia. Weigert is mentioned in note[9].

References Garrison/Morton (1970), Rather (1978), Silverman et al (2006).

12 Rudolph Virchow (1821–1902), b in Schievelbein, Pomerania, entered the Gymnasium in Köslin in 1835, and the Royal Medical-Surgical School, Friedrich Wilhelms Institute, Berlin, in 1839; worked in Müller's laboratory (see note[7] above). Virchow was appointed Assistant Physician at the Charité April 1843; awarded Doctor of Medicine October 1843, became voluntary assistant to Friorep (see above) in the Autopsy department of the Charité in 1844, and passed the State Examination in March 1846. He was appointed acting Demonstrator/Prosector (after Friorep's resignation) May 1846 and was released from clinical duties at the Friedrich Wilhelms Institut and further military obligations in April 1847. Later in the same year appeared the first issue of *Archive f. path. Anat. (etc)* which he published with Reinhardt, and is now known as "Virchow's Archives".

A forceful intellect and disputant, he was a favourite of students in his youth, and held markedly liberal views. These opinions were manifest by his condemnation of living conditions in Silesian towns (in an officially-commissioned report), his editorship of a Liberal journal "Medical Reform" (1846–1850), and his involvement on the side of the revolutionaries in the Revolution of 1848 (in which Hansemann's grandfather was a principal – see main text of this chapter).

After the suppression of the political uprising of 1848–9 in Berlin, Virchow lost his lectureship (above) and was forced to go to Würzburg (in the less repressive state of Bavaria). Outcry against his banishment caused Virchow's return to Berlin, where construction of a new Institute Building was begun (completed in 1865, but requiring many additions in subsequent years). Virchow entered the City Council of Berlin in 1859; became a member of the Prussian House of Representatives (*Abgeordnetenhaus*) in 1862, and from 1880–1893, was a member of the Imperial Assembly (*Reichstag*). He was a founder of the Progress Party (*Fortschrittspartei*) in the Prussian Assembly from 1861. Later, during the period of secular-Catholic religious struggle (*Kulturkampf* – see chapter 2) he was forced to acknowledge the separation of medical science from religion in society (see pages 35-40 in Schipperges, 1983). Bismarck challenged Virchow to a duel in 1865 (the challenge was not accepted) but the two adversaries later cooperated on the issue of the *Kulturkampf*. (A cartoon and other illustrations from the period are reproduced in the guide book of the Berlin Museum of Medical History at the Charité).

Virchow's interest in anthropology developed in the late 1860s and he founded a journal (*Zeitschrift für Ethnologie*). Virchow abandoned the fourth volume of his work on "Disease-related Tumours" (*Die Krankhaften Geschwülste*, 1862–1866; see also chapter 4). In anthropology, he spent much of his time studying skeletal remnants claimed by their discoverers as of "prehistoric races". Virchow did not decide that any examples of these were proven to be of any "prehistoric" peoples. Unfortunately for his reputation, one specimen on which he pronounced "normal European with disease" was the Neanderthal skull (discovered in the Neander valley in what is now North Rhine-Westphalia). This has come to be recognised as indeed an example of a different race of man (Harvati et al, 2004). Perhaps his anti-evolutionary stance (Virchow, 1886) contributed to his mistake in this regard. Virchow also conducted anthropological studies of Jews, showing that there were no significant physical differences between this group and Gentiles, and hence suggesting that a concept of European Jews being of a different "race" of man is without foundation (Ackerknecht, 1953).

Sadly, in recent years, Virchow is alleged to have contributed to an "anti-humanist" turn in German science in the nineteenth century (Zimmerman, 2001), characterised by the accumulation of collections of specimens in museums. However, to a pathology educator, the value of museums of specimens is so manifestly obvious (as could be seen in either preserved specimens or as casts in any medical school since the seventeenth century) that a museum of anthropology for the purposes of maintaining and furthering knowledge in this discipline would have been unchallenged (museums of Natural History were being established as public and private institutions throughout the Western World at this time). For an account of anti-vivisectionism, Darwinism and Wagnerism in Berlin, see Rather (1990b). Furthermore, Virchow's reputation as a Liberal, an anti-racist and a spokesman for Science should not be tarnished by such narrow considerations. Virchow continued to edit his Archives (only officially renamed "Virchow's Archives" after his death) and the museum for a new Institute building was erected in 1901 in time for his 80th birthday. He remained a teacher of Pathology at the Institute of the Charité until he died from complications of a fall from a tram in Berlin in 1902.

Additional references: Israel (1903), Lubarsch, (1921); Ackerknecht (1953), Rather (1971), Schipperges (1994), Taddey (1977), Zimmerman (2001), Goschler (2002), Andree (2002).

13 The Charité Hospital was founded in 1710 beyond the city limits, and was intended to be a "pest house" for potential cases of plague during an epidemic in the region. However, the epidemic did not reach Berlin, and it served as a "work house" (destitute asylum). In 1713, an anatomy school for military doctors was attached; in 1727 the complex became a hospital, was given its current name and became the centre for the more extensive teaching and research of the "Medical and Surgical College" (military medical school). From 1785 to 1797 there was an extensive building programme. In 1831 an autopsy department (separate from the University Department under Rodolphi, see note[7] above) under Probius was formed in the hospital. The second prosector of the department was Friorep, during which time, academic pathology was taught at the Medical School by J. Müller (see above). Virchow (see above) was appointed both head of the Hospital Department and Professor of Pathology in 1856. A new Institute building was erected in 1865, and an even larger one was begun in 1899, in association with great expansion of the site. The Charité was Berlin's largest hospital until the end of W.W. II. During the period of the German Democratic Republic few improvements were made, but a substantial rebuilding programme has been instituted since reunification of Germany in 1990.

References: Ackerknecht (1953), Ludewig (1986), Kreitsch (1990), Schattenfroh (2002).

14 Oskar Israel (1854–1907) studied in Leipzig, became *Assistent* (following Orth) to Virchow in 1874; State (registration) Examination (*Staatsexamen*), 1878 and *Dr habil.* (note[16], below) in 1885. He remained in Virchow's Institute as teacher and Prosector and published a practical guide to pathological histology in 1889. He was appointed *Professor Extraordinarius* (note[6] above) in 1893, and after Virchow's death, he remained Prosector under the new Director, Orth.

Reference: Dhom (2001).

Notes to chapter 1

15 Elie Metchnikoff (1845–1916), son of rural landowners in the Ukraine near Kharkov, graduated in biology from the University there in 1863. He subsequently studied in various universities in Germany, as well as at Naples, St Petersburg and Odessa. Metchnikoff began work on phagocytic theory in 1883 which essentially established that the main function of neutrophil and monocyte-type leukocytes is the phagocytosis and intracellular destruction of bacteria. He moved to Paris in 1888, published "Lectures on the Comparative Pathology of Inflammation" (1892) and continued studies of immunity and phagocytosis. He was awarded the Nobel Prize for Medicine and Physiology in 1908.

Reference: Metchnikoff (1921), Ghislein and Groeben (1997).

16 In Germany a Faculty Doctorate (e.g. Doctor of Medicine) can be obtained by approximately one year of post-undergraduate research work. The *Dr habil.* is a higher doctorate which is awarded following successful presentation of the *Habilitationsschrift*. It usually follows several years as a professional assistant (*Assistent*) and often lecturer (*Privatdozent*) in a University Department, and is the prerequisite for any professorial appointment. It therefore usually indicates a higher level of education and experience than a Doctor of Philosophy (Ph D) in the English-speaking systems.

17 Building of the Friedrichshain ("Friedrich's Heath") Hospital, at that time an outlying area of the city, began in 1864, and the institution opened in 1874 as the first hospital established in Berlin by the City administration, rather than by the monarch. The pathology department was originally led by the distinguished researcher Friedländer (1847-1887) until his early death. The position of Prosector was then left vacant until 1895 (due to the influence of Virchow) until Hansemann was appointed to it (while Virchow was away from Berlin on a visit to Egypt).

References: Obituary by Ostertag (Appendix D), Wolf (1999), Wirth (2005).

18 This college (the "Empress Friedrich Foundation" – *Kaiserin-Friedrich-Stiftung*) was established adjacent to the Charité Hospital at No 7 Luisen Platz (now "Robert Koch Place"), as a post-graduate medical educational institute in 1906. The leading figures in its foundation were the surgeon von Bergmann (1836–1907); the urologist Kutner (1867–1913) and Friedrich Theodor Althoff (1839-1908) who was departmental head for universities (*Universitätsreferat*) in the Ministry of Education from 1897. The College was named after its major supporter, the widow of Emperor Friedrich III (1831–1888). Victoria (1840–1901) was daughter of Queen Victoria, Princess Royal of England and mother of Wilhelm II. The Institute had a lecture theatre, and rooms occupied by displays of contemporary medical equipment of all types. It served these purposes until it was taken over by the Russian occupying military forces in 1945, and after that, housed the Academy of Arts (*Akademie der Wissenschaften*) of the German Democratic Republican (D. D. R.). Since 1992, the building has been elegantly restored, and re-established as a centre for post-graduate medical education, although many of the rooms are let to private medical practitioners.

References: Bergmann (1906); Sachse (1927), discussions with Prof. Dr. Jurgen Hammerstein, Director of the Institute, personal observation (LPB).

19 The Rudolph-Virchow Hospital was founded in Wedding in 1906 to the design of Ludwig Hoffmann. Architecturally it was famous for its parallel pavilions, with the pathology department at the end of a long central avenue. Hansemann was appointed as the first Prosector, and was made *Ordinary Honorarius Professor* of Pathology in 1912. It has since become a modern general hospital with numerous specialist clinics. In 1989 the original pathology department building was converted into a library, especially for medical students and little now remains of the original internal design of the building.

References: Schattenfroh (2002); guide book of Berlin Medical Museum at the Charité.

20 The "Ultramontane" movement referred to the activities of German Catholics under the influence of the Papal assertion of infallability, and the power of the Pope over local secular political leaders. In Germany resistance (anti-Ultramontanism) to this Catholic initiative was mainly by liberal nationalist Protestants, and took the form of Associations having activities as indicated in Hansemann's letter (Appendix 1). The struggle was conducted in the political and cultural arenas, and there were no civil disorders or significant illegal actions by either side.

Reference: Clark and Kaiser (2003).

Figures

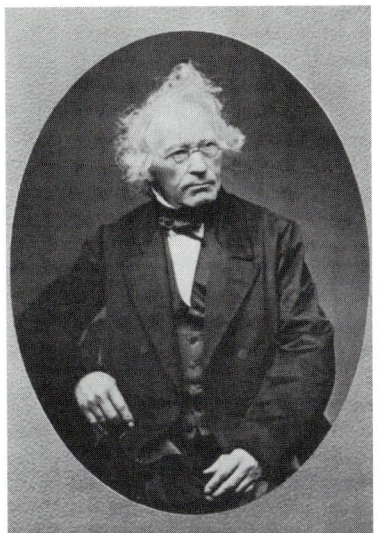

Figure 1. Portrait of David Justus Hansemann (1790–1864). Courtesy of Mr Wolfgang von Hansemann.

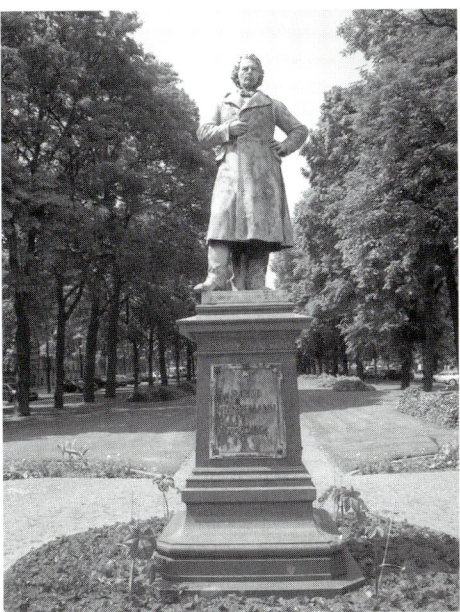

Figure 2. Statue of David Justus Hansemann, located in Hansemann Platz, Aachen. Photographed in 2006 by Dr Bignold.

The inscription on the base (four panels) reads

"David Hansemann 1790–1864.

To a meritorious citizen of the city of Aachen 1820–1848.

To the founder of the Aachen and Munich Fire Insurance Society and the Aachen Society for the Promotion of Industriousness (*Arbeitsamkeit*) 1825.

To the leading campaigner (*Vorkämpfer*) for the development of railways in the Rhineland Province."

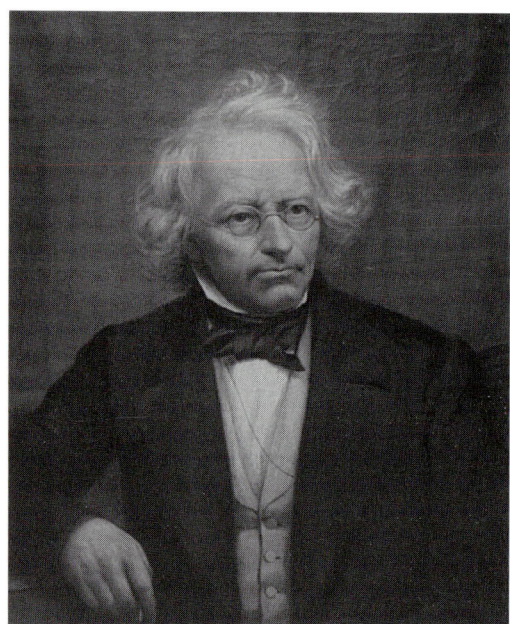

Figure 3. Portrait of Gustav Hansemann (1829–1902). Courtesy of Mr Wolfgang von Hansemann.

Figure 4. Buildings (thought to be original) on the site labeled "Dye-works of Gustav Hansemann" on the Town Plan of Eupen, 1860s. Photographed 2006 by Dr Bignold.

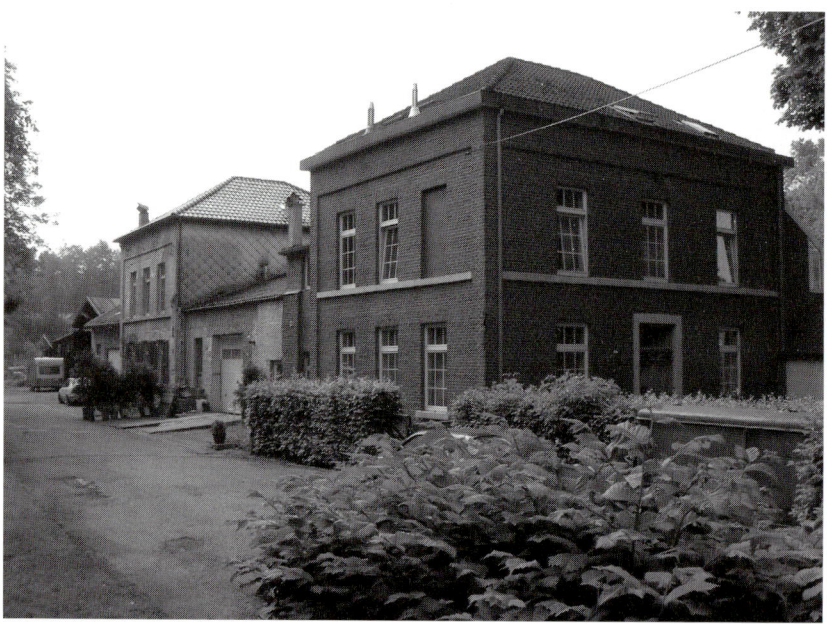

Figures

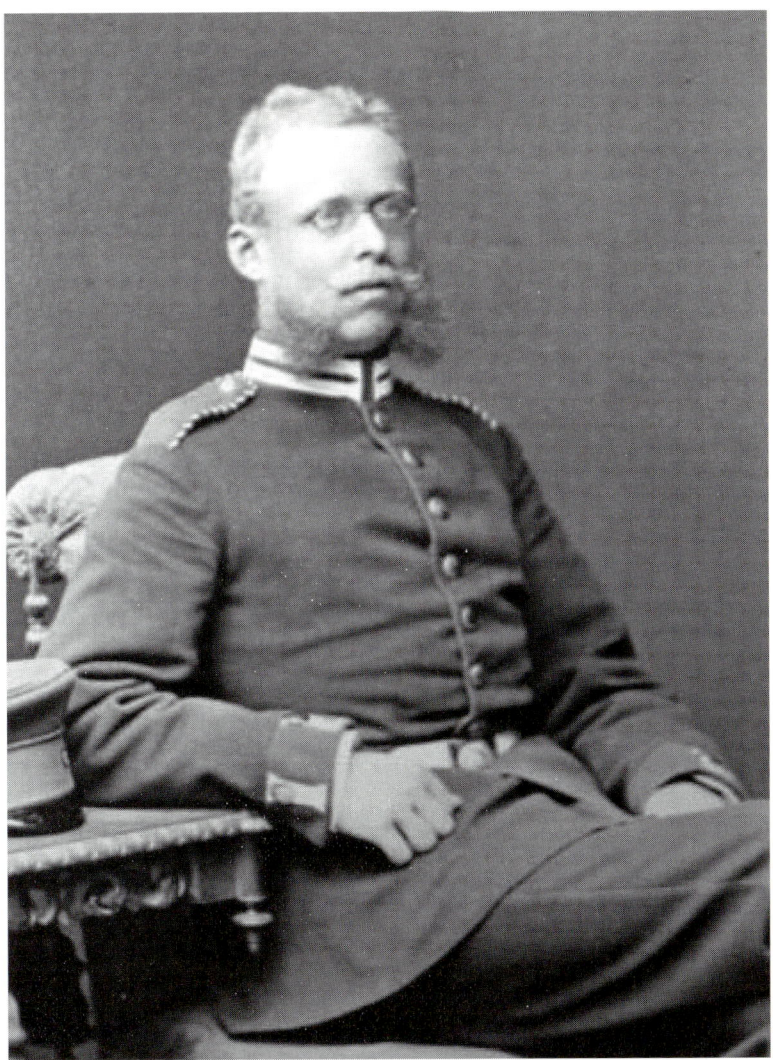

Figure 5. David Paul Hansemann in 1882, the year of his military service. Courtesy Mr Wolfgang von Hansemann.

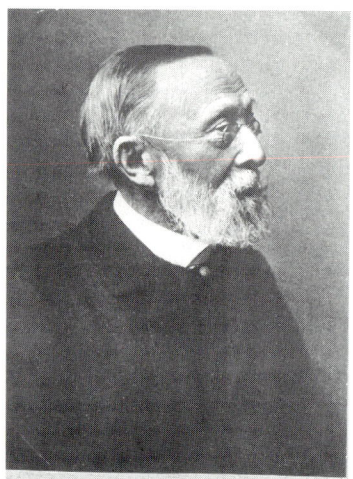

Figure 6. Rudolph Virchow (1821–1902) in 1890. Courtesy Ms Elke-Barbara Peschke, Director of the Historic Book Collection of Library of the Humboldt-Universität, Berlin.

Figure 7. Virchow's Institute Building, as it appeared in the late 1880s. (Reproduced from Virchow's Arch. vol. 235, 1921)

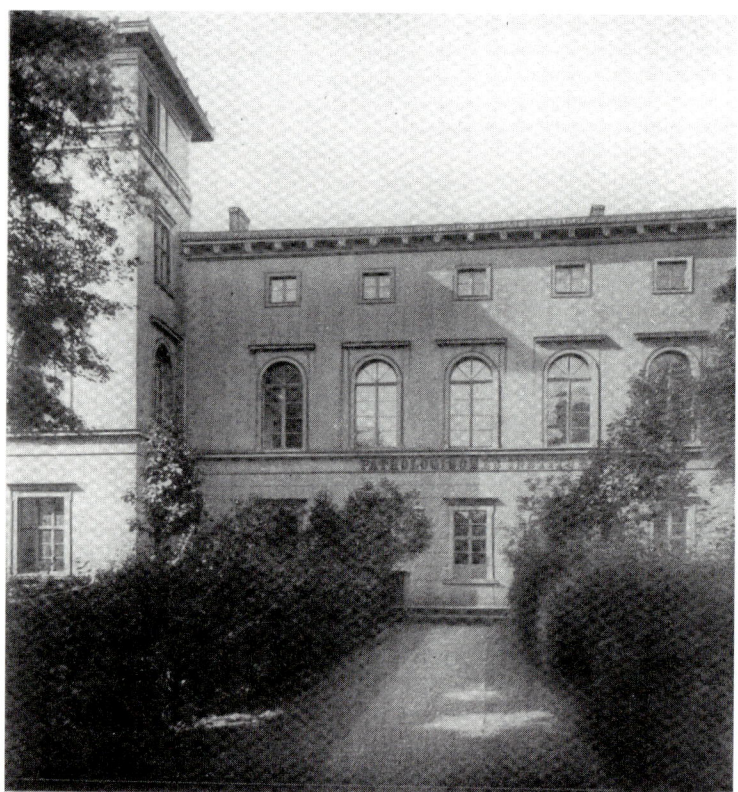

Figures

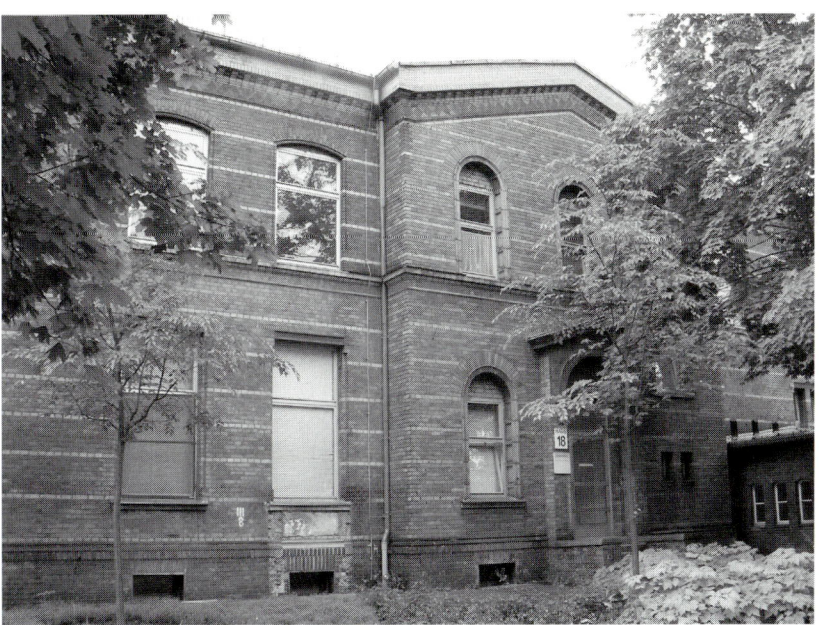

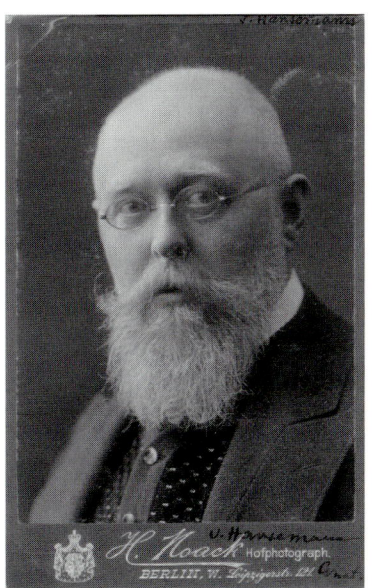

Figure 8. Facade of Pathology building at the Friedrichshain Hospital now, and probably little changed since Hansemann's day. The interior, however, was altered in the 1950s. Photographed by Dr Bignold, 2006.

Figure 9. Hansemann in early middle age (date not known, but possibly in 1897). Courtesy Ms Peschke, Director of the Historic Book Collection of Humboldt-Universität Library, Berlin.

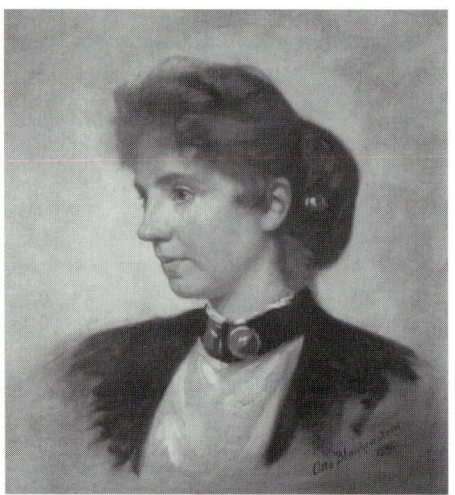
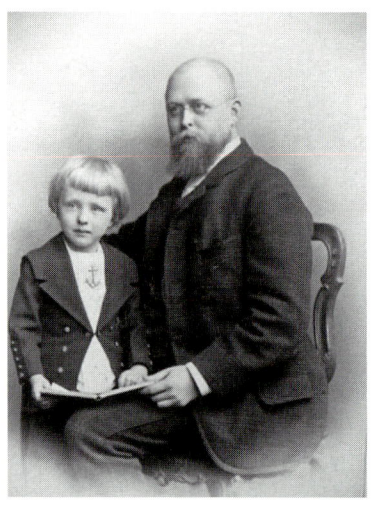

Figure 10. Portrait, dated 1895, of Elizabeth Hansemann (nee Walter, 1863–1935). Courtesy Mr Wolfgang von Hansemann.

Figure 11. David Paul Hanseman and his son Fritz, about 1892. Courtesy Mr Wolfgang von Hansemann.

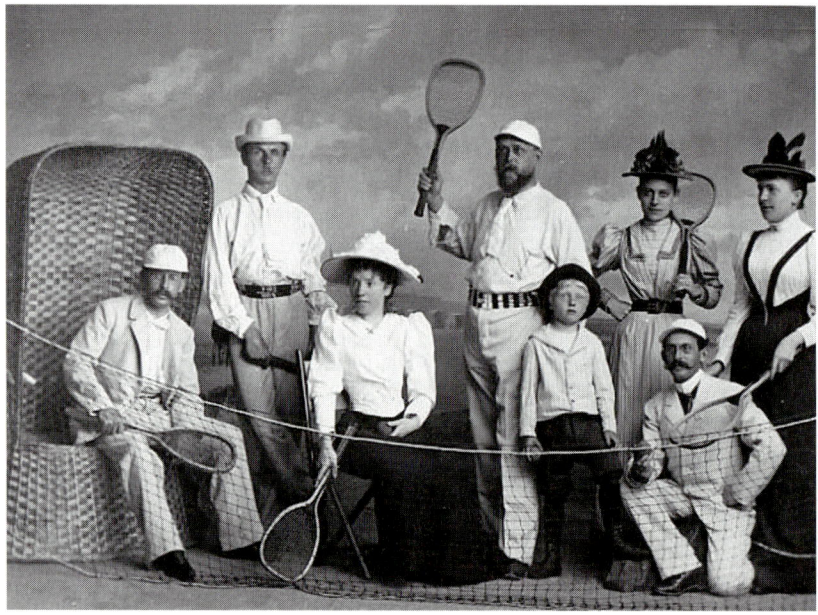

Figure 12. Hansemann family on holiday, about 1892. Courtesy Mr Wolfgang von Hansemann.

Figures

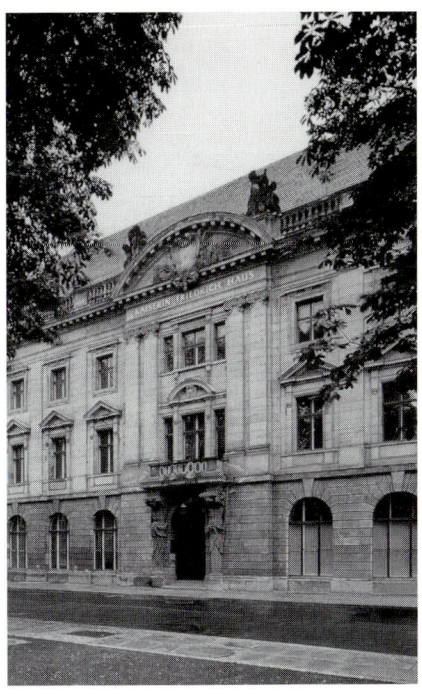

Figure 13. Facade of the *Kaiserin-Friedrich-Stiftung* (1906) restored to its original appearance in the 1990s. Courtesy Professor Dr. med. Jürgen Hammerstein.

Figure 14. Facade of the Pathology Building of the Rudolph Virchow Hospital photographed 2006. This aspect of the building is probably little changed since Hansemann's time, but the interior is now the library of the Campus Virchow Klinikum. Courtesy Ms Mary Peterson.

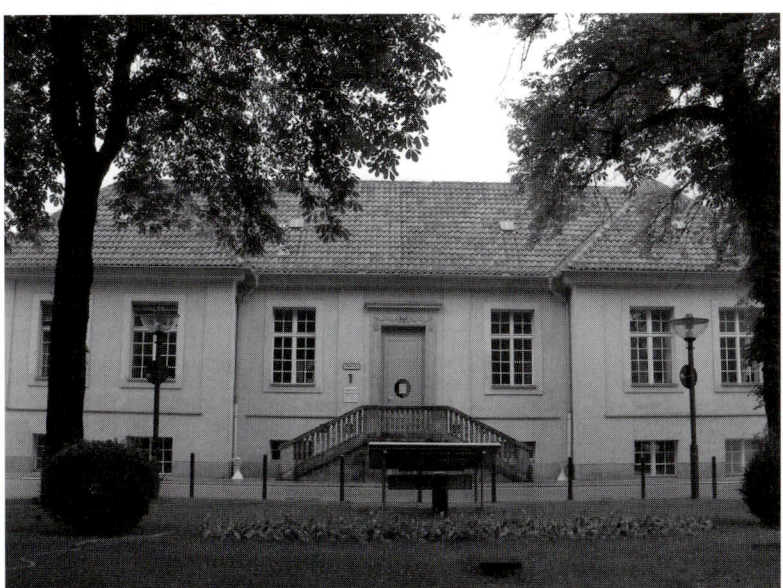

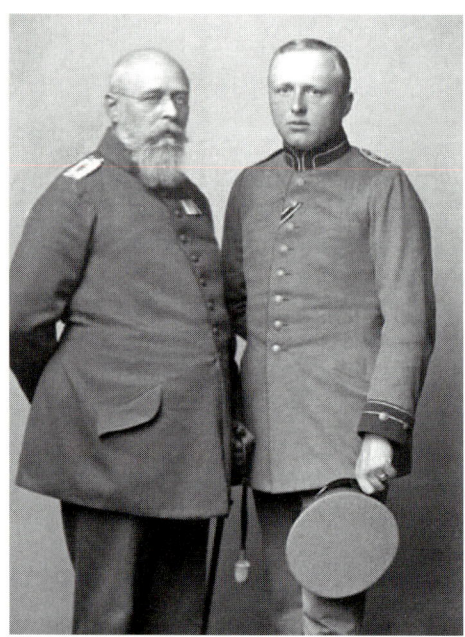

Figure 15. David Paul von Hansemann and his son Fritz in 1914. Courtesy Mr Wolfgang von Hansemann.

Figure 16. The Hansemann Mausoleum, in Schöneberg, Berlin, photographed in 2006. A plaque on its wall reads:

"Family vault of the von Hansemann family,
Built in 1876 by Friedrich Hitzig,
Extended in 1901 by Walter Ende,
Restored in 1986 by the Deutsche Bank AG".

Courtesy Ms Mary Peterson.

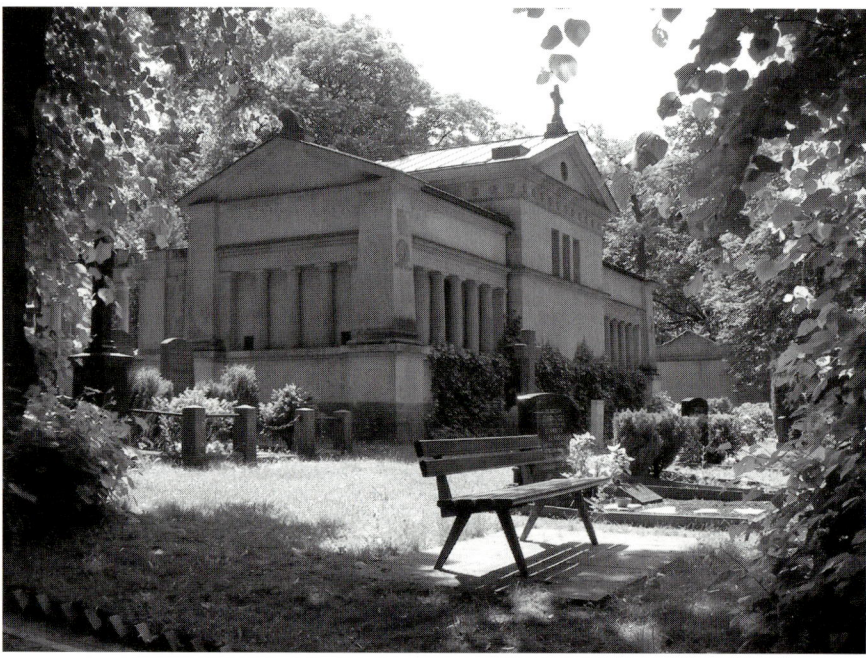

Chapter 2

Aspects of philosophy in the culture and science of Germany in the nineteenth century

Introduction

There is a clear philosophical component to Hansemann's works on cancer and other medical topics. The most obvious is the application of the concept of "altruism" in relation to cell biology in his article (1890a) and in "Studies …" (1893c). Further, his books "Origin and Pathology" (1909f) and "On conditional Thinking …" (1912f) include overtly philosophical discussions. The philosophical strands in Hansemann's cancer writings sometimes make his work difficult to understand, especially for those readers with an English-speaking background. Moreover, it was probably one reason for the later forgetting of Hansemann's ideas (chapter 6), not least because the "philosophical" approach to the analysis of biological issues was rapidly becoming obsolete in the 1890s.

Hansemann's philosophy of cancer (chapter 5) also probably contributed to some of his arguments with colleagues, for example Ribbert and Lubarsch, concerning the nature of the tumourous abnormality of cells (chapter 6). Finally, Hansemann's philosophical inclinations allowed later authors, such as Borst (chapter 6) and Ostertag (Appendix C) to discount all Hansemann's writings as "too philosophical", and thus ignore his valid contributions to the mechanistic analysis of the formation and characteristics of tumours.

The purpose of this chapter is to sketch those aspects of German philosophy, including the ideas of Rudolph Virchow (Hansemann's teacher) which are relevant to the formation and expression of Hansemann's ideas, as well as those aspects which influenced views of Hansemann's contemporaries.

Influence of the Ancient Greeks

The influence of specific Ancient ideas in biology, physiology and medicine (for example, those of Aristotle, Hippocrates and Galen) began to decline with the discovery of the circulation of the blood by Harvey in the 1640s, and with the advent of reliable microscopy in the early nineteenth century. Nevertheless, the general concepts of the Ancients did not lose their influence so quickly. For example, the edition of the Hippocratic writings published in 1849 in London was said by Garrison/Morton (1970) to have been for possible practical use by medical practitioners at the time. According to Virchow, in the 1850s the Viennese school of tumour theorists was essentially "neohumoralist" in type. By Hansemann's time, only some ritualistic introductory mention of the Ancients persisted in academic medical and biological writing. Hansemann himself mentioned Pliny the Younger[1] in the Introduction to "Studies ..." (1893c) and Aristotle's "Four Causes"[2] in the Introduction to his "On Conditional Thinking ..." (1912f).

These persistent influences of the Ancient Greek legacy had negative effects on science even in the nineteenth century (Nordenskiöld, 1928; Singer and Underwood, 1962) which were probably relevant to Hansemann and his opus.

The first negative influence was the continuing acceptability of supernatural/irrational/mystical mechanisms of biological phenomena and disease to many nineteenth century authors. Although specifically "rational/mechanist" ideas of biology and disease appeared in anti-Aristotelian publications during the Reformation[3], and were the essence of Descartes'[4] work in biology, direct use of specific irrational mechanisms, especially Plato's concept of "forces" (Nordenskiöld, 1928) and Aristotle's notion of "spirits" (Singer and Underwood, 1962; Hall, 1972; Carter, 1983), continued well after that. For example, in the nineteenth century, "forces" were still being used as explanatory biological mechanisms; for example, "organic forces" by Müller in his "Elements of Physiology" (1838), "life forces" by Virchow in 1854 (Rather, 1990a) and "plastic forces" by Charles Darwin, in his "Variation in Plants and Animals under Domestication" (1868). There were also indirect applications of irrational Graeco-Roman ideas in the eighteenth and nineteenth centuries, for example, by Stahl in his concepts of "Anima" and by Barthez in his idea of "Vitalism" (Daremberg, 1870; Driesch, 1914; Schubert-Soldern, 1962; Williams, 2002). By the 1890s vitalist and similar notions were losing popularity. This was especially because the proofs that fermentation occurs by catalysis (not by "vital forces") and that chromosomes are the vehicle of the transference of heredity (chapter 3) made valueless most of those non-mechanistic theories of biology which had been associated with philosophy since Ancient times (Nordenskiöld, 1928).

There is no evidence of Hansemann himself embracing any vitalist or similar ideas to explain cancer or any other biomedical phenomenon. Hansemann's work was probably affected only in so far as he was opposed to the vitalist and other mystical notions still espoused by some of his contemporaries.

Second was the particular belief in the significance of "harmonies" and "balances" for "normal" existence and health. Many subsequent medical writers used "balances" of various factors in their theories (Singer and Underwood, 1962). Virchow (see section on "Cellular Pathology" below) thought of disease in terms of "harmonies" and "balances" in actions of cell types in relation to one another. In his early papers Hansemann analysed the possible effects of asymmetric nuclear division on the daughter cells in terms of "balances of chromosomes" and also balances of hereditary units ("plasmas", "ids", "gemmules", see chapter 4). However, in later works, Hansemann hardly mentioned this principle at all.

Third, there was the tendency to over-abstraction, often in association with over-inclusion of disparate phenomena, in the search for all embracing systems or concepts. This was notable in Germany as "excess conceptuality" ("*übermässige*

Begrifflichkeit"). In medical science, Henle (1853) appears particularly to have had this tendency.

Fourth, there was a tendency to look for progress to truth through argument, rather than fresh observation, for example in the dialogues of Plato (Allbutt, 1921; Barnes, 2003). Such disputation is perhaps less conducive than quiet discussion to development of experimentally testable hypotheses in the natural sciences (Nordenskiöld, 1928). This argumentative tendency may have passed via Lessing's *Streitkultur* (below) to Hansemann and his contemporaries (see chapter 6).

German philosophy and literature after the Reformation; *Streitkultur*

A specific "German Philosophy" is considered to have emerged only after the Thirty Years War[5], perhaps particularly with Thomasius[6] (1655–1724), and Caspar Wolff[7] (1679–1754). These thinkers probably constituted a preliminary phase of the Enlightenment, which was largely concerned with attempts to secularise, liberalise, constitutionalise and perhaps most urgently de-brutalise European society. Progressively, the later German philosophers indulged more and more in metaphysics, and their use of conceptuality for clarity and classification resulted in ever more all-embracing concepts and complicated "systems" of thought. Conceptuality is identifiable especially in the works of Kant[8] (1724–1804) but also in those of Fichte[9] (1762–1814), Hegel[10] (1770–1831), Schopenhauer[11] (1788–1860) and even Richard Wagner[12] (1813–1883). In these works, the usage may or may not be considered excessive – and perhaps should be determined in each case by different opinions and different perspectives.

However, most German scientists were probably not affected by these developments to any great degree. In particular, Albrecht von Haller (1757) conducted and reported strictly experimentally-based studies of the "Motion of the Blood". This mode of experimentation was followed by nineteenth century physiologists, notably Carl Ludwig (1816–1895) but, as shown below, to only lesser degrees by contemporaneous German pathologists.

From this, Hansemann's "Studies..." (1893) can be interpreted as marked by *"übermässige Begrifflichkeit"*, because of the very extensive series of ideas which he included under each of his conceptual groupings of "Specificity", "Altruism" and "Anaplasia". Further in attempting to use this triad of concepts (Specificity, Altruism, Anaplasia) to categorise all aspects of tumour cell morphology and behaviour, he was in fact creating a "System of Cancer" or at least a "systematisation of cancer" in the German philosophical tradition (chapter 5).

In the middle period of the Enlightenment, Gotthold Ephraim Lessing (1729–1781)[13] stood out as an "even-handed rationalist". His idea of *Streitkultur* involved the use of open, vigorous public debate to address issues for the benefit of all (Mauser and Sasse, 1993). This seems to be, indirectly if not directly, a model for how Hansemann approached his chosen area of medical research, and also for the interpretations published by his contemporaries of his writing (chapter 6).

"Romantic biology" and *Naturphilosophie*

"Romantic biology" was a strand of nineteenth century philosophy which probably represented an off-shoot of the Romantic Movement[14] (Poggi and Maurizio, 1994; Maienschein and Ruse, 1999). Yet another strand in German thinking in the early nineteenth century was *Naturphilosophie*[15] which F.W. von Schelling (1775–1854) used as a counterpoint to his ideas of *Transzendentalphilosophie*. The latter was perhaps a forerunner of "biologistic sociology" (see below). Both of these included metaphysical concepts in their systems, and except for Hansemann's attempt to "systematise" cancer, there is no evidence of either Romantic philosophy or *Naturphilosophie* affecting his writings.

Characteristics of Virchow's thinking

Virchow did not write any exclusively philosophical texts, and hence he is not often regarded as a philosopher in the conventional sense. However, the "Cellular Pathology" had the characteristics of a "philosophy of pathology", as discussed in the next section. The general characteristics of Virchow's thinking included:

(i) Persistent influence of the Ancient Greeks, which was evident in his acceptance of "life forces" as a biological mechanism (see above).

(ii) Inclination to overarching concepts. In general this is evident in Virchow's use of phrases such as "Law of …" or the "Doctrine of …".

(iii) Romantic notions of the role of medicine in society, and the dramatic moments which "turn" medical history. These are to be found especially in his articles in his journal "Medical Reform" (1848-9) (Ackerknecht, 1957, Rather, 1962, 1971; Virchow, 1907).

(iv) Perceptions of cross-disciplinary analogies, especially the attempts to link social processes and disease processes (as in his version of Cell Theory, above). Early in his career Virchow intended to achieve a philosophical construction involving both the biological and the social worlds; he was not just using the comparison in a metaphorical sense in political debates (Rather, 1962; Schipperges, 1994; Goschler, 2002). In this Virchow saw a philosophical analogy with human society to underpin his humanitarian objectives. Thus Virchow has to be included with Haeckel (see below) among the contributors to "biologistic sociology" (see below).

In relation specifically to Virchow's "scientific method", Rather (1962) stated:

> "With a remarkably clear idea of scientific method, avoiding both the halting gait of narrowly conceived Baconian induction and the erratic flights of the less critical nature-philosophers, he stated that hypotheses and analogies should be firmly based on phenomena of general occurrence." And also: "Systems, according to Virchow, were to be avoided until a sufficient quantity of empirical data could be accumulated".

Hansemann praised Virchow's adherence to "scientific method" in a few articles (Hansemann, 1891c, 1895d), but his own thinking does not seem to have been particularly affected by it. Hansemann's mental processes seem simply and solely to have been in accordance with the general "scrupulous intellectual tradition of *Bildung*" (chapter 1).

Virchow's "Cellular Pathology" as a philosophy of pathology

Because Hansemann defended Virchow's "Cellular Pathology" in several articles (1891b; 1893a; 1895d), some indication of the nature of Virchow's concepts is relevant here.

An analysis of "Cellular Pathology" in anatomical and pathological terms is given in chapter 3. Discussion in this section is limited to views of "Cellular Pathology" as a philosophy.

Rather (1962) believed that Virchow's "Cellular Pathology" represented a system of pathology in the tradition of eighteenth century philosophers. Rather (1962) also noted that Virchow attempted to discuss "the nature of disease" in ontological terms (i.e. do diseases have real existence? – "ontology" is the part of metaphysics concerned with being).

Bölsche (1906, p. 152) thought Virchow's ideas amounted to the following:

> "Health was the harmonious cooperation of (the various cell types within – eds) the cell-state; disease was the falling away of some of the cells to special work that injured or destroyed the whole community."

Schipperges (1994, pp 58-9) expressed the matter as follows:

> "With the dictum '*omnis cellula e cellula*', the principle lines of the entire concept can also be sketched, namely,
> 1) the genetic (*genetische*) principle which rejects all earlier theories of alien, ontological or parasitical causes of disease, and points on the contrary, wholly to the unified developmental line of the healthy as also of the diseased, life;
> 2) the social-political moment, which does not wish to see in the cell complex anything other than a democratically ordered constitution of balance;
> 3) the scientific method, which, via an empirical path, with morphological presuppositions and the help of experimentation, leads further to the verification and falsification of the theories."

Overall, the "Cellular Pathology" can be interpreted as a philosophical system of thought, especially because it approved some modes of contemplation and scientific investigation, and it specifically excluded others. In fact, the great weakness of "Cellular Pathology" was that it declared that any significant external causes of disease are impossible. It also denied any possible role of blood-borne pathogenic factors, whether they were circulating whole bacteria (as in septicaemia) or circulating toxins ("toxaemias"). Possibly it was partly on the basis of this philosophical component of "Cellular Pathology" that Virchow opposed Cohnheim's work on the leukocytic origin of pus cells (Rather, 1972); Klebs' work on bacteriology in general, and Koch's work on anthrax and miliary tuberculosis (both of which involve blood-born microorganisms) – see also Malkin (1990) and chapter 6.

Early in his career, Hansemann was doubtful about the pathogenic nature of microorganisms. In fact, his defence of "Cellular Pathology" against bacteriology, serology and immunology (Hansemann 1891c; 1895a; etc – chapter 12) probably damaged his own reputation in the profession, and may even have cost him appointment to Virchow's chair of Pathology in 1902 (chapter 6).

Darwinism in Germany

Much "Darwinism" preceded Darwin[16] (Glass et al, 1959). Suggestions that species may change into other species were made by various authors as early as the Ancient Greek Xenophanes. In the period immediately relevant to Hansemann, Charles Darwin's grandfather, Erasmus[17] challenged the Christian dogma of immutability of the (God-created) species in "Zoonomia" (1796). This idea was rejected at the time, but after Erasmus Darwin's death, the study of geology (which, like the biological sciences, was assisted enormously by better microscopes – chapter 3) led to a better understanding of the great age of the earth, and of life upon it.

Meanwhile, expeditions to all parts of the globe to collect specimens accumulated biogeographical data of increasing significance. The concept of mutability of species nevertheless was resisted. The idea that living things could be altered by human beings (either by hybridizing plants or by selectively breeding domesticated animals with particular characteristics of economic value) was incontrovertible but largely ignored. The major cause of dispute was the proposal that species in the wild change under the influence of a pitiless, never-ending natural struggle for survival, in which no God ever intervened (Hodge and Radick, 2003).

In the discussion of the fact of mutability of species (see above), comparative embryology became an important consideration. The early embryologists (chapter 3) had found similarities between the adult morphology of "lower" animals and the early embryos of "higher" animals. It is clearly of little value for the survival of (say) a species of placental animal for its embryos to have (at any stage) gills like those of a fish. The only explanation of such developmental features common to many species is that a gradual evolutionary change of species has occurred over time, by some process of "modifications and add-ons" to earlier and simpler species, leading to the formation of "later", "higher" and more complex species. Darwin (1868) emphasised that evolution must occur by these "small changes" but could not establish their mechanism (chapter 3).

In Germany the most prominent Darwinist was Ernst Haeckel[18] (1834–1919). Having conducted significant research on the biology of *Radiolaria*, published in 1862, Haeckel became absorbed in Darwin's theory of evolution and launched the Darwinian phase of his career with a lecture at a scientific meeting at Stettin in 1863. In this he affirmed the development of Man from apes; the emergence of "higher" forms from "lower" forms in sequence over a long period of time; and described the "tree model" of evolution, in which species branch off from one another with the passage of time. Haeckel also included the observations that evolution results in greater degrees of "perfection" of the individual, and also greater sophistication of the relationships between the cells in the "Cell State" of the body (quoting Virchow's conception of Cell Theory – above and chapter 3).

Haeckel then proceeded further to analyse zoology in his "General Morphology" published in 1866. Bölsche (1906) summarised Haeckel's work as follows. First, Haeckel identified unicellular organisms as a separate "Kingdom" ("Protista", now known as Protozoa); second, he described his notion of subcellular units of life (*Monera*); third, he emphasised his "Biogenic Law": "Ontogeny recapitulates Phylogeny"; and fourth, he attempted to find mathematical laws for animal morphology, such as the angles between the arms of starfish.

Philosophical tendencies are obvious in the chapters of "General Morphology" dealing with methodology, and in the approaches to the mental and social aspects of human life presented by Haeckel in the later volumes. These parts of his work can be seen to be a component of the "biologistic sociology" of the later nineteenth century (see below).

In Britain and the United States, Darwinism was attacked in various ways, and underwent a period of eclipse until the 1920s (Bowler, 1983). Some of Darwin's supporters took intellectual paths which diverged to varying degrees from the utterly rational and secular nature of Darwin's theory. Wallace[19] (1823–1913), who had a similar idea of the mechanism of the developments of species, later adopted spiritualist ideas. Haeckel[18] (see above and chapter 3) in later life accepted "psychic" experiences as valid. However, T. H. Huxley[20] (1825–1895), widely referred to as "Darwin's bulldog", remained committed to evolution to the end of his life, although he was concerned with what he saw as the dubious moral and ethical ideas which some authors were deriving from Darwin's theory.

In Germany generally, Darwin's theory did not cause such great controversy as it did in England, perhaps because the Lutheran Church was less interested in biological matters, and further, perhaps because the tolerant attitude to diversity of religious beliefs in the era of Fredrick the Great (1712–1786) may not have faded. Another factor may have been that religious concerns in Germany at the time were dominated by the secular-Catholic struggle of the *Kulturkampf*[21].

Virchow certainly attacked Haeckel's views on evolution at a congress in 1877 (Bölsche, 1906) and later published a formal critique of evolution (Virchow, 1886). However, there is little evidence that Virchow's views were very influential, and they were certainly little discussed in Britain or the United States.

Hansemann was concerned with Darwinism and embryology insofar as he was concerned with heredity and variation among cells of any type. Furthermore, his theory of tumours involved a "hereditary modification/loss or add-on" of the normal cells, and he cites Darwin's "Variation of Plants and Animals" (1868) in this regard. However, Darwin's theory was not essential for Hansemann's theory, perhaps because Hansemann relies so much on chromosomes for his mechanism of genetic alteration, and these structures were not known in Darwin's time. Furthermore, the "new differentiation pathway" implied in "anaplasia" was not related to any contemporaneous ideas of mechanisms of evolutionary change of species. Nevertheless, the resistance to evolutionary ideas, especially mutability of species, is possibly relevant to the fate of Hansemann's ideas. This is because, at the same time and possibly as a result of this opposition to Darwinism, "somatic cell mutation" was widely disbelieved for no conclusive reasons (chapter 6).

Altruism, "cellular altruism" and "biologistic sociology"

The fact that, under certain circumstances, individuals of a species will fight to their own death for the good of the species (e.g. a female deer protecting its fawn) was noted by the Ancients, but not perceived as having any particular philosophical significance. The discoveries in the 1840s of the cellular nature of larger living organisms, and the cooperative, and particularly self-sacrificing behaviour of the cells of tissues (e.g. epidermal cells being generated to die for the protection of the "interior milieu") in relation to the whole body, was greeted with some interest. The discoveries were made at the same time as new social arrangements involving cooperation of individuals for the benefit of "society" were occurring in the industrialising European countries. Virchow, in particular, saw some significance in this analogy (above). A new field of philosophy developed to explore social ideas to parallel the scientifically verified behaviour of the cells. In the writings of some authors biological phenomena were used to "justify", or at least give added credibility to, the social ideas.

Perhaps the first relevant figure in this field was Auguste Comte[22] (1798–1857) whose major works were published during the period 1843–1862. He saw societies as progressing through three stages: religious, metaphysical and scientific, the last being "positive". Later, Comte was largely concerned with developing a "science of society" in the sense of an entirely secular system for analysis and management of human societies. He invented the word "sociology", and wrote on the methodology of sociology, the progress of human societies, the progress of the intellect of the individual, and the hierarchy of the sciences. In later work he suggested a new system of management of society, based on a priestly class of "sociologists" who would monitor and foster correct "positive" behaviour, including "altruism" (a moral obligation of individuals to put the interests of others before their own) among the citizenry.

Although Hansemann used "Altruism" in his work, he did not refer to Comte or "positivism".

Perhaps the major figure in later "biologistic sociology" was Herbert Spencer[23] (1820–1903) to whom Hansemann does refer (Hansemann, 1912d). Initially a "Radical" with ideas derived from the English philosophers Bentham and J. S. Mill, Spencer's thoughts gradually became influenced by Comte and more centred on "social philosophy" (see above). Ultimately Spencer was attracted mainly to Darwin's theory of evolution by natural selection. Spencer used biological phenomena to support his views as "biologistic-sociological analogies" which were a significant part of his nine-volume work "A System of Synthetic Philosophy" (1862-93). Thus his phrase "survival of the fittest" was a use of Darwinism to support *laissez faire* government policies in the field of what are now called "social services".

Spencer[23] also used "differentiation" in relation to societies, and adopted "altruism" from Comte (Cosner 1977). Spencer's works were translated into German (Spencer, 1875), so that von Hansemann probably obtained his ideas from there.

Militarism and *Junkertum*

The *Junkers*, who were the land-owning class of north-eastern Germany and particularly of Pomerania and East Prussia, dated from the early feudal period. From the time of the Great Elector in the 17th century the Junker ethos evolved, characterized by a strong sense of prerogative and obligation to the state in the person of the King of Prussia, or later, the German Emperor. They had no avenue of direct political influence as did both the English peerage (by automatic membership of the House of Lords) and the English squire class (which could contest elections for the House of Commons). The ethos of *Junkertum* therefore tended to exaggerate (by the standards of English-speaking nationalities) some feudal sentiments of patriotism, loyalty to the monarch, "personal honour", and *noblesse oblige* to the tenants and workers of the estates.

Although Prussia had been a militarised state from its inception (taken as the inception of the programme of settlement of the southern Baltic shores by the Teutonic Knights in the thirteenth century), the particular dominance of the military over civilian life is particularly associated with the period after the Revolution of 1848. The popularity of militarism was enormously enhanced by the success of Prussia under Bismarck (1815–1898; Prussian Minister-President 1862–1870; Chancellor of the Second Empire (*Reich*), 1871–1890) in the three wars. The first was against Denmark (1864, after which Denmark lost Schleswig-Holstein to Prussia), the second against Austria (1866) and the third against France (1870–1, after which France lost Alsace and Lorraine to Germany).

For the German bourgeois intellectuals the failure of the 1848 revolution, and the continuing exclusion of their social group from political power, led to degrees of despair and resignation. After 1871, the ascendancy of Prussia over the previously more liberal western German states was even more pronounced, and this prolonged period of autocracy and rising illiberalism caused many of this social group to emigrate (Hochstadt, 1999). Many went to the U.S.A. (especially Chicago in this period), but others settled in the U.K. In Manchester for example, there were a substantial number of Germans in the business class (Engels' father owned a factory in the city) and the "Halle Orchestra" (after Karl Halle, the first conductor) was founded there by the same group. As another example, many Germans migrated to South Australia, where they formed a large distinct group until the First World War. Bourgeois Germans remaining in Germany tended to withdraw into private, professional pursuits. Thus, in (1933) Thomas Mann wrote of Richard Wagner:

> "So he went the way of the bourgeoisie from failure, to resignation to non-involvement".

All this is well known, but can be seen as context for three biomedical sidelights on militarism in German society at the time.

First, after 1865, nationalism in Germany was such that a feeling of "German Science" as opposed to "French-" or "English Science" had developed (Ackerknecht, 1953). This tendency led to increasing isolation of German intellectual life, so that the Germans excluded themselves from the potential benefits of the American bioscientific revolution (of 1890–1910, see Maienschein, 1986) especially in genetics (Bonner, 1963).

As a second example, Virchow's involvement in politics was significant for Germany. In the period when he was a bitter opponent of Bismarck (above) Virchow wrote in a report of 1866 (Ackerknecht, 1953):

> "It is clear that absolutism has been re-established in Prussia, and without the limitations it imposed on itself before March 1848. There is no control of public finances, no budget law anymore; instead of laws we have decrees; the control court (sic) is without subject; treasury and property of the state are at the free disposal of the government."

As a third example, Billroth (1924, p. 240) gave what must have been the then-"standard" justification of militarism while trying to support government expenditure on medical science. He compared the costs of a medical school with those of an infantry regiment. Having pointed out that the running costs of a medical school are similar to those of an infantry regiment, Billroth goes on:

> "By no means would I presume to criticise these (military) expenditures. I am so thoroughly convinced of the high cultural value of compulsory service and of the importance of these (military) institutions in the development and the maintenance of a spirit of national patri-

otism, that no sacrifice seems too high to maintain these forces at their minimum strength. Moreover, the money which is spent on them remains in circulation within the country and millions of factory workers and artisans gain employment thereby. Without a strong, thoroughly trained army it is in our day not so easy to promote the progress of civilization in the various states, and to maintain the present political and social order. For without the restraint of the army, the ever-increasing clamour for individual rights and liberties would soon lead to a reversion to primitive conditions in which the strong would be strengthened and the weak enslaved.

My only object, as I have already pointed out, is to show by way of comparison that the sacrifices which the state is called upon to make for the development of science are by no means so great as they seem to be at first glance, if we compare them with other national expenditures."

Hansemann used, very briefly, a military analogy in one article (1891c), but there is no evidence of any "militaristic thinking" in his works on cancer or philosophy.

Notes to chapter 2

1 Pliny the Younger (c63–113 AD) nephew of Pliny the Elder (a biologist), was of the senatorial class in Ancient Rome, and became a lawyer, subsequently holding various civil and military positions. He is renowned for his letters which were collected and have been preserved.

Reference: Sherwin-White (1967).

2 One looks in vain for methods of investigative science in Aristotle's "Four Causes", mainly because these "causes" are little more than "four considerations". Thus "material cause" is composition, "formal cause" is plan, "efficient cause(s)" are the effector agents of all types and the "final cause" is purpose (for which the plan was drawn up). This is little help in investigation of the nature and aetiology of disease. For Aristotle, natural phenomena offered the most likely field for useful contribution. His exhortations to further study were ignored for nearly two-thousand years.

Reference: Gotthelf and Lennox (1987).

3 As part of the Reformation, invention of a "new", non-Catholic science was attempted, especially by Paracelsus, Van Helmont, Campanella, Glanvill, Glisson and Descartes (Pagel, 1953). Van Helmont (1577–1644) in particular laced his writings with expressions of (Protestant) Christian consciousness, together with the opinion that the teachings of Aristotele are "heathen". His general modes of thought, however, were very similar to those of the Ancient Graeco-Romans, even if he intended the works to be critical of those philosophers. The other type of anti-Aristotelianism was based on a taste for evidence of fresh observation and experimental results to support hypotheses in the areas of natural science, notable also in the countries affected by the Reformation. Particular scientists to note in this regard were Francis Bacon (1561–1626), William Harvey (1578–1657), Robert Boyle (1627–1691), Isaac Newton (1643–1727).

References: Pagel (1944, 1953, 1982), Crowther (1960), Hall (1983), Vickers (1987).

4 Descartes (1596-1650) believed in God and a soul, but maintained his early purpose of explaining natural phenomena in terms of "mechanisms". Descartes' use of "animal spirits" is misleading, because by this he meant physical events, later conceivable as analogous or equivalent to electrical impulses, not Aristotelian "spirits" (Cottingham, 1993). Descartes' mechanistic theory of tissue formation was applied to tumour formation by the later French school, as is outlined in chapter 4.

5 The Reformation may perhaps not be an entirely appropriate marker for the beginnings of a German philosophy. The great medieval Mystics, Meister Eckhart (c.1260–1327), Heinrich Seuse (Suso, 1295–1366) and Johannes Tauler (c.1300–1361) contributed a mystic strand, which was vital to the mode of contemplation (*Betrachtungsweise*) for the Lutheran Reformation. Specifically, they contributed to the development of the tendency to abstraction and inwardness (*Innerlichkeit*). A later contributor was Jacob Böhme (1575–1624), who was foremost among the Silesian Pietist Mystics after the Reformation.

6 Christian Thomasius (1655–1724) was a lawyer and a professor of philosophy (in Leipzig and after being proscribed there, as a Foundation Professor at the University of Halle). Initially he sought to divorce natural law from theology. This was similar to Descartes' purpose (see note 2 above). Thomasius was opposed to prejudice, belief in superstitions, religious persecution, witch-hunts and the use of torture.

Reference: Mauntner (1995), Audi (1999).

7 Caspar Wolff (1679–1754) Professor of Mathematics and Natural Science at the University of Halle, conceived a system of philosophy based on a world-wisdom (*Welt-Weisheit*) as the means to public enlightenment. For this reason he wrote in German, at least during his Halle years. His democratic views expressed in essays such as in "German Theology" in 1724 caused Friedrich Wilhelm I in Berlin to expel him from Prussia on threat of hanging. Of relevance to the over-inclusive tendency of German philosophers (see main text, this chapter), his systematizing philosophy integrated different ideas from the philosophical tradition according to the model of mathematics.

Reference: Mauntner (1995), Audi (1999).

8 In his "Universal Natural History" Immanuel Kant (1724–1804) did indeed "out-Newton" Newton in relation to "reason". Newton thought that cosmic organization required the hand of God, and that God regularly infuses nature with new motion to keep the world machine from running down. Newton also accepted the notion of final causes as ways in which God makes himself known. Kant eliminated God from the workings of the Universe. In Kant's system, a principle of nature streams outward in a wavefront of organization, generating worlds, biological systems and finally Reason (human and otherwise).

Reference: Neiman (1994).

9 Johann Gottlieb Fichte (1762–1814) who was Professor of Philosophy at Jena (1794–1799) and eventually (1810) at the University of Berlin, developed during the final decade of the eighteenth century a radically revised and rigorously systematic version of transcendental idealism, which he called *Wissenschaftslehre*.

Reference: Mauntner (1995), Audi (1999).

10 Georg Wilhelm Friedrich Hegel (1770–1831) who was one of the most influential of German philosophers, made one of the last great attempts (following on from Aristotle, Aquinas, Spinoza, Kant and others) to develop philosophy as an all-embracing scientific system. His system was based on a "Philosophy of Spirit" and a "Science of Logic". In our present context, we cannot present the precise meanings of this, which would doubtless be "a field too far"/*ein zu weites Feld* (Fontane, *Effi Briest*).

Reference: Kainz (1998).

11 Arthur Schopenhauer (1788–1860) believed that the world is not primarily a rational place, but could be understood by the introspections of the sentient individual. He thus became a philosopher of the late Romantic period. His "system" was outlined in "The World as Will and Idea" (1819, 2nd edn 1844).

Reference: Mann (1939).

Notes to chapter 2

12 Richard Wagner (1813–1883, composer notably of music dramas, including the "Ring" tetralogy), consciously attempted to assemble vast, comprehensive, multiform structures referred to as "The Total Work of Art" (*Gesamtkunstwerk*).

   Reference: Newman (1976).

13 Gotthold Ephraim Lessing (1729–1781) was a liberal, humanist publicist and playwright who was the first German to earn his living by his pen. Only towards the end of his life did he accept an official appointment as Court Librarian for the Duke of Braunschweig. Lessing took up the disputative model of the Ancient Greeks (see below) as *Streitkultur* for the German "Age of Reason", but insisted on absolute self-control in argument and the avoidance of dogmatism. He was comfortable with "flux" as an acceptable condition for unresolved issues. His particularly careful, fair, honest and temperate mode of expression was to be ignored subsequently by the Romantic philosophers (see below).

   Reference: Mauser and Sasse (1993).

14 A preliminary feature of the German Romantic movement was the creation of a near-mythological history of the German Medieval period. This myth-making began in the eighteenth century especially with Johann Gottfried Herder (1744–1803), who identified an original national "folk spirit" (*Volksseele*) with a "better" German past. Perhaps definitively, German Romanticism began in the early 1770s with the *Sturm und Drang* movement (involving Goethe in early life, Schiller and others). A progression from this is perhaps traceable in German cultural history through Wagner to Freud. *Sturm und Drang* developed into a "movement" characterised by dramatised heroics, emotional excess, lack of control, zealotry and abstraction. Individualism, ideas of infinite personal potentialities, introspection, celebration of nature and mysticism are additional aspects of the ethos of this movement.

   References: Pascal (1954), Reinhard (1961), Taylor (1997).

15 *Naturphilosophie* is particularly associated with Friedrich Wilhelm Joseph von Schelling (1775–1854) and to a lesser extent Georg Wilhelm Friedrich Hegel (1770–1831). This thread of German idealism exhibited a search for an all-embracing "system" in which "Nature" – as an abstraction of the body of facts which was accumulating from biology, geology and the physical sciences etc – could be seen as being more than the sum of that which is objective. Because it amounted to more than the objective facts, the system (if found) would thus have had a significance which was not restricted to that which can be established about it in scientific terms. On the other hand, "intelligence" was seen as the complex of all the activities making up self-consciousness – these being denoted "transcendental" facts. According to Schelling, the philosophy of nature and transcendental philosophy are the two complementary portions of philosophy as a whole.

   Reference: Audi (1999), Pinkard (2002).

16 Charles Darwin (1809–1882), considered the most important biologist since Aristotle, grandson of Erasmus Darwin (see below), studied at Cambridge and Edinburgh Universities, travelled on the "Beagle" expedition (1831–1836) and published his "Origin of Species Based on Natural Selection" (1859, with many subsequent editions). In several later works he enhanced his argument and reputation concerning the mechanisms of evolution. Darwin neither taught at nor held an appointment in a University.

   References: Browne (2002), Hodge and Radick (2003).

17 Erasmus Darwin (1731–1802) was a physician, medical and botanical author, poet; graduate of Cambridge (St John's) and the University of Edinburgh Medical School. His most famous work is "Zoonomia" (1795) in which the great age of the Earth and the mutability of species were both supported. His work was successfully attacked, mainly by William Paley in the latter's "Natural

37

Theology" (1803). The fate of "Zoonomia" probably contributed to the reluctance of his grandson Charles to publish similar ideas without detailed supporting evidence.

References: Haber (1958), King-Hele (1963, 1983).

18 Ernst Heinrich Philipp August Haeckel (1834–1919), b Potsdam, studied medicine under Müller, Virchow and Kölliker, graduating at Berlin in 1857. He took up zoology at Jena, and was appointed to the Chair there in 1865. For an account of the high degree of his admiration for Darwin and Darwinism, see Desmond and Moore (1992). Later, Haeckel's ideas became more "philosophical", arguing a fundamental unity of animate and inanimate matter ("Monism"). He rejected conventional religious beliefs, but accepted "psychic" phenomena as valid, and believed all living things to be susceptible to them.

Reference: Haeckel (1903), Bölsche (1906), Richardson and Keuck (2002).

19 Alfred Russell Wallace (1823–1913), b Usk, Monmouthshire U.K., became a surveyor and school teacher. From age 25, he joined naturalist expeditions to collect biological specimens in South America and later the Malay Archipelago. By 1855 he had arrived at broadly the same conclusions concerning the origins of species as had Charles Darwin. Wallace, like Darwin, lost faith in formal religion as a result of his studies, but later became a spiritualist because he could not see how evolution could explain aspects of human mental life, such as philosophical musings, artistic feeling, and humour. Darwin disagreed with this, believing that evolution of these aspects can occur by their effect of influencing sexual selection.

References: Wallace (1889), Raby (2001).

20 Thomas Henry Huxley (1825–1895), son of a teacher of mathematics in Ealing, London, studied medicine (becoming a naval surgeon), while pursuing his interests in biology and zoology. At 26, he was elected Fellow of the Royal Society for his work on invertebrates. A supporter of Darwin from the start, he is famous for his defence of the theory of evolution against Samuel Wilberforce, Bishop of Oxford at a Union Debate there in 1860. In later life he became concerned with ethics, morals and evolution, inventing the word "agnosticism". He is said to have strongly supported the teaching of Christianity in schools, and resisted any fully "gladiatorial" theory of existence.

Reference: Barr (1997).

21 The *Kulturkampf* (the "conflict of cultures") began with the "Catalogue of the Principal Errors of Our Time", published by Pope Pius IX in 1864, and was followed by the promulgation of the Doctrine of Papal Infallibility in 1870. Bismarck saw this as a threat to the secular basis of Prussian government, and responded with various laws, including for the direct control of schools by the government, the expulsion of Jesuits, state supervision of clergy and compulsory civil marriage ceremonies. He was supported on this issue by Virchow (Schipperges, 1994). The issues involved were still significant in Germany throughout Hansemann's lifetime (see chapter 1) and beyond.

References: Taylor (1951), Ross (1998).

22 Isidore Marie Auguste François Xavier Comte (1798–1857), born Montpellier, France, studied science and medicine, but ultimately became a secretary, writer and philosopher. Coser (1977) stated that:

"Although Comte conceived of society by analogy with a biological organism, he was aware of the difficulties that such analogical thinking brings in its wake. A biological organism is, so to speak, encased in a skin and hence has material boundaries. The body social, however, cannot be held together by physical mean, but only spiritual ties."

Additional references: Marvin (1936), Bryant (1985), Pickering (1993).

Notes to chapter 2

23 Herbert Spencer was son of a school teacher in Derby, England and became a journalist, political writer and philosopher. Coser's (1977, p. 90) general view of Spencer's philosophy is:

"It is axiomatic to Spencer that ultimately all aspects of the Universe, whether organic or inorganic, social or nonsocial, are subject to the law of evolution. His sociological reflections concentrate, however, on the parallels between organic and social evolution, between similarities in the structure and evolution of organic and social units. Biological analogies occupy a privileged position in all of Spencer's sociological reasoning, although he was moved to draw attention to the limitations of such analogies."

Spencer used "differentiation" for the increase in complexity of societies, such that individuals in it divide labour (Coser, 1977 p. 92) as follows.

"As the parts of a social whole become more unlike and the roles individuals play become in consequence more differentiated, their mutual dependence increases. 'The consensus of functions becomes closer as evolution advances. In low aggregates, both individual and social, the actions of the parts are but little dependent on one another, whereas in developed aggregates of both kinds that combination of actions which constitutes the life of the whole makes possible the component actions which constitute the lives of the parts' (original ref 16). It follows as a corollary that 'where parts are little differentiated they can readily perform one another's functions, but where much differentiated they can perform one another's functions very imperfectly, or not at all.' (original ref 17)".

This was Hansemann's view of normal and tumour cells.

Coser (1977) went on:

"The increasing mutual dependence of unlike parts in complex societies, and the vulnerability it brings in its wake necessitate the emergence of a "regulating system" that controls the actions of the parts and insures their coordination."

Additional references: Peel (1971), Andreski (1972).

Chapter 3

Aspects of biomedical science in the nineteenth century

Introduction

One of Hansemann's major ideas was that the abnormalities of tumour cells are the result of abnormalities in the inherited material of the cell, arising through abnormalities in their chromosomes. This idea was original because before the 1870s, the chromosomes had not been discovered – because they could not be seen. No optical apparatus existed for visualising anything much smaller than about half an erythrocyte (magnification of 500 times). The nucleus was considered to be the probable repository of most of the hereditary material in the cell, but little had been achieved in the understanding of nuclear division other than to note that it necessarily accompanied cell division. Sub-nuclear detail, and especially the definite equality of distribution of nuclear material during nuclear division, could not be appreciated.

Nevertheless, the ideas and theories concerning the biology of cancer which had been derived during the pre-chromosomal period remained dominant throughout Hansemann's time and for several decades afterwards. This present chapter first sketches the development of microscopy up to Hansemann's time, and in particular the invention of the techniques which allowed the chromosomes to be studied. At the University of Berlin, Hansemann had the highest quality equipment for his studies involving microscopy as soon as it became available. Then we mention briefly the changes which these advances in microscopy made to concepts of histology, embryology and genetics.

It should be noted that in the middle of the nineteenth century, physiology and biochemistry underwent great development, especially under the influence of two very notable Frenchmen. First, Claude Bernard (1813–1878) discovered – among many other things – the glycogenic function of the liver, and hence that the liver "internally secretes" glucose into the *milieu interieur* (which he named). Second, Louis Pasteur (1822–1895) discovered – again among many things – that fermentation is due to micro-organisms. Thus by this alone, Pasteur made a great contribution to the discipline of metabolism. However, Virchow paid little attention to Bernard – although his "Cellular Pathology" (1858) was "based on physiological and pathological histology" – and ignored Pasteur, whose work contradicted the essential element of Virchow's philosophy of pathology (see below and chapter 2). Hansemann was doubtless familiar with concepts of "internal secretion" and "fermentation" from his undergraduate education, and acknowledged Bernard in "Studies ..." (Hansemann, 1893c, original p. 53). No further details are mentioned here of physiology and biochemistry, because the works of Hansemann, and of Virchow before him, were not further directly influenced by them.

Microscopy

Successful microscopy using visible light depends on two things: (i) satisfactory preparation of the object (usually as thin slices called "sections") by processes of fixation, hardening, embedding, sectioning, staining and mounting of the specimen, and (ii) the quality of the microscope which is used to examine the sections. Microscopes comprise not only the main lenses but also the secondary optical components for condensing and restricting the path of light through the object and to the main lenses (substage condensers, diaphragms and oil immersion).

Attempts at fixation of biological specimens originally involved boiling or application of acids and/or alcohol (Bracegirdle, 1978). Chromium trioxide was used as a fixative from 1840 and was used by some authors for the study of chromosomes in the 1870s. Mercuric chloride ("sublimat") had been used by Blanchard as early as 1846, but only after 1878 did its use become widespread (Bracegirdle, 1978). "Sublimat" was Hansemann's preferred tissue fixative (Hansemann 1893c), and is still recognised as an excellent fixative of chromatin.

Various means of holding fixed specimens firmly for sectioning had been used since the beginnings of microscopy. However, paraffin embedding, as described in 1869 by Klebs was much superior to other techniques and had become widely used in the 1880s (Bracegirdle, 1978). Sectioning with microtomes has a history dating from the eighteenth century, and by the 1880s various satisfactory models were sold by manufacturers in Germany, Britain and France, including (in Germany) by the Zeiss, Reichert and Schiefferdecker companies (Bracegirdle, 1978).

Staining of histological sections had been attempted from the beginnings of microscopy (Clark and Kasten, 1983). Raspail[1], in the 1820s, used alcoholic solutions of iodine, which was probably the best technique at that time (Weiner, 1968; Clark and Kasten, 1983), and was used by Lebert in the 1840s (Rather, 1978). Later carmine (from cochineal), safranin and indigo were popular stains (Clark and Kasten, 1983), being used by authors such as Julius Arnold in the 1870s (see chapter 4).

Haematoxylin (produced from aqueous extracts of logwood by subsequent ether extraction) and eosin (an aniline dye) were introduced in the 1860s and by the 1880s had become popular general stains for nuclei and cytoplasm respectively. However, even up to the twentieth century, there was little standardisation of preparations of haematoxylin, so that some variability of results did occur from laboratory to laboratory (Clark and Kasten, 1983).

Various mounting media (the transparent substance applied between the specimen or section and the coverslip of a microscopic slide) had been used for over a century. Canada balsam, which has a refractive index similar to that of the glass used for lenses and microscopic slides, was introduced for this purpose in 1832 (Bracegirdle, 1978). Various immersion liquids (which are used to fill the space between the specimen/coverslip and the objective lens) had been used by Robert Hooke (Gunther, 1961), but the specific iso-refractory oil now in use was only introduced in the 1870s by Abbe at the Zeiss company (Bradbury, 1967).

The story of the development of microscopes has been well-told elsewhere (Carpenter, 1891; Bradbury, 1967) and will be only summarised here. Briefly, the first magnifying instruments were made in the late seventeenth century with simple crude single glass-lenses. Their magnification depended on the quality of the lens-making, but was rarely better than 50X. In the 1830s, the first "achromatic" lenses (two or more crown- and flint glasses together) were made, allowing magnifications of 200-300X. The "apochromatic" ("away from colour") lenses were invented by Abbe at the Zeiss works and consisted of various composites of new glass types which included especially borate glass. These, with oil immersion, give magnifications of approximately 1000X.

Hansemann does not state the manufacturer of the oil-immersion oil which he used. Nor does he state the manufacturer of his microscope. However, his microscope was fitted with apochromatic Zeiss lenses although the date of their manufacture is not given. Hansemann's photomicrographic equipment involved a Zeiss model. In "Studies ..." (1893c, chapter 11) he mentioned that he had shown his micrographs at a scientific meeting. These may well be the first photomicrographs of mitotic figures shown in public. Nevertheless, photomicrography itself was not new. Among the first photomicrographs of any type were probably those of Donné in Paris, who pioneered the use of prints of Daguerrotype micrographs for teaching purposes (La Berge, 1994). Oskar Israel (note[14] of chapter 1) is mentioned by Dhom (2001) as being particularly competent in photomicrography.

Thus Hansemann possessed all the latest technical developments in all fields of light microscopy which were available. These have not changed in principle to the present day.

Normal histology

The structure of multicellular organisms was discussed by the Ancients, but little attention was paid to the actual structure of organs until the seventeenth century[2]. A small number of microscopists, working independently of each other, especially Malpighi (1628–1694), Leeuwenhoek (1632–1723) and Swammerdam (1637–1680), identified erythrocytes, white blood cells, cells in lymph, "fibres" of muscle, as well as specific structures including spermatozoa, but with little understanding of their functions (Nordenskiöld, 1928; Cameron, 1952; Hughes, 1959; Harris, 1999). Especially after the discovery of the circulation of the blood by

Harvey, there was a decline in the influence of the Galenic "humouralist" theory of disease, which considered all diseases as due to imbalances of diffusely-spread "humours" and thus implied that local circumstances might have little to do with these conditions. The trend to consider local causes of disease was promoted by the study of clinico-pathological correlation, emphasised most notably by Morgagni (1682–1771). Nevertheless, even in the late eighteenth century, the relative significance of "fibres", "globules" and "accretions" in the tissues of multicellular organisms was unclear, so that anatomists could still ignore the existence of these structures more or less completely. In France, Bichat[3] (1771–1802) introduced the classification of the tissues (such "textures" of the organs which could be identified with the naked eye, together with a little simple mechanical and chemical testing) with little use of microscopy. After the invention of effective achromatic lenses (late 1830s), the primary physiological significance of cells in the body became evident, and was propounded as the "Cell Theory" by Schwann (1810–1882) and Schleiden (1804–1881) (see Cameron, 1952; Hughes, 1959; Harris, 1999). The primary concept of the "Cell Theory" as elaborated by Schwann and Schleiden was not just that cells exist, but also that they are the metabolic units of the body. Its corollary was that metabolic changes do not occur to any significant extent in the intercellular space (i.e. between cells). Therefore, an appropriate slogan for the Cell Theory as it was originally expounded, and which would be consistent with other slogans for biology at the time (see below), could be

"omnes metabolica per cellulae" ("all metabolism through cells").

After the acceptance of the primacy of the cell in the lives of organisms, a major debate began concerning the origin of cells. Schwann, Schleiden and Müller thought that cells precipitate from suitably-altered intercellular material, which they called "blastema" (Rather, 1972; Rather et al, 1986). In fact, Raspail[1] had noted in 1825 that vegetable cells reproduce themselves, and invented the phrase *"omnis cellula e cellula"*. His work, however, was largely ignored. In effect, by the early 1840s, the situation was as described by Lonsdale (1868):

"Granted cells and their membranes, cytoplasm, nuclei and nucleoli, what then?"

The next step was provided by John Goodsir[4] who noted that some animal tissues are made up of specific cell types, which reproduce themselves within anatomically specific sites. Because all growth of tissues at that time was thought to be controlled by the supply of nutrition, he called these cell-forming sites "nutritive foci". Goodsir's second blow to the "precipitation theories" of cell growth or formation was that bone forms by the actions of local cells. This idea – that cells control what happens in the immediate environment and can even cause solid materials (even bone matrix) to precipitate around themselves (see also below) – was a considerable departure from the previous idea, which was that cells precipitate out of the intercellular material.

Other histologists, such as Kölliker and Henle, made further contributions to the microscopic study of the tissues. By the time Kölliker's text appeared (1846) it was clear that each whole multicellular organism consists of a "cooperative" mass of mutually supportive and self-renewing tissues, and that many tissues consist of cells which change their morphological features while undergoing "differentiation" in the sense of specialisation.

Virchow's "Cellular Pathology" – an analysis

Views on the philosophical essence (*Wesen*) of Virchow's "Cellular Pathology" are mentioned in chapter 2. The following is an analysis of "Cellular Pathology" in the context of the anatomical and pathological knowledge of the 1850s (see also Malkin, 1990; Wagner, 1999).

There were probably two paramount issues relevant to Virchow's biomedical thinking at the time. First, the "Cell Theory" of Schwann and Schleiden (published in 1839) implied that all metabolism occurs in living cells (above). Another relevant issue was the view of Rokitansky and the Viennese School that disease is the result of blood-borne disturbances ("neohumoralism" according to Virchow) affecting local parts of the body.

Virchow's contribution was to realise that, if the metabolism of the cells in a tissue is responsible for the normal function of the part, then disturbances of the metabolism of the same cells (that is, the cells at the local site) are probably responsible for the manifestations of the disease. As noted in chapter 2, Virchow went even further: he declared that the "harmonious mutual support of local tissue types" is the essence of health, and that loss of such "harmony" is the cause of disease. Probably because of his strident opposition (*Streitkultur!*) to Rokitansky, Virchow adopted the incorrect opinion that all diseases are caused by local factors, and that circulating disease-causing agents are impossible.

This opinion that the metabolism of the local cells is all-important in the causation of disease occurred at precisely the same time (mid 1850s) at which Virchow was "converted" from his earlier faith in the "blastema" theory of the spontaneous generation of cells to the idea that each cell only arises from another cell (Wolff, 1907; Long, 1958; Weiner, 1968; Rather, 1971, 1978; Schmeidebach, 1990; Malkin, 1990; Wolpert, 1995; Harris, 1995, 1999).

Virchow then used the slogan of that idea (*"omnis cellula e cellula"*) to popularise his concept of "Cellular Pathology" (Rather, 1971; 1978; Schipperges, 1994). While the slogan could encompass his anti-Rokitansky/anti-neohumoural view that disease comes from circulating agents in the body, it was nevertheless an imprecise and imperfect summary of Virchow's contribution. Virchow's significant idea – being that all diseases are caused by disturbances of local, fixed living cells – is not appropriately indicated by *"omnis cellula e cellula"* but is summarised by *"omnes rera pathologica per cellulae locis"* ("all things pathological through local cells").

Virchow and the origin and lineage fidelity (an aspect of "specificity") of cells

After the identification of cells as the metabolic units of the body, and the acceptance of the idea that cells beget themselves, a major issue in biology and pathology became the degree to which cell types can change their form, especially in adult life. Because Hansemann discussed this as a component of his over-arching concept of "specificity" of cells (1893c), Virchow's ideas on this subject are relevant here.

In "Cellular Pathology" (1858), Virchow called these changes "histological substitution" and believed them to be common events in normal tissues. Later he divided the phenomenon into "metaplasia" and "cellular adaptation" (Virchow, 1870; 1884; Adami, 1908; Bignold, 2005), but still considered them common and important. The contrary view was proposed by Remak, Bard and others, and finally expressed (after a vast effort in the study of the "pedigrees" of cell layers – see Hertwig, 1890; Rather, 1978) as *"omnis cellula e cellula ejustum generis"* ("each cell from a cell like itself"). This concept was developed to its most extreme and detailed form by Bard, who supposed that the germ layers are not simply the original tissues of the organs, but are complex structures in which particular parts of each are destined to provide the various organs which derive from them (e.g. the breasts from ectoderm, and the liver from endoderm) from very early in the development of the embryo – see below. This "specificity of the cellular elements" (see Rather, 1978, pp 176–8) was vital to Hansemann's concept that "specificity" is one general aspect of the nature of cancer, and indeed (we suggest) one concept of the triad of concepts in his "system of cancer" (chapter 5).

Embryology

The nature of sexual fertilization and the question of how adult organisms form from eggs (especially chicks from hens' eggs) was addressed by the Ancients and by Aristotle in particular (Needham, 1934; Gasking, 1967; Oppenheimer, 1967; Farley, 1982; Horder et al., 1980; Churchill, 1991). Progress was slow until the eighteenth century and the overthrow of the so-called "preformationist" theories (Gilbert, 1994). This left the alternative view (the "developmentalist" theory[5]) dominant. Thus, the fact that formation of adults from eggs depends on "differentiation" of less differentiated structures to more differentiated ones during embryonic development was established by the work of early embryologists, including Caspar Wolff (1733—1794) and Oken (1779–1851). Even Goethe[6] (1749–1832) expressed views along these lines. However, it was Pander and independently von Baer[7] who identified the precise phases through which embryos pass to develop into adults forms and also identified the development of organs from "germ layers" (ectoderm, mesoderm and endoderm). Von Baer (1827), who had already provided the first description of an egg in a mammal, also noted that there are relationships between the type and grade of development, and the taxonomic position of the species to which the embryo belongs (see Churchill, 1991). As well as leading to the ideas of Bard (above and chapter 4) this became a starting point for the role of embryological data in the debates which were to follow concerning evolution (see chapter 2 and Ospovat, 1981).

Through the subsequent nineteenth century, the following additional advances of observation and interpretation in embryology (Oppenheimer, 1967) were made: (i) that the egg is a single cell, by Schwann in 1839; (ii) that spermatozoa are cells of the organism arising in the testis (and thus are not parasites, as von Baer had thought), by Kölliker in 1841; (iii) that fertilisation is associated with a sperm entering the egg, by Martin Barry in 1843 (Farley, 1982) and (iv) that the processes of germ layer formation and gastrulation are common to all animal phyla, by Kowalevski in 1867. At the time Hansemann produced his theory of "anaplasia", the manner of production of gametes, especially of the egg by the ovary was under active consideration. The "polar bodies" had been identified as early as 1848 (Hertwig, 1890), but their significance was still unclear. For the details of this, see the excellent historical sections in the relevant chapters of Hertwig (1890) and the references cited above.

Another particularly important issue of embryology was the mechanism of the regulation of the growth of tissues and parts of the body. Since Descartes in the seventeenth century (see chapter 4), growth had been considered to be controlled by the delivery of nutrients, and hence in turn, under the control of the vascular system. In the nineteenth century, growth was being seen in terms of the balance of opposite metabolic processes *viz*:- "anabolism" and "catabolism". In 1866, Haeckel (see chapter 2) had used the word "anaplasia" for the growing phases of life (ana = upwards, plasia = "fit for moulding" – Wolff, 1907), and "cataplasia" was for the older age characterised by retrogression. "Anaplastic substances" had a meaning of "adding to a formation", and therefore "ana-" was being used in the same way as it is used in the modern word "anabolic".

Finally, experimental embryology was introduced as a new approach to embryological research by Wilhelm Roux[8] (1850–1924). A good overview of the intentions of Roux can be identified in a translation of his introduction to the *Archiv für Entwicklungsmechanik des Organismus* which is included in Maienschein (1986). The effort of these biologists was concerned to explore the mechanisms of embryological development (*Entwicklungsmechanik*), rather than just document the phenomena of normal development. The methods of Roux's experiments were crude, and the significance of the results and Roux's interpretations of them were rightly considered with some scepticism (see Baltzer, 1967; and chapter 4).

Hansemann based his main theory on the process of "differentiation" (see chapter 4) and hence was interested in its relation to all these topics, especially in relation to the experimental embryological results of Roux (above). Hansemann was also concerned with cell function and, to a lesser degree, with the formation of eggs. However, he was not particularly concerned with germ layer theory except in the context of his general concept of "Specificity".

Genetics – general considerations

Because Hansemann was proposing that normal cells become cancer cells because of a primary alteration in their hereditary material, we shall discuss here the various concepts of heredity as they were then understood. The era is well described in various books (Wilson, 1924; Dunn, 1962; Allen, 1978; Farley 1982; Harris, 1995; Carlson, 2004), but the main points of the matter are so central to understanding von Hansemann's opus that they are reviewed here.

There are four circumstances in living things in which transfer of heredity is relevant. The circumstances are:

(i) in the context of the continuity of characteristics of a species (ancestral heredity);

(ii) during sexual reproduction, during which the degree of influence of each parent on the phenotypic features of the offspring is determined;

(iii) during embryological development, when cells deriving from the zygote give rise to progressively more and more specialised cell types (see also "differentiation");

(iv) in the tissues of the adult, where the "germinative cells" (now known as "stem cells") of any particular cell type reproduce (usually) only daughter cells of the same particular cell type.

In all of this, Hansemann was among the first to discuss the roles of mitoses and these hereditary processes in pathological lesions. However, in his various works he did not state whether or not he considered that the same mechanisms underlie them all.

Heredity at the level of the whole individual (ancestral heredity)

Heredity at this level was discussed by the Ancients including Aristotle, although because spontaneous generation of life was accepted as well at the time, there was little of significance in these discussions (Dunn, 1962). With the recognition of "*omnis cellula e cellula*" (marking the overthrow of theories of spontaneous generation of cells – see above), a question arose as to why some features (e.g. gender) of children are inherited entirely from one parent but not the other, while other features such as the skin colour of a child appear to result from contributions of both parents. Considering only the rational theories which were current at the time, it can be noted that before the era of Cell Theory, Maupertuis[9] had suggested that each organ contributed one or more "particles" to the sperm and/or ovum, and that the amalgamation of these masses led to the beginning of the formation of the embryo. In the nineteenth century, the idea that all parts of the body contribute to the hereditary material of the individual, i.e. to either the egg or "seminal material" during adult life, was in accord with the Lamarckian notion that traits acquired by the individual during adult life can be transmitted to offspring[10].

The three major nineteenth century authors on this topic before von Hansemann used essentially the same idea in principle: Charles Darwin (1868) as "gemmules"[11], August Weismann (1892) as "plasmas" and Nägeli (1884) as "ids".

In contrast to Darwin (whose ideas on the mechanism of ancestral heredity were Lamarckian), Weismann made the major contribution by pointing out that the "drawing of units from all parts of the adult body to the gamete" is unlikely (Allen, 1975; Farley, 1982). In a famous experiment, Weismann showed that the offspring of mice which have had their tails amputated before mating, have tails. Thus he suggested that the "gemmules" etc for the tails of the offspring must be coming from a site other than the parents' tails. He proposed that a separate line of cells (in the "germ plasm") must be present in the body which preserved all the hereditary units ("plasmas") for packaging in gametes. In human embryology, this separate line was obviously the gonadal precursor cells which develop in the retroperitoneum of the embryo in about the sixth week after fertilisation.

Heredity material in sexual reproduction

By Hansemann's time, the nature of the egg and sperm as gametes was established (see "embryology" above), and the fact that fertilisation involves only one sperm entering an egg had been established (see above). However, exactly what happens to the chromosomes during the production of the gametes was unclear at that time. Generally, in 1890, the cell divisions in the gametes were not fully recognised as different from those of ordinary cell replication. The term "meiosis" lay in the future. Furthermore, whether or not all species used the same mechanisms for production of gametes was unclear. The topic is well covered in Gasking (1967) and Farley (1982) and there are several valuable original essays from the period in Maienschein (1986).

Cellular heredity in embryonic development

Even with simple microscopes, it was clear that embryonic cells undergo strikingly regular changes in type (i.e. one of the forms of "differentiation", see below).

For example, Müller (1840) fully illustrated subdivision of the zygote (i.e. blastula formation) in the frog. Having established that these changes occur (see section on histology, above) the question became: how is it that particular daughter cells in the embryo proceed by an unfailingly regular process to only specific types of "more differentiated" cells according to the part of the adult body in which the whole process occurs?

Microscopy with the new (apoachromatic) microscopes in the late 1880s allowed the replication of chromosomes and their subsequent movements in these cells to be studied. However, a controversy arose concerning to what degree equality of distribution of chromosomes occurs during this embryonic developmental change of cell types. Weismann (see above) suggested that the changes in cell functions are associated with loss of hereditary material (the "quantitative" theory). On the other hand, Hertwig (see above) considered that it involved alterations in the functional status (equivalent to the current term "gene activity status") of the hereditary units (Farley, 1982).

The field of experimental embryology was of considerable importance to Hansemann, because potentially it provided data concerning the mechanism of differentiation in relation to cellular genetics in embryos. But the results available at the time were not satisfactory (see above).

Thus Hansemann formulated his theory at just the time when the major issue of the mechanism of the functions of chromosomes (number versus activity status) was in flux. Worth noting here is that Hansemann (1893c) considered that cells replicate their chromosomes after nuclear division, not before (chapter 11).

Heredity in cell populations which turn over in adults

The existence of a regular turnover of cells in normal tissues was suggested by Goodsir[5] (1843, 1868) (see above) and accepted by Virchow (see above), but the achromatic lenses which were the best available at the time could not reveal mitoses at all. Because of this, all the details of the site of the proliferation of the local stem cells could not be established with certainty. As a result, the degree to which cell types turn over in normal adult tissues, and the mechanism of the turnover, was a very controversial in the early phase of Hansemann's career.

Hansemann in fact spent considerable time on this issue from the beginning of his career, by studying the origin of cells of the human epidermis [and published in his contribution to the Festschrift for Virchow by his Professional Assistants (*Assistenten*), Hansemann, 1891h]. As will be described more fully in chapter 5, Hansemann found that the occurrence of mitoses in the lower layers of the epidermis is consistent with basal production of new cells which then mature as they rise to the surface. Hansemann believed Weismann's theory of quantitative reduction of chromosomal material as the basis of embryonic differentiation, but apparently never found proof of this (either as loss of chromosomal material from dividing basal-layer cells, or as asymmetric division) in his studies of normal human epidermis. Thus Hansemann referred to the issue only briefly in his papers, and seems to have considered that the mechanism of "tissue differentiation" might be via variable influences of "main plasmas" and "auxiliary plasmas" (*Hauptplasmen* and *Nebenplasmen*) (chapter 5).

We can note that the current general classification of cell types in adults into "labile", "stable" and "permanent" was made by Bizzozero (1894). However, the mechanism of how a local stem cell divides such that one daughter cell continues as a stem cell, and the other goes on to specialise (for example, one daughter cell of basal epidermal cell continues as a basal cell, while the other matures into a keratinocyte in epidermis) has still not been solved today.

Applications of the word "differentiation"

Hansemann described the changes of tumour cells in comparison with the mother cells in terms of "loss of differentiation" or "de-differentiation" (*Entdifferenzierung*). In all his papers, Hansemann did not define exactly his use of the word, although he used "differentiation" in referring to the same phenomena to which the term is applied today. Here, therefore, we will consider all five phenomena to which the term "differentiation" had been applied by the time Hansemann formulated his theory. Further, we will discuss the "capacity for independent existence" of various types of cells, and the "survivability after transplantation" of cells, and tumour cells in particular. This is because Hansemann discussed both issues at the same time, and he may have included both of them among his usages of "differentiation". In general though, it seems probable that Hansemann was using "differentiation" as a convenient generalisation, rather than for one of the various specific processes which he mentioned in his first paper (1890a).

First of all, many of the nineteenth century biological research workers were probably familiar with the term "differentia" (similar in meaning to the modern use of "criteria") as it was used by Ancient Greek philosophers, especially Aristotle, in theories of Categorisation[12].

By the end of the nineteenth century, the term was used in relation to five separate biological issues:

(i) the process by which embryonic cells change into adult cells (e.g. by von Baer, see above).

(ii) the process of change which the daughter cells of basal cells undergo in their progress into specialised cells. For example, the division of each basal cell results in a continuing basal cell, and a daughter cell which progresses (after what are now called "amplifying" divisions – Alison et al, 2002) to keratinocytes of the epidermis (see Hansemann, 1891; and above). In both cases, the word was used both for the fact that differences between two things are present, and also for the process during which, and also by which, the differences are achieved.

(iii) With the formalisation of evolutionary theory in the mid-nineteenth century, "differentiation" was used in reference to the changes which may occur in whole species, and more particularly, for the process by which populations of more "primitive" species might be the source of populations of "higher" species. This is essentially the process of mutability of species being applied to the transition from less complex to more complex types.
Charles Darwin defined "differentiation" in the glossary in the "Origin of Species ...", 6th edition (1872) according to embryological-evolutionary phenomena:

> "The separation or discrimination of parts or organs which in simpler forms of life are more or less united."

From the following passage on p. 156 of the "Origin of Species...", it is clear that for Darwin, "differentiation" is part of evolution:

> "... for in a district where many species of a genus are found – that is, where there has been much former variation and differentiation, or where the manufactory of new specific forms has been actively at work – in that district and amongst these species, we now find, on an average, most varieties".

(iv) "Differentiation" was applied in experimental pathological studies of regeneration of injured cells and tissues. The fact that various "lower" animals can regenerate their body parts had been noted by Aristotle, and various experiments on a macroscopic level had been conducted through the centuries. After the beginnings of histology, regeneration of tissues was investigated by microscopy (e.g. Müller, 1840). By Hansemann's time, the cellular events, and in particular the role of mitoses in these changes, were only just being investigated with the new microscopic techniques. English language summaries of the understanding of regeneration at the time can be found especially in Morgan (1901), in an article by Morgan republished in Maienschein (1986) and in chapter XII of Adami (1908).

(v) Another group of pathological situations in which "differentiation" was considered to be relevant was that in which the type of cell normally found at a site altered to one of a cell type normally found at another site in the body. Virchow identified this as "histological substitution" in the second edition of the "Cellular Pathology" (1858), but by the fourth edition (1870, see also Virchow, 1884) he had realised that such changes of cells include two phenomena. The first of these arises simply by external factors acting on otherwise unchanged cells. This Virchow called "adaptation" (see chapter IX of Adami, 1908). In the second type of change, there was a change in the type of functional specialisation of the cells, for example, from mucus-producing glandular cells to keratin-producing squamous cells. Virchow, and those who followed, considered that for this change to happen, the local cells must undergo a "de-differentiation", and then a "re-differentiation" along another line of development to the new type of adult cell. Hansemann addressed this issue particularly when using "de-differentiation" (*Entdifferenzierung*), although he generally down-played the phenomenon of metaplasia (see chapter 11).

"Capacity for independent existence"; in normal, pathological and experimental studies

In Hansemann's writings, he discusses "capacity of cells for independent existence" in a variety of circumstances. This issue was not a major one in the biology of the time, and its relationship to "differentiation" was not widely considered except in Hansemann's writings. The mention of "capacity for independent existence" by Langenbeck in 1840 (Rather, 1975) is discussed in chapters 4 and 5.

Here, we can note briefly that in Hansemann's thinking, "capacity for independent existence" encompassed four phenomena, two of which relate to normal processes and two are relevant to apparently separate aspects of cancer biology.

(i) In normal biology, the ripe egg (i.e. at the end of the process of oogenesis) is capable of existing in the Fallopian tube, which the oogonium is not. Thus the egg has acquired through oogenesis a greater capacity for independent existence in comparison with the oogonium.

(ii) In normal biology, individual cells of the early blastula (according to species) can, when separated from the blastula, develop into whole individuals, whereas the individual cells of later-stage blastulae cannot, and die. The later blastula cells have therefore lost a capacity for independent existence.

(iii) Cancer cells from a site can grow in remote parts of the body (i.e as in the process of metastasis – see next chapter), whilst the "normal mother cells" from which the tumour cells arise are not able to grow in these distant locations. In this situation, the tumour cells appear to have acquired an increased capacity for independent existence at the remote site compared to the normal cell type from which they arose.

(iv) Cancer cells can grow in the tissues of another member of the same species of animal (now: "homologous grafting"), whereas normal cells from the original donor of the tumour cells cannot. This was seen to be further confirmation of the phenomenon of "increased capacity for independent existence".

In "Studies ..." (1893c) Hansemann included reference to the experiments of Roux[9] (see above) concerning the exact stage of embryonic development at which the capacity to form a complete, normal foetus is lost (see Allen, 1975). Hansemann clearly saw this as relevant to the process by which cells lose capacity for independent existence and gain increased functional specialisation. Because this combination of changes is characteristic of embryonic "differentiation", it is not surprising that Hansemann's proposal that the tumourous change which he called "anaplasia" was often confused with Fol's theory of embryonic reversion. For discussion of this problem in relation to Hansemann's theory of cancer see chapters 5 and 6.

Notes to chapter 3

1. François-Vincent Raspail (1794–1878) worked in Paris. He received little formal University education, and in his early career, was a largely self-taught botanist and plant physiologist. He was the first histochemist, and described his techniques and coined the phrase "*omnis cellula e cellula*" in a paper in 1825. In 1828, Raspail described the mite responsible for scabies. In the 1830s, he was gaoled by the government of Louis-Philippe for his anti-Monarchist activities. Later he took up issues in medical care, without any formal medical education. His "Health Annual", 1845 (a simplified version of his "History of Health", 1843) was very successful. In it, he advocated utter cleanliness and the use of an antiseptic (a camphor oil-alcohol mixture) for the treatment of wounds, thus predating Semmelweiss, Pasteur and Lister by many years. His radical republican political activities inhibited public recognition of his efforts until the end of monarchism in France in 1871.
   Reference: Weiner (1968).

2. For an account of the development of ideas regarding the structure of tissues, dating from Aristotle's "homoeomerous parts" to Bichat's "membranes and tissues" see Forrester (1994).

3. Xavier Bichat, although not using any microscope, divided tissues (which he called "membranes") into twenty-one categories in his "General Anatomy" (1801). He included a short section on pathology in his "Treatise on Membranes" (1800).

4. John Goodsir (1814–1867), Professor of Anatomy (1846–1867) at the University of Edinburgh. This author wrote several essays on a variety of human and comparative anatomical topics, including "Microscopical Observations" (1843). He is celebrated for being the person to whom Virchow dedicated his "Cellular Pathology" (1858). Lonsdale, the author of the biographical section in Goodsir's collected works ("Anatomical Memoirs", 1868) points out that Virchow makes scant reference to any of Goodsir's work in the text of the great work. However, that is perhaps a little unfair, since Virchow had already given Goodsir great credit in an article on parenchymatous inflammation (Virchow, 1852). Certainly, Goodsir's observation that cells of some tissues "turn over" in a controlled fashion is a major support of the concept of "*omnis cellula e cellula*". The consequence of this observation was to raise the issues that the reproduction of cells is not only controlled as to number, but also as to the specific type of the tissue to maintain the function of the tissue. This set the stage for the still-unsolved issue of local tissue lineage fidelity: or how does a particular basal cell only reproduce the right type of specialised cell.
   Goodsir made yet another observation of particular relevance to Virchow's thinking. It was that the extracellular material is made by cells, and especially that osteoid is made by bone cells. Virchow used the "model" of the healing of fractures as the major observation in support of his generalisation that "connective tissue cells" can inter-convert with epithelial cells, and thence that carcinomas come from connective tissue cells, not epithelial cells. The tumour aspect of this part

of Virchow's thought is further developed in chapter 4. This twofold debt to Goodsir is a possible explanation for the fact that Virchow dedicated "Cellular Pathology ..." to this author (see also Rather, 1971).

References: Goodsir (1845, 1868), Cameron (1952), Jacyna (1983).

5. The debate concerning preformationists versus developmentalists virtually ended with the realisation of the great age of the earth. How millions of generations of individuals could be "preformed" for the millions of years of life on earth was unaccountable by preformationist ideas. Gasking (1968) points out that the very often-reproduced drawing of a speculative "homunuclus" by Dalenpatius in 1699 was disbelieved by most of his contemporaries. The microscopes of the day could not have given the necessary resolution for anyone to see such details in a sperm head.

6. Johann Wolfgang von Goethe (1749–1832), Germany's most famous *littérateur*, was also a scientist involved particularly in chemistry, geology and biology. His ideas on evolution were published in an essay "The Metamorphosis of Plants" in 1790.

7. Karl Ernst von Baer (1792–1876) b Piep, Estonia, graduated in medicine from the University of Dorpat in 1814, but then pursued a career in zoology, studying in Germany, Austria, working at the University of Königsberg, where most of his work in embryology was done (1817–1834) and then St Petersburg (1835–1862).

   Reference: Gilbert (2003).

8. Wilhelm Roux (1850–1924) trained under Haeckel in Jena and later was professor of anatomy (1895–1921) at Halle. His most famous experiment, supposedly showing that the first-stage blastomere cannot develop into a normal individual, was flawed because his method of destroying the second blastomere (with a hot wire) damaged the first. Virchow had previously pointed out that in humans, the existence of identical twins meant that both blastomeres, after the first division of the zygote, must be able to develop into a full, normal individual (cited by Hansemann).

   References: Allen (1978), Farley (1982), Maienschein (1991).

9. Pierre-Louis Moreau de Maupertuis (1698–1759), mathematician and physicist with interests in physical geography and biology, was made Fellow of the Royal Society (1728), Director of the Académie Française (1743) and then President of the Berlin Academy (1746–1753, courtesy of the "westernising" activities of Frederick the Great). Maupertuis' suggestion concerning "particulate" hereditary factors was contained in a work *Système de la Nature*, published in 1751, in which he documented hereditary polydactyly in a family in Berlin.

   Reference: Glass et al. (1959), Sandler (1983).

10. Jean Baptiste Lamarck (1744–1829), biologist, believed until about 1800 that species are immutable. However, in 1809 he published *Zoologie Philosophique*, in which he accepted mutability of species, and proposed that the changes occur because alterations which parental individuals undergo during their adult lifetimes can be transmitted to their offspring.

    References to Darwin's Lamarckianism are given in Paul (2003) but there are many related insights in other chapters of Hodge and Radick (2003).

    Additional references: Packard (1901), Corsi (1998).

11. Darwin introduced the idea of "gemmules" in his "Variation of Plants and Animals under Domestication" (1868). The word "gemma" = a bud (which develops by asexual reproduction) was used by Müller in his "Elements of Physiology" (1840), so that gemmules were meant as "budlets".

12. For Aristotle on the Categories, see entries in Organ (1949).

Chapter 4

Theories of tumours prior to Hansemann

Introduction

This chapter deals only with theories of tumours related to Hansemann's opus. Other theories popular at the time, such as that local parasites or microorganisms stimulate local cells to behave in tumourous fashion – von Leyden, Blumenthal etc – are not mentioned. For these theories, readers are referred especially to Section VII in Wolff (1907) and also to Triolo (1956), Shimkin (1977), Rather (1978), Cremer (1985), Fitzgerald (2000) and Dhom (2001).

The concept of "plasias"

Hansemann chose the term "anaplasia" for the essential process which he proposed characterises the abnormal morphology and behaviour of tumour cells and which he perceived as similar to the process which occurs when a germinal epithelial cell in the ovary develops into an ovum (see chapter 5). The following outlines the derivation and history of the use of "-plasia" in the biological literature.

According to the biological philosophy of Plato and Aristotle (see above), changes in biological systems were caused by the actions of poorly-specified, and probably supernatural "forces" of different types, for example "animal" and "vegetative" (Barnes, 2005). The phrase "plastic force" (from *plasos* Gk "forming" or "formative" force) was probably introduced by Plotinus[1] (c 205–270 AD). This idea was supported by Avicenna (980–1037) in his medical works (the "Canon") and thus the concept became part of European learning in the Middle Ages. Subsequently the idea of a "plastic force" was also used to explain, variously, some aspects of theology, the formation of fossils, the development from eggs of adult living organisms, and as a descriptive phrase in philosophy and art[2].

As a separate development in relation to the biology, Descartes[3] asserted that growth of individual tissues occurs because material ("white threads") leaves the blood vessels (extravasate) and accumulates at these sites[4]. In accordance with his "mechanist" principles (see also chapter 2) Descartes excluded supernatural "forces" from his explanations of physiological phenomena, and did not use the term "plastic force", or "force" at all except in a strictly mechanical sense[5]. In Cambridge, England, however, a school of philosophers including Cudworth, More and others adopted many of Descartes' ideas, but retained belief in mystical concepts and "plastic forces". This group became known as the "Cambridge (Neo-) Platonists" (Patrides, 1980).

Meanwhile the first evidence of a vascular system which is distinct from the blood-vascular system came from discovery of lacteals by Aselli (1581–1626) in 1626. Subsequently, investigations of the role of movements and composition of blood and lymph fluids in medicine and pathology were carried out in Italy, especially by Malpighi, Borelli and others[6]; in Germany by Stahl and Hoffmann[4] and in France, where many authors, especially Le Dran, Petit and others came to believe that tumours begin in material which is deposited out of the lymph rather than extravasated from the blood (Wolff, 1907).

The Hunterian school[7] in London, and particularly William Hewson (1739–1774) and William Cruikshank (1745–1800), carried out extensive investigations of lymphatics. However, John Hunter[7] (1728–1793 – the most famous member of the school) used the phrase "coagulating lymph" for the clear liquid component of blood which has the inherent property of coagulating, and thus not exclusively for the material in lymphatic vessels (Hunter, 1794, pp 16–17). Hunter (1794) thought that coagulum from blood has a "living principal" (*materia vitae*) in its composition, and that greater amounts of this principal might be transferred from the local blood vessels to the "coagulating lymph" at the site of inflammation and cause formation of new tissue, including tumours.

With respect to increased size of tissues, Laennec had introduced the term "hypertrophy" in 1802 (Wolff, 1907), indicating that local changes of nutrition (and thus presumably extra-vascular deposition in some form) were responsible for these increases. This term continues to be used in medicine.

However, according to Wolff (1907), the only author who supported the role of lymphatic material in disease, and who used the suffix "-plasia" in relation to tumor formation was Lobstein (1777–1835)[8] in his "Treatise on Pathological Anatomy" (1829). Lobstein's account of the role of lymph in the formation of tumours was rather vague, but he quite clearly described the idea of a "plasia" as a pathogenetic (not aetiological) process which is identifiable by its morphological and physiological characteristics. Lobstein did not mention any *materia vitae* but described the formation of new tissues in terms of a biological process which results from the action of presumed specific aetiological "viruses or specific agents". These agents, he thought, attack particularly the local lymphatic system changing that system's vital properties. Because of this alteration the nature of the locally deposited material is altered too.

Lobstein was vague also on the different types of "-plasia" which might occur. From the relevant sections of the "Treatise" (especially article 11 of chapter IV, article 6 of chapter V and all of chapter VII) it seems that Lobstein classified the natures of the deposited material and associated process of development of the lesions as either "euplastic/euplasia" (associated with normal developmental growth), "homeoplastic/ homeoplasia" (fibrosis), "heteroplastic/heteroplasia" (most swellings) or "cacoplastic/cacoplasia" ("harmful" swellings, mainly comprising malignant tumours). All local processes were thought to be under the influence of locally-acting "plastic forces". Nevertheless, while in many parts of the text Lobstein implied that the nature of the deposited material determines the nature of the lesion, in section 408 Lobstein suggests that the (plastic) forces may act with variable speed and intensity at various times and sites. Thus Lobstein never quite determined whether it is the nature of the matter deposited by the locally-disordered lymphatic system, or whether it is the changes in the natures, intensities or effects of locally acting "plastic forces", which determine what type of "plasia" occurs at a particular site.

Lobstein's ideas initially received little support in France, Germany or England[9], but "fibro-plasia" was used by Lebert in 1845 (Wolff, 1907) and in a book (Lebert, 1851).

Virchow (1854) used both "neoplasia" and "hyperplasia" in relation to enlargements of tissues due to increased numbers of cells. He only used "hypertrophy" for increased size tissues due to increased size of the cells of the region. His usages of these terms have been general ever since.

Haeckel's use of the word "anaplasia" is noted in chapter 2, but no author of a pathology text read by the present authors has adopted this usage.

In the 4th edition of the "Cellular Pathology …", Virchow (1870) introduced "metaplasia" as a type of "histological substitution" which he had used in the second edition (Virchow, 1858, "adaptation" was the other type of histological substitution, see above).

Lanceraux (1875) used the term "neoplasia" extensively, but did not provide any history of its usage. This author used "-plasia" in the same way as had Lobstein (1829) to indicate a growth, in all cases specified by a prefix to indicate its special features. This convention had not changed by the time of Hansemann (1890).

Virchow's concepts of tumours

Virchow' received his entire medical education in Berlin (chapter 1), and worked for Johannes Müller from 1843. Virchow seems to have derived most of his fundamental ideas from Müller, who was prominent in scientific circles, having already published his work on the microscopy of tumours (1838) and "Elements of Physiology" (1840) (Haggard and Smith, 1938; Rather et al 1983). Essentially, Müller described only "true" tumours, omitting tuberculosis and some cystic conditions. He found that the cells of tumours are generally similar to those of the surrounding "normal" cells, except that they exhibited degrees of variability of sizes and shapes of cells and nuclei, not only between the various tumour types, but also among the cells within individual tumours. Müller thought that tumour cells arose in the interstitial space (avoiding the word "lymph") from *seminum morbii*, ("seeds of disease"), a concept which presumably came from Gaub's account of three types of *seminum morbii*. Rather and co-workers (1983) published an account of Müller's work; this should be read in conjunction with the account of blastema in Rather (1972).

Because the comments by Ackerknecht (1957), David (1988) and Rather (1990) do not completely describe Virchow's thoughts on tumours, we shall discuss these in some detail.

In early writings Virchow (1847) followed Müller's opinions, but in 1855, at the same time as he was converted to *"omnis cellula e cellula"* (chapter 3), he came to believe that tumour cells were derived from the cells of the connective tissues (*Bindegewebe*). This view, therefore, simply substituted "cells in connective tissue" for "*seminum morbii* in blastema" in Müller's scheme. As a separate issue Virchow came to adopt the idea that there is no such thing as a "cancer specific cell" as had been suggested by Lebert (see Rather, 1978).

By his own subsequent account, Virchow (1858) was keen to establish tumours as locally-occurring lesions. This was in contrast to the Le Dran-Hunterian model of "ex-vascular deposits" (see above) in which tumours form from material delivered to the site by the blood or lymphatics. Thus Virchow's view established tumours on a "solidistic" or "local" basis, which was a considerable achievement.

In Virchow's "Cellular Pathology ..." (1858), there are views on cancer which have not stood the test of time. In particular, Virchow supported "chronic irritation" as the mechanism for induction of growth in tumours. He used as a "tumour analogy" the healing of fractures of bone through callus. In this phenomenon, there is not only transient growth, but also frequent changes of cell type among the connective tissue cells, especially from fibroblast to chondrocytic cells. Virchow had no explanation for the permanency of the proliferative change in his irritated cells (the effects of irritation normally subside when the irritant is removed), nor did he believe in trans-vascular travel of tumour cells as the basis of metastases. On the contrary, Virchow believed that the primary tumours liberated some unknown substance which "converted" distant connective tissue cells to the cell type of the primary tumour from which these "influences" came.

In 1863 Virchow began what was to have been his *magnum opus* on tumours ("Disease-Related Tumours"), but abandoned it before publication of the part (second part of vol III) on carcinomata[10]. He retained Lobstein's terms of "homeoplastic" and "heteroplastic" as late as the fourth edition of the "Cellular Pathology ..." (1870).

The following list summarises the views held by Virchow with which Hansemann could not agree. Probably because of Virchow's views and far-reaching influence, Hansemann included extensive justifications of his own opinions in his articles.

(i) That carcinoma cells arise from cells of the connective tissue (*Bindegewebe*) locally (not the local epithelial cells) – hence Hansemann's long account of the matter under "Specificity".

(ii) That cells in general, change their morphological type (see above) frequently, as in healing of fractures. Hansemann, to the contrary, believed that these changes are relatively uncommon, and hardly mentions healing of fractures in any of his works.

(iii) That the apparently separate foci at the edges of tumour masses are due merely to exclusion of the connecting parts from the particular section, and do not represent separated foci of tumour (which result from invasion). Hansemann believed to the contrary that tumour cells can invade connective tissue by their own motile activity.

(iv) That distant growths occur because some factor emanating from the main tumour mass recruits distant cells of the connective tissue (*Bindegewebe*) to the same tumourous behaviour. Hansemann took the opposite view, which was held by Langenbeck, Remak and most other authors of the time, that distant growths (metastases) grow only because physically-translocated cells from the main mass are able to grow at the distant site.

(v) That the pathogenesis of tumours is an abnormal healing reaction to chronic irritation (see above). Hansemann agreed with many other authors, including those who believed in parasitic theories, that many tumours arise without any evidence of previous chronic irritation at the site.

"Embryonal" theories of cancer

Before microscopy, students of tumours had only to explain excessive local growth, some macroscopic appearances, and the spread of tumours. Until the seventeenth century (before anything of cells was known), tumours were explained mainly in terms of local imbalances of "humours".

In the early period of microscopy with achromatic lenses, and with the advent of "Cell Theory", the problem became mainly one of explaining the local excess proliferation of cells, and the changes in the appearance of their nuclei and cytoplasm. Very quickly tumour cells were seen to be related to "embryonal" cells in some way, for example by Royer-Collard in 1826 (Wolff, 1907). This was because most tumour cells and embryonal cells grow rapidly and tend to have a greater nuclear volume compared to the cytoplasmic volume (higher "nuclear:cytoplasmic ratio").

Several variations in the "embryonic" idea of tumours developed over the next fifty years. The most important were, first that tumour cells represent the results of a reversal of embryonic differentiation occurring in the adult tissue (Fol, see Wolff, 1907). The second important idea was that tumour cells are embryonal cells; – but which have been left over from embryonic and foetal development, and which are stimulated by irritation to "embryonic-cell-like behaviour" (Cohnheim, 1882). Cohnheim suggested this idea of "cell rests", particularly because histology showed that some tumour types comprised cell types which are only found in embryos (e.g. myxomas). Subsequently the existence of "embryonal rests" could not be proven, and no natural mechanism of "embryological reversion" has been found (although it has been achieved experimentally, in the "cloning" of new individuals from adult cells – for example, in the sheep called "Dolly" – Wilmut et al., 1997). The abandonment of the cell-rest theory was only completed after the Second World War. Prominent twentieth century authors who gave it credence included Borst (chapter 6) and Ewing in the 4th edition of his work "Neoplastic Diseases" (1940).

"Egg-like" features of cancer cells

Perhaps the most relevant part of the literature for Hansemann's theory is the section in Langenbeck's article of 1840 (Rather, 1975, see Bignold et al., 2006b) concerning the egg-like nature of the capacity for independent existence of metastatic tumour cells. (Langenbeck's paper is mainly in support of his theory of the blood-borne nature of metastasis in general, and to the lung in particular). The relevant section is as follows:

> "To me it seems highly probable that cancer of the lung in most instances develops within the branches of the pulmonary artery from cancer-molecules that have gained access to the venous circulation from a primary carcinoma. Carcinomas in other parts of the body almost invariably precede the development of lung cancer, and instances of primary carcinoma of the lung appear to be extremely uncommon. Bayle saw only one and Bouillaud two instances of carcinoma of the lung in the absence of preceding similar disease in other parts, and Andral will have it that he has never observed one.
>
> That the smaller parts of a cancerous tumour, the carcinoma cells, still have the ability to develop independently into cancerous tumours, even though they have separated from their primal native soil, the carcinoma, and transplanted to a foreign one, may appear less surprising when we consider that the germ of the ovary, likewise no more than a cell and indeed one strikingly similar to a large carcinoma cell, separates itself from the ovary after fertilisation in order to develop independently in the uterus or quite outside the material body.
>
> Like the germ of the ovary, every single carcinoma cell must now appear as an organism endowed with life-force and developmental ability which, even though robbed of all organic connection with its primal native soil, can nevertheless continue to develop independently as long as it finds itself in the neighbourhood of and under the influence of living organic tissue. Despite its extremely great external resemblance, however, a cancer cell differs essentially from a cell of the ovary in that it requires no more than contact with and the enlivening effect of living organic substance, whereas the constrained life-force of the latter can come into living effectively only under the influence of a specific external stimulus, the male generative substance."

The substance of this idea is clearly repeated in Hansemann's works (1890a; 1893c etc), although with little acknowledgement (see section below). Further discussion is unnecessary here.

"Fecundation/fertilisation/fusion" theories

The basic idea in this group of ideas was that, if two cells fuse, the resulting cell will exhibit some of the properties of each of the original cells. Some authors (see Wolff 1907) provided early versions of this idea by suggesting that transferences of "influences" from one cell type to another might produce a cancerous change in the "target" cell. Simon (1878) suggested that such an "influence" might be the product of some enzymatic action, and (in the same paper) speculated that metastases might occur because "molecules" from the primary tumour exert a "spermatic force" on the tissues where a secondary growth occurs. Virchow (1880) suggested that the process of transference seemed analogous to the sperm "targeting" an egg, but without discussing this view in detail or committing himself to it in any way.

In chapter 11 of his "General Pathology" (1889) (see also Wolff, 1907), Klebs[11] devoted several pages to the suggestion that leukocyte nuclei fuse with a local cell to produce a cancerous change. Later in the same chapter Klebs referred to the "foetal characteristics" of cells after nuclear fusion. Thus Klebs perhaps favoured the embryonal model, at least in some ways.

Schleich and others produced variations of this view (see Wolff, 1907 pp 360 ff[12]). Finally, if a gamete were to fuse with an adult cell, the resultant cell might have a mixture of embryonal and adult-cell features. This idea was put forward by Farmer and Moore (1902) and briefly supported by Bashford (1905) but was never credited as likely. In particular, Bashford later withdrew his support for it (Bashford, 1908).

The role of mitosis in heredity at the time of Hansemann

Improved methods of histology (chapter 3) – especially with the use of haematoxylin and eosin – had been applied to the events of cell division by many authors, as outlined by Hansemann in references within his own book (1893c: chapter 11). These can be read in summary in Hertwig (1890; 1892), Wolff (1907) Wilson (1925), Hughes (1959), Farley (1982) and Lima-de-Faria (2003). The condensation of chromatin into "threads" (also termed "loops", "filaments" and later "chromosomes", or "nuclear segments") prior to nuclear division was discovered by many authors, including Strassburger, Waldeyer, Flemming, Boveri, van Beneden and others, although many different ways of describing the phases of nuclear division were used.

At the time of Hansemann's first cancer paper (1890), understanding of the following matters was lacking as follows:

(i) The differences between mitosis and what was later called "meiosis" (the sequence of divisions which support oogenesis and spermatogenesis) were not understood.

(ii) Whether or not the striking species-consistency in numbers of chromosomes, which had been found among lower animals, also applies to higher animals and especially to Man, had not been established.

(iii) The fact that the "gemmules/plasmas/ids" are integral to the chromosomes, not just associated with them in some way, was not known.

(iv) No even nearly-correct estimate of the number of chromosomes in human cells had been advanced (because the small ones cannot be seen except in "squash" preparations).

(v) That for any species, an individual sperm head contains the same number of chromosomes as the nucleus of the egg of that species was not understood.

(vi) As a corollary of (iv) it was not clear when during mitosis – especially in man – that the chromosomes replicated themselves.

The following summaries are of two major articles which were cited by Hansemann. Hansemann's own articles are very similar to these in style and lack of definite structure, which were in fact typical for the literature of pathology at the time.

Schottländer's (1886) article is long, and begins with a thorough review of the topic. He provides a general preamble, after which the author states his aim as "… to examine observations with special regard to normal typical karyokinesis in order to make statements as to whether there are any regular laws on what happens in various pathological conditions."

He then reviews nuclear division and reports of atypical karyokinesis since the 1840s. On pages 434-5 Schottländer reviews experimental corneal injury, followed by an account of his own experimental methods involving the cornea of the green frog. Methods are given in detail for how the eye is cut, the angle of knife, the platinum wire for scraping, the application of acid and so on. In particular he used picric or formic or chromic or acetic acid as fixative, and carmine or haematoxylin and eosin for staining. The main "results" involved the morphology of the mitoses and the time courses for the mitotic responses.

The obvious sources or errors in such a study are that secondary infection (not mentioned) could affect the outcomes; that the intensity of the injury is poorly controlled; that in early healing, the nuclei of damaged cells could resemble poorly-fixed mitoses; and that proliferation in macrophages close to capillaries might be confused with those of endothelia. The reliability of Schottländer's findings is questionable overall because he was unable to find any mitoses in corneal epithelium, as part of the healing response, at all. He was also unable to see how many threads there were in the metaphase figures of the cells. Thus the accuracy of his identification of any metaphase figure in his preparations must be treated with suspicion.

On p. 450 begins a description of nuclear division according to a 5-stage process. The author then comments "atypical" mitoses in these preparations.

1. These are mainly irregular deviations with the overall character of the mitosis preserved – referring to Flemming and Rabl. The abnormalities include changes in size shape and lie (position) of chromatin material, abnormal shrinkage, blurred delineation, occasional errant chromatin spheres. He could not tell how much this is due to variable fixation.
2. Some abnormalities have certain regular features (quoting Flemming), meaning especially multi-partite nuclear divisions.
3. Chaotic mitotic characters were not preserved.

After consideration of many aspects of the mitotic forms, which, in view of the possibility of fixation artefact and other sources of error cannot be assessed, Schottländer provides a seven-point summary:

1. After placing chlor zinc solution in the centre of the frog cornea, the epithelium decomposed, and histologically there was no slow degeneration or regeneration of cells.
2. If the irritation was massive and the animal strong, metamorphoses on day 2, as well as wandering cells, some with direct segmentation and some with direct fragmentation, were seen.
3. Not until day 7 are mitoses found near the acid area which undoubtedly serves regeneration – regeneration is complete by day 15.
4. The majority of mitoses are analogues of almost always 24 loops; the mode of cell division is reminiscent of cell plate formation in plants.
5. Aberrations from this can be irregular dual division figures.
6. The multiple nuclear division figure is a completely different phenomenon, and is undoubtedly meant to be a multinuclear division. As in normal mitosis, irregularities and atypias are found here, but more often.
7. Some cells show the phenomenon of indirect fragmentation.

Flemming's article (1887) followed three earlier long articles (1879, 1880, 1881) which had amounted to a full review of cell division. All these articles were written before meiosis was distinguished from mitosis, and thus difficulties with concepts are to be expected. The article (Flemming, 1887) begins by stating that some years before, the author had reviewed all relevant knowledge, but that the topic now (in 1887) has undergone so many new developments that a revision was in order. In addition, the author has new findings to communicate. Of particular interest are the obscure forms of mitoses which were found in the spermatocytic cells of *Salamandra*; these are different from all others known.

There are ten sections to the paper as follows.

Section I comprises a brief review of the literature, and description of sperm formation in the testis of the Salamander (an amphibian which has moist skin like that of the frog).

Section 2 concerns methods involving rapid plucking and spreading on glass, fixation with chromium acetic acid-osmium mixture and platinum chloride with chromic acid. Staining with safranin and Gentian are all recommended, but not Bismarck Brown and Methyl Green in acetic acid. Flemming found that alcohol fixation is satisfactory, as is counterstaining with haematoxylin. Celloidin was used for embedding to harden the tissue, then Bergamotte oil, then clove oil and Damar resin were applied for mounting.

Section 3 concerns dimorphism of mitoses in spermatocytes, section 4 is on "heterotypical" variants, section 5 describes the nuclear spindle (achromatic) and section 6 deals with "homeotypical" forms.

Section 7 deals with the number of chromatin "segments" (i.e. chromosomes). It is stated that the numbers are: spermatocyte 24, secondary cells have 48, all daughter cells 24, sperm cells "half".

Section 8 deals with deviations of mitoses from the norm in spermatocytes and various forms of degenerate nuclei; clear evidence is found of pluripolar nuclear divisions (p. 445). The hallmark is asymmetric, unilateral herniation of the spindle, which then attracts some of the chromatic segments in that direction to form an "abnormal tripolar spindle". In all segments, each "thigh" is swollen to the shape of a minisphere. Groups of four spheres, two of which are stuck together, are scattered irregularly through the spindle zone (Figs 48 and 50).

Section 9 discusses the relationship of mitotic forms described here to the usual scheme of mitosis. Section 10 concerns a comparison with the findings of Carnoy.

Flemming calls the abnormalities "pathological nuclear division", which is different from Hansemann's usage (1891a – chapter 8). There was no general conclusion.

By 1893, however, the specificity of the "reduction division" for gametogenic divisions had been described, especially by Hertwig (1892). Subsequently, when all chromosomes were shown to exist as pairs in adult cells, and gametes were shown to be haploid (contain one of each member of these pairs of chromosomes in the adult cells), Flemming's ideas of nuclear division in the testis were obsolete.

Chromosomes in tumour cells

The discovery of chromosomes through the use of better histological stains and lenses was documented in chapter 3. The first observers of atypical mitoses were most concerned with their frequency, and possible "physiological" role in either development of embryos or maturation of cell types in adult tissues. The methods of fixation and sectioning used by these authors caused such marked shrinking of the chromosomes that little could be seen but shrivelled dots. Three major articles (Arnold, 1879; Martin, 1881; Pfitzner, 1886) to which Hansemann refers will now be summarised in some detail.

Arnold (1879) begins his paper with the comment that in recent times much work has been done on cell division, especially in plants, and lists a number of authors who have published on this. Only a few of these works, however, have concerned pathological tissue. This paper reports Arnold's own work, and in particular, that in the tumour cells, some unusual metamorphosis of the nuclei takes place. For samples Arnold recommends carcinomas or sarcomas, especially the large-cell variants of tumours with soft and juicy nuclei, because division is too hard to see in small nuclei. His first technique involved incubation of fresh tumour fluid in small chambers made of hard rubber, sealed with Canada Balm, and using a drop of immersion oil for microscopy and aqueous safranin as a stain. There was no fixation to avoid artefact. He hoped to see movement of nuclear threads, but this was not seen. Arnold then cites von Pruden and Schleicher who claimed to have seen nuclear threads in cartilage. For other histological preparations he fixed the tissues with alcohol and chromatic acid (for up to 6–8 days), then cut the tumour into cubes, and then further hardened the tissues in methanol for 24 hrs: 2 changes of methanol, then ethanol over 72 hours. Sections were cut without embedding and stained with haematoxylin.

His results first concerned the appearances of interphase nuclei, and consisted mainly of the finding that the interphase cancer nuclei consisted of many small and large bodies with shiny surfaces within the chromatin of the nuclei. The editors' opinion is that Arnold's methods produced such marked shrinkage and coagulation of structures that artefact is the most likely cause of them.

The second part of the results begins on p. 290 of the original, and concerns nuclear division. Arnold notes that all phases of nuclear division known from other work are seen in tumours. Could the order of events be different? He is unable to tell. Then there is a systematic description, dividing nuclear division into four phases, *viz:*

1) preparation for nuclear division;
2) immediately pre-division;
3) during division;
4) after division.

Arnold concludes this section by stating that the threads are the "pivotal thing" in nuclear division.

Abnormal nuclear divisions are mentioned briefly (p298) (referring to the works of Strassburger and Ebert) but Arnold states that he has seen triple or quadruple division and illustrates these in Figs 17, 18, 19 and especially 35 and 36 (triples). Arnold also states that he has seen cells with 3 or 4 young nuclei (i.e. after such division) and that he saw fine threads between the nuclei. There is then a discussion of Flemming's work and his concept of indirect (requiring mitotic chromosomes) and direct (not requiring mitotic chromosomes) nuclear division. Flemming is stated to believe that the mechanisms of multi-nuclearity are difficult to understand. Arnold finishes with a wish that the pathological anatomists might realise that in pathological neoplasms, there is much opportunity for study.

Martin (1881) begins his paper with references to the works of others, including Arnold (1879, above) on "indirect" (i.e. mitotic) nuclear division in normal and pathological tissues. He notes that knowledge of it was still incomplete. Hence, he continues the structure of nuclei before division, how they come about, and the sequence of the phases all need further work.

Discussion is then presented of whether or not more than one nuclear division can occur simultaneously in a single cell, or whether one division can result in more than two daughter nuclei. A review of current literature (Eberth, Flemming, Strassburger, Hegelmeyer) follows. Martin's (1881) text then becomes a complicated account of the issue of four nuclei in one cell. He doubts that multipartite division occurs, and suggests that Hegelmeyer's example might be the result of the joining of 3 colliding daughter nuclei with one in the middle.

On p. 60, Martin begins a report of his own observations. These were derived from a single case of a breast carcinoma, which grew and replaced the whole breast in 7 months. On microscopic examination, the tumour was found to contain large numbers of all sorts of mitoses. His method involved fixation in methanol (*spiritus conservatio*) but the duration was not mentioned. For sectioning a Thoma sliding microtome was used, so that only one layer of cells was included. Martin justified this, because it was the preparation in which detecting mitoses and other structures was easiest. (This is the basis of the controversy concerning the proper thickness of sections, which Hansemann deals with in several articles and in 1893c – eds). Martin then stained the sections with haematoxylin, alum-carmine and borax-carmine which colour chromosomes intensely.

Spindle fibres, on the other hand, were best seen after embedding in resin (not further detailed) and staining with haematoxylin.

Martin's results consisted of observations of this in relation to the various stages of mitosis. There are numerous unremarkable observations, but on p. 61 he describes a nucleus which divided into more than 4 parts (Fig. 6). The shape of the nuclear plate was very complicated, and appears to be 7 or 8 parts, suggesting the phenomenon now known as "mitotic catastrophe" (Castedo et al,

2004). Subsequent description in the paper attempts to establish that the best explanation of the abnormalities seen is multipartite division.

Martin concludes:

> "I stress again that I have produced incontrovertible evidence of multiple divisions of the one nucleus in indirect division manner. Special emphasis is placed on the structure of the nuclear plate in early stages of division. Also the position of the nucleus in later division stages, and their relationship to the threads, as well as the way the cytoplasm divides, allow only multiple division as the explanation.
>
> Further investigations are needed as to whether these multiple divisions occur only in tumours, and in particular, in rapidly growing tumours, or whether this modality is more commonly found in physiological and pathophysiological conditions in plant or animal kingdoms."

Pfitzner (1886) begins with 15 pages of introduction, making the significant points that (i) studies of mitosis could allow proliferating cells, metamorphosing cells, fully viable and degenerate cells to be distinguished from each other, (ii) counting mitoses in tissues is difficult. Pfitzner then falls into error by stating that "The development of the chromatin is the measure for the developmental stage of the cell" and "paucity of chromatin is the hallmark for the embryonal character of a cell". (It is against this error that Hansemann had to struggle in his early articles – eds). There is also much comment on differences between mitoses under specific situations, and Hansemann's section in "Studies ..." (1893) can be considered in contrast to this section. Pfitzner also thought that the chromatin richness of cells relates to the age of the whole individual. On p. 289 of the original there is an account of division of nucleated erythroid cells, leading to the correct conclusion that anuclear state of human erythrocytes is due to the dissolution of pre-existing nuclei. There is a very brief account of methods (p. 296). On p. 297 Pfitzner states that the differences between the nuclei of regenerative and tumour cells are in the ratios of the amounts of nuclear parts and that the tumour cell nuclei are of "embryonal character". There was no summary.

Other authors immediately before Hansemann added little to these accounts. Cornil (1886) described the nuclear abnormalities in tumour cells, but did not suggest that they might have any pathogenetic significance.

Klebs[11] (1889) (see above) described a variety of abnormalities in chromosomes and mitoses in tumour cells. However, he was unsure of what they meant, and how they might be associated with the phenomenon of fusion of leukocyte and epithelial nuclei which he claimed to have seen (see above). In relation to atypical mitoses Klebs (1889 p. 529) stated:

"As far as the pathological significance of these different nuclear division processes is concerned, which in any case deviate substantially from the norm, establishing their relationship to the incipient cells and to the newly-formed tissue of tumours presents us with considerably more difficulty than recognising their origin. We can say at once that they appear for preference in very strongly proliferating tumours, perhaps even exclusively. Often, haemorrhagic conditions too have a particular relationship to the luxuriant development of abnormal (*anormalen*) nuclear proliferation. Within such haemorrhagic parts it is, quite specifically, unusually large and misshapen nuclei with coarse-grained content which appear, which, set free from their context, are situated in the blood masses."

Difficulties of diagnosis of tumours by histopathology in the 1890s: the case of the laryngeal cancer of Emperor Friedrich III

The microscopic appearances of human tumours provided most of the essential "raw data" of tumour research throughout the nineteenth century. Such considerations were important to academic pathologists (in university departments) for their theories on the nature of cancers. However, these appearances were not immediately of practical use for hospital pathologists examining biopsies.

First, microscopy is not really necessary for macroscopic masses which are obviously tumours by naked-eye examination. Thus large, irregular ulcerating-fungating masses of the stomach or colon are rarely due to anything but a tumourous process.

Second, for those cases of macroscopic masses which consist of excess fibrous-like tissue, those microscopic details which can be seen with an achromatic lens and simple nuclear stains (see above) are not enough to enable either infiltrating or "desmoplastic" cancerous lesions to be distinguished from non-tumourous disorders such as inflammatory and fibrosing processes. In particular, individual tumour cells, or small "lines" of tumour cells lying between collagen fibres, could not be distinguished from inflammatory cells. For this reason, most histopathologists, as explained by Virchow (1888) needed to see rounded clumps of tumour cells (say at least 20 cells – so-called "alveolar forms") before they could make a diagnosis of cancer.

The diagnostic difficulty was exemplified by the case of Emperor Friedrich III. The lesion itself was an infiltrating squamous cell carcinoma (caused no doubt by the Emperor's heavy smoking). Virchow's reports on the biopsies (Dhom, 2001) specifically state that none of the "alveolar forms" which were required for a diagnosis of malignancy could be seen (Dhom, 2001) so that the diagnosis of malignancy could not be made[13]. For further discussion, see chapter 5.

Notes to chapter 4

1. Plotinus (c 205-270 AD), b Egypt, but lived most of his life in Rome. He was generally a follower of Plato, hence a "neoplatonist". "Plastic forces" he considered to be emanations of the "world soul" which give rise to matter.

   References: Whittaker (1901), Russell (1956), Gerson (1996).

2. For example, Nieztsche in his essay "On the future of educational systems", 1872. See also entry in "The American Heritage Dictionary of the English Language", 4th edn (2000).

3. René Descartes (1596–1650) is considered by many to have been the first "modern" (in the sense of fully rational/mechanist) philosopher and was concerned with many issues including metaphysics, ethics, mathematics and the structure and function of the human body. He is most famous for his dictum "I think, therefore I am" (*"cogito ergo sum"*). It is said that he continued to state his belief in God and the Soul because of his knowledge of the fate of Galileo (1564–1642), who had stated opinions concerning the solar system which were unacceptable to the Church. His ideas of cardiovascular physiology were misguided because he refused to accept Harvey's account (published in 1628) of the circulation of the blood.

   References: Chavois (1966), Hall (1972), Carter (1983).

4. Mention of the concept of "white threads" is to be found in vol. XI, sections 265–276 of Adam and Tannery (1996).
   In relation to tumours, Wolff (1907) begins his discussion of the "lymphatic theory of cancer" with mention, as "heroes" of the overthrow of Galenic theory, of Francis Bacon and Descartes (see chapter 2). Wolff then has a paragraph:

   "As to the theory of cancer, Descartes' lymphatic theory was by far the most important. For almost 150 years, authors who dealt with cancer were under bondage to his theory, and all research work was directed to unravelling the nature of lymph. We shall now examine the progress of cancerology that is owed to the so-called Cartesian school."

   The present authors do not believe that this paragraph means that Descartes described a "lymphatic theory" in the modern sense. First of all, there had been no description of any generalised lymphatic system of the body before Descartes died (1654). Only lacteals in recently-fed dogs had been described (by Aselli in 1626, and this came to Descartes' notice only in 1640). Descartes did not use the word "lymph". Descartes did suggest a theory that solid organs form in spaces between blood vessels because of the ejection of minute threads from arterial branches (Adam and Tannery, 1996, XI S 265–276). In other writings he used the word "corpuscles" for such material. This is discussed by Hall (1972). Tumours are not mentioned in any writing by Descartes that we have examined.
   In the "Cartesian school" Wolff (1907) included many French authors, including the later author LeDran (1685–1770). Rather (1978) gave prominence to Stahl (1660–1732) and Hoffmann (1660–1742) (both at Halle). Dobson (1959) gave priority to Ledran (i.e Le Dran) as the author of the "lymphatic" theory.

   Additional references: Daremberg (1870), Hall (1972), Rather (1978), Carter (1983), Cottingham (1993).

5. This is based on our reading of Hall (1972) Carter (1983), and Adam and Tannery (1996) – "The Human Body" (*Du corps humain* – vol. XI pp 252–292), "Reproduction of Animals" (*Generationem animalium* – vol XI pp 505–538) and "Anatomy" (*Anatomica* – vol XI pp 252–292). See also Cottingham (1993).

6   For accounts of the dispute on priority concerning this issue, see Haviv (1999). There are also articles in Italian which we have not consulted: Bertoloni Meli D: The posthumous dispute between Borelli and Malpighi. In: "Marcello Malpighi, Anatomist and Physician". Firenze, L. Olschki, 1997, pp 247–275. In the same volume, Guerrini A: The varieties of mechanical medicine: Borelli, Malpighi, Bellini and Pitcairne, pp 111–128, and Gòmez Lòpez S: Marcello Malpighi and atomism, pp 175–189.

7   The Hunterian school consisted of its founder, William Hunter (1718–1783), his consecutive assistants William Hewson (1739–1774) and William Cruikshank (1745–1800); William Hunter's younger brother John (1728–1793); and finally John Hunter's brother-in-law Everard Home (1756–1832).

Both William and John Hunter were slow to publish their findings, and provided few references to previous authors. Hewson and Cruikshank themselves were competent investigators and authors. John Hunter's brother-in-law Everard Home is said to have published many of John Hunter's notes and manuscripts after the latter's death under his (Home's) own name, and burnt John Hunter's originals to conceal his deeds (Oppenheimer 1946; Livesley and Pentelow 1978). It is difficult, therefore, to be sure of the origins of particular ideas amongst this group, and also the extent to which their ideas were derived from European authors.

In the works of the Hunterian School:

(i) There is no mention of diseases or tumours in William Hunter's "Lectures of Anatomy" (Dowd, 1972), and none of the titles of publications by William Hunter listed on p. 240 of Mather (1893) suggest any consideration of tumours by this author.

(ii) In the "Complete Works of William Hewson" (original publications in the 1770s, collected and republished by the Sydenham Society in 1846) there are mentions of many aspects of blood, serum, and lymph; and of most relevance, the coagulability of the last of these. In the section on "Morbid Conditions" (pages 201-3, originally published in 1774), there is little mention of tumours, other than to note that the "humour" of them spreads to lymph nodes from primary sites. The therapeutic importance of surgical removal of both the primary tumour and the nodes is stated clearly. Whether or not tumours form from or in "lymph" is not stated.

(iii) John Hunter's "Lectures on Surgery" (1837; written after his death by others on the basis of notes taken by a student who attended his lectures in 1786-7), describe tumourous material as follows:

(In vol. 3 of these "Complete Works", p. 420): "The curdly substance is, we may suppose, the coagulating lymph deprived of its serum and the other or flaky is probably the same, only in smaller parts; it looks like the precipitate of animal matter from an acid or an alkali."

However, it is not clear whether scrofula or cancer or both are being referred to here.
On p. 619 of the same volume: "The tumefaction is from interstitial extravasation of coagulable lymph ..."

(iv) In his book (1790 pp 114-5) William Cruikshank noted that there might be different types of lymph, resulting in different types of lesions, as follows:

"In the last place, the lacteals and lymphatics become the cause of the most fatal diseases which attack the human body: this also puts these vessels in a very important point of view. These diseases may be divided into the following classes: In the first place, such as arise from these vessels not absorbing the healthy and sound fluids and solids of the body; secondly, such as arise from their absorbing too much of the healthy and apparently sound fluids and solids of the body; thirdly, such as arise from absorbing morbid fluids generated in the body; fourthly, such as arise from absorbing the diseased solids of the body; fifthly such as arise from their absorbing irritant substances not generated in the human body, the infectious matter of other persons, and poisons, animal, vegetable, and mineral, from whatever quarter."

Notes to chapter 4

In this section, there is no mention specifically of tumours. On a subsequent page, however, concerning cancers of the breast and testis, Cruikshank writes:

"… the poison is generated in the cells of the gland, or in the acini; the external absorbents may sometimes carry it from these cells, to the intermediate (lymph) glands described between the nipple and axilla … The poison remains in the cells of the mamma, perhaps a year or two, before it infects any gland in the axilla".

Thus Cruikshank does not clearly state that tumours come from a component of lymph.

(v) In his "Blood, Inflammation and Gunshot Wounds" (1794), John Hunter was mainly concerned with inflammation. Its great value is that it showed that blood vessels play an active part in the inflammatory process, and that inflammation is not due to obstruction of blood vessels, as Boerhaave had thought. There is little mention of tumours in this book.

(vi) Everard Home (1820) published microscopical examinations of cancer in which he suggested that tumour cells look like blood "globules" and so are probably derived from them. Therefore, at least by 1820, he seems to have abandoned the "lymph-origin" of tumours if he ever subscribed to it. The illustrations in Home (1820) are reprinted in Home's book of 1832 (not consulted by the present authors), and in Shimkin (1977).

Additional reference: Dobson (1959).

8 Jean Georges Chrétien Fréderic Martin Lobstein, nephew of a distinguished surgeon (Johann Friedrich Lobstein the elder 1736–1784) became a noted surgeon and pathologist in Strasbourg, but apparently had a disastrous later career, and went to the United States (Wolff, 1907).

9 We have found no mention of any "-plasia" in any of the following: Pinel (1818), Andral (1836), Magendie F. (1836), Meckel J.F. (1837), Walshe (1846), Vogel J. (1847), Bennett (1849), Paget (1853), Wedl (1855) or Velpeau (1856).
Williams (1856), however, used the terms "euplastic", "cacoplastic", although with meanings which were different from those of Lobstein, and "aplastic" (which seems to have meant non-progressive alterations thought to be in the nature of deposits from the blood).

10 This issue has been discussed elsewhere (Ackerknecht, 1953). Garrison and Morton (1970) suggested that Virchow may have abandoned "Disease-related Tumours" (1863) because of an apparent unwillingness to change his belief that carcinomas arise from connective tissue cells, not from epithelial cells. Perhaps his political interests in the 1860s, not to mention the challenge to a duel by Bismarck, was a greater factor in his failure to complete the work. Virchow did produce a fourth edition of the "Cellular Pathology …" (1870) without changing his views on tumours, but there were few other changes in the book either.

11 Edwin Klebs (1834–1913) b Königsberg, studied medicine in Berlin and was Professorial Assistant *(Assistent)* to Virchow in the early 1860s, until being called to Bern as *Professor Extraordinarius* in 1865. He was appointed *Professor Ordinarius* there in 1866, and studied mainly bacteriology, working on anthrax, and wound infection (in the Franco-Prussian War). His work made a major contribution to the establishment of the bacterial causation of disease, and his four "basic essentials" (*Grundversuche*) of infectious disease were a major influence on the "postulates" formulated by Robert Koch. The foreword of Klebs' book (1876) was directed to Rudolf Virchow, as if simultaneously making an acknowledgment and recognising a legacy (*Vermächtnis*). Klebs remarked: " 'Cellular Pathology …' is said to have demonstrated 'the disturbances of the inner mechanism of the animal body'. The new direction has the task is 'of becoming familiar with those intruders and their biological behaviour' ".
A productive period in Prague (1873–1882) was followed by a period in Zurich (1882–1893) where Klebs neglected his academic duties in favour of research on tuberculosis. As a result the students there threatened an exodus to Strasbourg unless changes were made, and Klebs was forced to

resign. He went to the U.S.A. as Professor of Pathology at the Rush Medical College in Chicago, returning to Europe in 1900 and to Bern in 1913 shortly before his death.

Reference: Dhom (2001), Carter (2001).

12 But note that Wolff (1907 p. 361) wrongly describes Hansemann as supporting Klebs' theory.

13 The details of this diagnostic difficulty are given by Dhom (2001). Unfortunately the glass slides of the case disappeared and cannot be re-studied. They would be of great historical interest if they were ever to be re-discovered.

The Emperor Friedrich's widow (Victoria) was apparently already dissatisfied with German medical practice at the time. She blamed her obstetricians for causing the left-sided Erb's palsy (an obstetric mishap which damages the brachial nerve plexus, so that the corresponding arm does not develop properly) in her first-born son (later Kaiser Wilhelm II). The diagnostic confusion concerning her husband's disease, especially the view that the emperor may have had syphylis, probably provided another reason. Both these experiences may also have caused her to support the formation of the post-graduate medical college (*Kaiserin-Friedrich-Stiftung*, 1906) (chapter 1) at which Hansemann gave lectures.

References: Ober (1992).

Chapter 5

Hansemann's ideas of the nature of cancer: description and analysis

Introduction

Throughout his lifetime von Hansemann's theory represented only one of many ideas concerning the nature of cancer, none of which even now has gained universal acceptance. Hansemann made numerous contributions to oncology, however, and many of them are accepted today. Especially, he emphasised the fact that changes in the hereditable material of a cell can occur entirely endo-cellularly (i.e. without addition of hereditable material from outside the cell) through abnormalities of the chromosomes, and that such changes might in turn change the morphology and behaviour of the affected cells in various ways, according to the "quality" of the hereditable material affected. Since the 1960s this has come to be understood as probably the correct view. Hansemann's suggestions as to the nature of the change in the hereditable material, and the nature of the process which follows on from that change, are of greatest interest but are also the most difficult of his ideas to understand. Moreover, Hansemann's ideas remain of interest at the present time (2006) when the phenomena of mutation, aneuploidy and genomic instability are being so thoroughly investigated in relation to the pathogenesis of tumours (Bignold et al, 2006a).

This chapter first describes the elements of Hansemann' theories, and then provides some critical analysis of them. It should be noted that Hansemann's theories applied to malignant tumours only. Hansemann was not able to explain "benign" tumours according to the same ideas. At the end of the chapter there is a discussion of Hansemann's highly successful application of his theory to the problem of diagnosis of malignant tumours. An analysis of Hansemann's philosophical inclinations is also included

The original version of the theory (Hansemann 1890a)

By the late 1880s it was generally agreed that malignant tumour cells differ from normal cells principally by (i) excessive growth, (ii) showing (usually) evidence of reduced specialised function, and (iii) being liable to be followed by the appearance of similar growths at distant parts of the body. It was also agreed (iv) that cancer cells do not arise from any "specific cancer cell" (as had been suggested by Lebert – see Rather, 1978) or from "lymph" (meaning coagulating material from blood; as had been suggested by John Hunter – see chapter 4).

Except for Virchow's views (see below), it was further agreed (v) that the distant growths (iii, above) occur first by physical displacement (usually through vessels) of tumour cells from the primary site to the distant site, and second, their growth at the distant site and (vi) that tumour cells are derived from the normal type of cell which they resemble most. That is to say, if a tumour cell looks like an epithelial cell it probably is derived from an epithelial "mother cell" (*Mutterzelle*) in the region, or has metastasised from such a tumour elsewhere to the site in which it was found.

The essential components of Hansemann's theory (1890a – translation in chapter 7) are as follows:

(i) Cancer cells are usually characterised by loss of some specialised functions.

(ii) Cancer cells exhibit a greater capacity for independent existence in the tissues of the host. That is to say, the cancerous derivatives of a normal cell could grow in anatomical sites where the original normal cell could not. This greater capacity was seen to be necessary for the formation of metastases, in the way that Hansemann described from the results of previously reported transplantation experiments.

(iii) The cancerous process begins with an asymmetric division of chromosomes after metaphase in a local tissue cell.

(iv) In at least one of the daughter cells, the resulting abnormal number of chromosomes causes an abnormality in differentiation. This assertion was based on Weismann's hypothesis – which was current in 1890 – that normal differentiation in embryos occurs by changes in the number of chromosomes – see chapter 3.

(v) Tumour cells do not behave physiologically like embryonal cells because they rarely differentiate into other cell types, as do the cells of the zygote. This reinforced Hansemann's acceptance of the (lineage) "specificity" of cells. Thus he could not accept Virchow's contrary view (above). Moreover, the abnormality induced in the tumour cells is not one of embryonic reversion.

(vi) The formation of tumour cells is like that of the production of the ovum from oogonia in the mammalian ovary. In his view, this was apparently supported by two facts. The first fact was that chromosomal material is ejected from each developing ovum as "polar bodies", although no further information was available concerning the significance of this phenomenon. In particular, it was not known in 1890 that "polar bodies" are surplus haploid nuclei. The second fact was that ova exhibit an increased capacity for independent existence manifest by survival in the Fallopian tube and endometrial cavity, at least for a few days.

(vii) The combination "loss of differentiation" and "increased capacity for independent existence" is a single real biological process manifest in the process of formation of an egg from "germinal epithelium" of the ovary. Hansemann supplied the name "anaplasia" for this process.

Although Hansemann (1890a) expressed his thoughts in a highly convoluted way, in effect he meant that malignant tumours arise when the process of oogenesis occurs in a non-egg-progenitor cell and that the process is particularly manifest by the continuing oogenesis-like chromosomal mal-distributions (as in the ejection of the polar body).

On further analysis, however, there were immediately obvious problems with this proposal. First, asymmetric mitoses in carcinomas are not all of the same degree, so that they could not all be exactly of the same type as the mitoses which resulted in ejection of polar bodies. Even in 1890 the ejected bodies were known to have approximately the same amount of chromatin for each species. Although Hansemann did not state this clearly, it may be that because of this fact he chose to include Weismann's theory of "differentiation through loss of chromosomal material" (chapter 3) in his scheme. Weismann's theory stated that "differentiation" occurred by loss of chromatin, by any cause: Hansemann amended this to "loss by asymmetric division"; hence, because each stage of "differentiation" might involve loss of different amounts of chromatin, so too would variable degrees of asymmetric mitosis occur in a mass of cells, if they were imitating the different stages of "differentiation".

The second problem was that throughout his writings, Hansemann insisted that "differentiation" is any progress which a cell line makes towards producing cells having less capacity for independent existence and greater specialised function (embryological or histological). "Un-differentiated" referred to cells which have not started this process, but "de-differentiated" refers to a cell line originating from a cell which was in a differentiated state, but lost its differentiation. This fine distinction has not been clear to many authors[1] (see also chapter 6). Hansemann wanted to indicate that his idea of "de-differentiation" was not just loss of specialisation of cells in the adult animal; this occurs regularly in regeneration – for example in the epidermis during healing of skin wounds – and is thus without any general significance. Hansemann also wanted to avoid any implication of embryonic reversion (chapter 4), although this process would be a "de-differentiation" according to his own general definition of the word. Logically, if Weismann's system was to be followed, "de-differentiation" in an adult cell should be accompanied by a gain of chromosomes; hence the "most de-differentiated" cells in a tumour should be the larger ones (with the hyperchromatic nuclei). This question is discussed in "Further analysis of de-differentiation" (below).

Further analysis of the oogenic model

Originally Hansemann identified oogenesis as a process which completes the differentiation cycle begun by normal embryological development and completed with the start of reproduction of a new individual. The process of oogenesis could be a model for Hansemann's ideas according to the following rationale.

First, the egg was considered **less** differentiated than the oogonium because it is susceptible to fertilisation by a sperm, after which it continues to **be** the undifferentiated basis for a new individual. Eggs of frogs were known to be able to develop into normal individuals by certain types of stimulation which do not involve fertilisation (i.e. parthenogenesis[2]). The idea of the egg as an "undifferentiated" cell could also be seen as having some validity if all "differentiated" cells are resistant to the entry of other genetic material.

However, the "model" does not survive further logical analysis for the following reasons. From the late 1840s it had been known that egg formation involves ejection of chromosomal material as "polar bodies" (Hertwig, 1890). Therefore, if Weismann's model of differentiation (chapter 3 and above) were to be applied, oogenesis would have to be considered a "gain of differentiation" simply on the basis of the loss of chromosomal material. Furthermore, in terms of physiology, the question of whether or not the egg is "differentiated" or "de-differentiated" is debatable. An egg might be considered "de-differentiated" in the embryological sense, because it is to be the precursor of a new individual (as above), but it could also be considered as fully differentiated in the histological sense because of its unique capacity to permit the entry of a single sperm. In the context of this debate the sperm is certainly highly "differentiated" because of its unique, highly specialised morphology and motile apparatus. In this debate, it would be difficult to accept one gamete as "differentiated" and the other as "undifferentiated".

To take this line of thought to a conclusion: fertilisation (which had been described by Hertwig in the 1880s – Hertwig, 1890) becomes the act by which all previous differentiation is abolished, and a new individual begins. By this line of thought it is not during oogenesis but during fertilisation that "de-differentiation" occurs. Hansemann's "logic" on this point therefore falls down.

What of the "increased capacity for independent existence" component of "differentiation" in all this? A modest degree of increase in this capacity is manifested by the egg, because it is able to survive in the Fallopian tube for several days. However, a similar degree of this capacity is demonstrated by the zygote, which can survive in the uterus until it finds the vascular support in oestrogen- and-progesterone-primed endometrium. Thus the act of abolition of "differentiation" occurs not only with the conversion of a germinal epithelial cell to an egg (in oogenesis) but also during the conversion of an egg into a zygote (by fertilisation). Hansemann avoided this point, although in later articles he was careful to define anaplasia as "loss of differentiation *and* increased capacity for independent existence".

From all this, it can be concluded that Hansemann's attempt to hammer all these facts together with Weismann's theoretical suggestions into a coherent theory failed because the "working concept" of "differentiation" does not extend to all the relevant cell biological phenomena; and also because chromosomal changes are not the mechanism of embryonic differentiation.

Hansemann's oogenic model has been given little serious consideration since its publication. However, insofar as cancerous phenomena are often considered in terms of de-repression of "normal" genes, the following questions might be asked:

Does the initiation of the "cancerous state" involve the "normal mother cell" acquiring "oogonium-like properties"? At the present time some expressions by cancers of sperm-germinal cell-specific antigens are documented (Simpson et al, 2005). But changes in expression of oogenesis-related genes have not been reported. Next, could there be an element of "meiotic" events in cancer? Further, could cancer begin with a triggering of the cytoplasmic factors normally found only in eggs which lead to embryonic-type growth?

Some further ideas may spring from this. Could the greater transplantability of tumour cells (chapter 4) be related to the greater transplantability of gametes and embryos in comparison with other adult tissues? Thus embryo transplants between members of the same species and even between species are possible. These extensions of Hansemann's thoughts have rarely been considered in relation to tumours in this way. Perhaps these questions deserve some modern investigation.

Further analysis of de-differentiation and numbers of chromosomes in tumour cells

Involving "differentiation" in the analysis of tumours created even more difficulties for Hansemann's theory than are mentioned above. In fact they added to the complexity which was to overwhelm his chromosomal concept of the pathogenesis of tumours. Our speculation as to why he involved "differentiation" at all was presented in the previous section. It is clear that Hansemann thought he had discovered the mechanism of the "normal" loss of chromosomes; Weismann had implied that this occurs in normal embryological differentiation. Hansemann in fact went further than Weismann by suggesting that there are successive "phases" of differentiation, each triggered by an asymmetric division of a cell from the previous phase (see above).

What now follows is an analysis of Hansemann's probable further thoughts on the problems in his theory at this point, although we recognise that nowhere did he express himself as succinctly as we do for him now.

After asymmetric mitosis, Hansemann was not certain which of the two daughter cells is the tumourous one (Hansemann 1891c, 1904c, 1904q). On the one hand, if "differentiation" occurs with loss of chromosomes, then "de-differentiation" should occur with gain of chromosomes. This would indicate that the larger cells are the tumourous ones (see above). However, according to his idea that "balances of chromosomes are necessary for viability" the larger cells should die. On the other hand, however, the fact that the egg has fewer chromosomes and has less differentiation (according to Hansemann) than the normal tissue cell was difficult to reconcile with the oogenic model of anaplasia. This is because, if the egg and the tumour cell are derived according to the same process, it would follow that the tumourous cells should be the smaller ones. But the smaller cells are liable to die, and many common epithelial tumours are in fact comprised mainly of large cells. These issues are major problems for his theory. In his books (1893c; 1897o) Hansemann's ideas on the question of which particular chromosome numbers are important for tumourous conversion became less clear. In later papers Hansemann (1904c, 1904q) provided a complex solution which attempted to accommodate the idea that neither the large nor the small cells are permanently viable. In this scheme, only cells with "normochromic" nuclei (with a "balance of chromosomes") could be viable in the long term. Hansemann suggested that the large cells might undergo subsequent asymmetric mitoses. The smaller of the daughter cells from this second asymmetric mitosis might have a normal total number of chromosomes, although the numbers of particular chromosome types would be abnormal. These cells, Hansemann speculated, are the on-going tumourous cells.

The answer to this problem came in the middle of the twentieth century, when it was found that most of the "permanent" cancer cell lines which have ever been obtained and are held in the American Type Culture Collection[3] have excess numbers of chromosomes per nucleus (i.e. are "hyperploid"). Thus, the large cells in most tumour types are probably the viable ones; certain "imbalances of chromosomes" affect the physiology and morphology of tumour cells, but not necessarily their viability.

Later modifications to the detail of the theories

The first new problem with Hansemann's theory after 1890 was that ejections of polar bodies during oogenesis were found not to have anything to do with "differentiation" but to be simply discards of surplus haploid sets of chromosomes during the reduction divisions in oogenesis. Because of this, and especially in view of the other problems of the oogenic model (see above), Hansemann was forced to change his views in some ways. Although he introduced "anaplasia" as

(i) a "normal process" which might be manifest in oogenesis (above),

he later defined anaplasia as

(ii) the abnormal process which leads to tumours.

Later modifications to the detail of the theories

This, however, initially at least, would have meant that the "de-differentiation leading to tumours" is "abnormal anaplasia"[4]; Hansemann then described anaplasia as

(iii) the effects on the cell of the process of abnormal de-differentiation and later

(iv) "de-differentiation" plus "loss of capacity for independent existence" (occurring in the one cell at the one time) and finally

(v) in later papers, "de-specialisation" of the cells of adult tissues.

Especially the distinction between "anaplasia" as a process (by which two phenomena become associated), and "anaplasia" as the simple association itself (ignoring the putative underlying process), became necessary because the proposed process, which he suggested causes it (abnormalities of chromosomes by the known mechanisms in oogenesis), became untenable.

As time passed, and as Wolff (1907, pp 404–5) noted, Hansemann decided to defend mainly his notion of "anaplasia". For example, in his later volume "The Diagnosis of Malignant Tumours" (1897o) he defended his view of the chromosomal basis of neoplastic change to only a slight degree. Hansemann seems to have retreated somewhat from the chromosomal biology of tumours; he did not publish any further original studies of the topic. In later years, he seems to have relied on changes of definition, which some might consider a "philosophical" activity.

Further modifications of Hansemann's views can be understood from his writings up to 1920 as follows. We stress, however, that Hansemann never consolidated his opinions in this precise way. Also, unfortunately, Hansemann was not always clear whether he meant "anaplasia" to be the initial event of tumour formation, or the process set in train by this initial event, or indeed, the morphological consequences of the process. Here in summary are Hansemann's later views:

(i) Anaplasia is a process causing genomic alteration in a normal cell. It determines the morphology and behaviour of the tumour cells which derive from the altered normal cell

(ii) Anaplasia can have delayed morphological effects. That is to say, the event which begins the "anaplastic" change, and the early anaplastic changes themselves, can leave the original cell (*Urtumorzelle*) morphologically unchanged.

(iii) The primary "anaplastic" change may be a change of chromosomes, but also may be too subtle to produce morphological abnormalities in the cell at all. When second changes occur to produce the tumour, perhaps due to growth stimulants, further chromosomal abnormalities may occur to inflict new characteristics on the cell.

(iv) The anaplastic change can vary quantitatively from case to case of the same tumour type.

(v) The mechanisms by which known carcinogens (e.g. paraffin, aniline dyes, irradiation) might cause anaplasia were unknown (in Hansemann's time).

Hansemann on mitoses and chromosomes in general

When analysing Hansemann's contributions to this field it can be observed that his techniques for examining mitoses microscopically (see especially "Studies...." 1893c) are very precise, and worth noting today by anyone interested in this particular area.

Hansemann's first work documented the location and appearances of mitoses and chromosomes in normal and pathological human epidermis (1891h), as well as their presence in carcinomas (see below). Perhaps nowadays, his later descriptions of the cell-type specificity of mitotic appearances (1893c; 1894i) seem excessively detailed, but at the time, this was new information. In the 1890s, Hansemann probably hoped that these mitotic differences between cell types might provide a basis for tissue-specific differences in the chromosomal composition of the nuclei according to the theory of differentiation he espoused in his book (1893c). It is now known of course that there is no tissue-specific distribution of chromosomes in cells during embryonic development. This is because it has been shown possible to "clone" whole animals from adult cells (for example, of a sheep – "Dolly" – from a mammary gland cell)[5] and because DNA analyses specifying an individual are the same whatever cell type (squamous epithelium of mouth, leukocyte, hair cell etc) in the individual is studied.

Nevertheless, the fact that differences in histological appearances of mitoses according to cell type are known at all underlines our current lack of knowledge of the exact events in the formation and movement of chromosomes in mitosis. The usual methods of fixation and embedding of samples for electron microscopy are physico-chemically so harsh that the structure of the chromosomes, and the morphology of the attachments of the centromeres to the spindles, do not survive such processing. Current studies with fluorescent-labelled proteins give an indication as to which macromolecules are associated with each intracellular event, but do not illuminate the exact relationship which the structures identifiable by light microscopy have to each other.

Currently (in 2006), most biologists would probably consider that the cell-type-related differences in mitoses, which Hansemann documented, are related to differences in the cytoplasmic milieu in which the chromosomes replicate, form and separate. Nevertheless there is one broader issue here. Cell-type-specific differences in mitoses might result in different susceptibilities of the "target cells" to carcinogens which act on chromatin during cell replication. From this might be explained the different cell-type-specific susceptibilities to tumours where all cells are presumably equally exposed to carcinogens. For example, tumours of fibrocytes are commoner than tumours of skeletal muscle cells, although both are presumably exposed to similar doses of carcinogens. To our knowledge, this issue has been little discussed in the literature.

Hansemann on abnormal mitoses and chromosomes in pathological cells

From his studies of mitoses in normal and injured or inflamed tissues, Hansemann was able to distinguish the abnormalities of chromosomes which arise from non-specific injury to a cell while it is undergoing mitosis from the abnormalities of chromosomes which are associated with an abnormal mitosis in an otherwise healthy cell. In particular, in "On pathological mitoses" (1891a – complete translation in chapter 9) Hansemann defended his theory against the view that abnormalities of mitoses in tumour cells are not due to a cancer-associated change in the mitotic apparatus at all, but are simply part of general cellular damage. Other authors, for example Ribbert and Lubarsch (see chapter 6), did not seem to think that this distinction was possible. Hansemann (1897o), however, provided the counter argument to the idea that all abnormal mitoses in tumour cells occur only in degenerate tumour cells: he pointed out that cancer cells go on proliferating and producing further asymmetric mitoses indefinitely (and hence hyperchromatic and hypochromatic nuclei), even in metastases. It was unlikely, he thought, that conventional "damage" to cells would permit them to grow excessively at all; the effects would not be evident in subsequent generations deriving from survivors of the damage without alteration of inherited material (usually a mutation). Thus whatever may have caused the initial lesion cannot any longer be operative (in the metastases) – thus the tendency to asymmetric mitosis is part of the inherited morphological/behavioural abnormality in the cells of the cancer. All this was implicit in, and can be deduced from, Hansemann's writings dealing with hyperchromatism (especially 1891c, 1893c, 1897o, 1904c, 1904q), although it was perhaps presented less clearly at the time.

Hansemann's findings on pathological mitoses have never been disputed since. On the contrary they have always been confirmed (Ludford, 1925, 1930a, 1930c, 1930c, 1934; Levine 1931; Koller, 1957). Experimentally, Lea (1962) noted that irradiated cells suffered a tendency to further mitotic abnormalities and that, although the most severely affected cells tended to die out with successive mitoses, some cells with apparently minor chromosomal changes could persist apparently indefinitely. Similar events were found to occur with alkylating agents[6] (reviewed Bignold, 2006). The mechanisms and significance of aneuploidy is still a major issue in tumour cell biology (Büchner, 1985; Epstein, 1986; Sandberg, 1990; Pathak and Multani, 2005). It can also be noted that "clastogenesis" is used to refer to the onset of mitotic abnormalities. "Aneuploidy", however, refers to the fact of abnormal numbers of chromosomes in cells, whether constant in degree in an individual cell line, or – with time – variable and progressive in a cell line. "Chromosomal instability" is used for the latter of these two phenomena; "mitotic catastrophe" (Castedo et al, 2004) denotes the latter when it runs a rapid course ending with death of the cell line.

Another of Hansemann's insights, indeed perhaps the most overlooked, is the constancy of asymmetric mitosis in many types of malignant tumours. For many common malignant tumours, such as adenocarcinomas of the stomach, colon and lung, **all cases** of the cell type show nuclear pleomorphism, that is to say, the nuclei of the individual tumours vary in size and avidity for stains; the average nucleus is larger and equally – or more – "stain-avid" ("chromatic") than the corresponding normal nucleus. These are in turn due to nucleus-to-nucleus variation in the chromatin content; the latter, on average, increased. The bases of these variations could be either (i) asymmetric division, with selective death of the daughter cells with the smaller number of chromosomes, (ii) complete mitosis not followed by nuclear division but loss of some chromosomes, or (iii) partial replication of some chromosomes ("partial mitosis") without nuclear division. "Partial mitosis" (some of the chromosomes being duplicated, but not others in a mitotic figure) of a nucleus is never seen, so Hansemann was correct in asserting that either asymmetric division or complete replication with failed nuclear division and partial loss of chromosomes are the possible mechanisms. It can be accepted, on the basis of simplicity, that asymmetric mitoses are likely to be the commonest mechanism of aneuploidy.

In relation to chromosomal instability and "tumour progression", it is worth noting here that Hansemann documented greater abnormalities of mitoses occurring with progressively increasing morphological abnormality of cancer cells, and that the reverse never occurs (1893c). While most authors considered this to indicate that both the behaviour of the cells and the mitotic processes were being adversely affected at the same time by some undefined "neoplastic process, or "deeper disorder" (Israel, 1902), the idea that the greater chromosomal abnormalities cause the greater degrees of cellular dysfunction was promulgated by Hansemann. This observation was revived in the 1970s, especially by Ohno (1971), Nowell (1976) and Fidler (1986) (see also Bignold, 2002, 2003a, 2003b, 2004). What may be of particular interest is that in chronic myelogenous leukaemia, where a chromosomal lesion is known to initiate the process, the progression of the disease ("blast transformation") is associated with further chromosomal abnormalities, although a consistent chromosomal lesion for this "blastic" change has not yet been identified.

Finally there is the argument as to whether or not asymmetric mitoses occur in sarcomas as well as carcinomas (Hansemann, 1892a; 1893c). Now (in 2006), it seems to be of no great importance; it is difficult to understand why so much was written on the subject. The problem may have been that the diagnostic distinction of sarcoma from carcinoma was an issue because of Virchow's idea that both types of tumour come from the one type of connective tissue cell, and are therefore likely to be similar. If no asymmetric mitoses occur in sarcomas, then perhaps they would more likely be different from carcinomas than otherwise. Another possible significance of the argument may have been that if the same biological changes (of malignancy) occur in a tumour type without asymmetric mitoses, then perhaps asymmetric mitoses are less likely to be universally important for malignancy. In fact, Hansemann's early statement that sarcomas were not known to contain asymmetric mitoses was **against** the general application of his own theory concerning the involvement of chromosomes. Was this the perfect scientist, able to argue against himself? Hansemann does not tell us exactly why this issue was so important to him.

Hauptplasmen and *Nebenplasmen*

In the article (1890a) and in "Studies ..." (1893c), Hansemann offered the idea that Weismann's plasmas might be of two types. Thus to explain events such as metaplasia (the change of morphology in a local cell type, for example, of mucus-producing cells into squamous cells of the bronchi) Hansemann suggested that the "plasmas" controlling the morphology of the cell (i.e. its phenotype) might be considered *Hauptplasmen*/"main plasmas", while those for the latent other morphology might be considered *Nebenplasmen*/"auxiliary plasmas". While this notion has some obvious similarity to concepts of gene activation and suppression, Hansemann did not develop the idea any further. In the context of Hertwig's and Nägeli's widely-known theories of activation and suppression of hereditary elements to account for developmental changes in animals and plants (which were referred to by Hansemann), Hansemann's sub-classification of "plasmas" does not seem very original. His *Hauptplasmen* and *Nebenplasmen* were perhaps an attempt to provide a synthesis of Hertwig's and Nägeli's ideas of the functioning of the hereditary units with Weismann's ideas and terminology.

Of course all these ideas could not be put into perspective until (i) Mendelian genetics was rediscovered (in the 1900s), and (ii) the chemical nature of genetic material (i.e. DNA) was established in the 1950s.

The problem of excessive growth of tumour cells

In the article (1890a) Hansemann attempted to invoke simple "change of phase" in a cell as a source of stimulus to excessive growth in tumour cells. He cited Virchow to support this. Thus, whatever the change was, the daughter cells were supposed to grow more quickly. Once he introduced the concept of "de-differentiation" however, growth became a problem. Thus, for embryonal de-differentiation and adult-tissue-type de-differentiation it could be accepted that the resulting cells would undergo more mitoses. However, in the oogenic model the resulting cell (the egg) has no proliferative capacity at all; therefore the applicability of the oogenic model to tumours was reduced even further than it had been by other problems (see above).

Thus one of the ironies of Hansemann's effort was that his concept of "anaplasia" cannot account for the excessive growth of tumours, but his postulated chromosomal mechanism can. Hansemann himself had suggested that "genetic units" may be inactive in some circumstances and "come to the fore" in others (see previous section). However, he remained convinced of Weismann's idea of progressive genetic loss in tissue development, and could not fully accept the Hertwig/Nägeli view that **all** changes of morphology in normal development are due to alterations in activity of genes.

The modern era probably began when Morgan demonstrated that some genes affect the activity of other genes ("modifier genes" – Morgan et al, 1915). We now know that mechanisms of excess growth can include loss of "tumour suppressor" genes (as in retinoblastoma) and also simple increase in the number ("amplification") of "copies" of growth-factor genes. One asymmetric mitosis in a cell line might occasionally produce cells which have gained copies of growth factors genes, or alternatively, two consecutive asymmetric mitoses might produce a cell which has lost both copies of a tumour suppressor gene. Both mechanisms are currently regarded as probably relevant to tumour types.

We also know now that most of the "growth factor genes" which are overexpressed in tumours, by comparison with adjacent normal adult tissues, are in fact, highly expressed in embryonic tissues, although not necessarily in the embryonic precursor of the adult cell type from which the tumour arises in the adult. Thus, in relation to the de-repression of embryonic growth-factor genes as the basis of tumours, it seems that in most cases "any embryonic growth factor will do" (see Bignold, 2005). Excessive growth in tumour cells may therefore be a much simpler phenomenon than the "embryonalist theoreticians" (such as Fol, Cohnheim and especially Hansemann) seem to have expected.

The application of anaplasia and de-differentiation to the diagnosis of malignant tumours

Hansemann's first contribution to tumour histopathology was to incorporate his observation that hyper- and hypochromatism of nuclei have their origin in asymmetric mitoses. In addition to this he asserted that because such asymmetric mitoses are uncommon in non-tumourous diseases, these nuclear changes are *per se* of diagnostic value. As Hansemann stated (1897o), while small numbers of atypical nuclei can be seen in non-neoplastic conditions, large numbers of such nuclei, especially if uniformly spread through the biopsy tissue, indicate malignancy. Thus the entire discipline of "diagnostic cytology" could begin.

Hansemann's second contribution concerned the application of the "differentiation" to the terminology and classification of tumours. As Hansemann pointed out in the early 1890s, there was no consistent terminology among histopathologists for the nomenclature of tumours. Terms such as "cancroid" were applied to "cancer-like" lesions, mainly of squamous type. The problem which most authors tried to avoid is that many cases of tumour have different appearances in different areas (intra-tumoural morphological heterogeneity). Thus, in the skin, a tumour may have areas of "cancroid" and of "round cell carcinoma". A very illuminating paper on this matter is Virchow's (1888) article "On the Diagnosis and Prognosis of malignant tumours". Here, Virchow was forced to refer to such lesions as "mixed tumours".

Hansemann's observation that the degree of manifestation (i.e. de-differentiation) of an underlying tumourous process (i.e. anaplasia) can be more severe in metastases than in the original tumour, and can in fact vary from area to area in either the original tumour or the metastasis, greatly simplified the problem of "mixed tumours". If most areas in a "round cell" malignant lesion could be considered "markedly de-differentiated"/ "of high anaplasia", then finding an area of "less de-differentiation"/ "low anaplasia" would still allow a single diagnosis to apply to the whole lesion. Thus "mixed round cell carcinoma and cancroid" could then become "squamous cell carcinoma with well- and poorly-differentiated areas". Hansemann's view, as expressed in "The Microscopic Diagnosis …" (1897o/1902) and in the "Atlas …" (1910k), has become standard opinion among diagnostic histopathologists from that time. Academic pathologists, however, have generally ignored this fundamental aspect of tumour biology – that individual tumours can vary considerably from area to area – and along with that, have not discussed any possibility that it might be of any theoretical significance. This can be seen in textbooks of "general pathology" throughout the twentieth century, from Adami (1908) to Robbins and Cotran (2004). Academic texts have almost always repeated lists of "theories of tumour formation", "classifications of tumours" and "characteristics of tumour cells" and have rarely emphasised area-to-area variation in tumours, or how it might be explained.

Hansemann's philosophy

It is clear that there are several strands of German philosophy in Hansemann's various works. The first of these was the rationalist and mechanist approach to biological science which – in the late nineteenth century – was the dominant mode of thought for German Natural Science (*Naturwissenschaft*). Thus Hansemann's accounts, both of the theory of the derivation of "adult" cell types from earlier embryonal cell types and of the development of cancer cells from normal adult cells, are completely in accord with this tradition. Although Hansemann's views on these matters were opposed to Virchow's, the weight of scientific evidence made Hansemann's views undeniable by the 1890s. Further Hansemann's hypotheses concerning the role of abnormal chromosomes in cancer, as expressed from his first article on the topic (1890 – complete translation in chapter 7) to his last (1920 – abstract in chapter 12), were consistently rational and mechanistic.

However, "altruism" demonstrated a different philosophical approach. Hansemann sought to describe a particular and all-embracing phenomenon of cells, and applied a concept which had originated in sociology (chapter 2). For this there were many precedents. Several "biologistic-sociological" theories were popular at the time, especially those of Haeckel and Herbert Spencer (see chapter 2). Perhaps more significant, however, was the "biologistic sociology" which Virchow had included in his "philosophy of pathology" (chapter 2). Specifically, Virchow had asserted that the different behaviours of the types of cells – and especially their metabolism – occur in a mutually cooperative manner, which human societies could take as a model.

Perhaps a more complete examination of Virchow's and Hansemann's personal papers (not available to us) might shed more light on the matter, but the facts already clearly suggest a strong influence of this aspect of Virchow's "philosophy of pathology" on Hansemann's. The supposition here is based on the fact that the term "altruism" was only invented (by Comte) in the 1840s, and only discussed in detail by authors such as Spencer two decades later. By this time (1860s), Virchow had abandoned further development of his "philosophy of pathology". There is an obvious closeness between (i) Virchow's use of "cooperativeness" among individuals in a society and (ii) Hansemann's emphasis on the "altruism" of the individuals in the society which makes such cooperation more likely and thus enhances the success of the society as a whole.

By way of further background, Hansemann may have developed the idea of the applicability of "altruism" to cells from the contemporaneous work by many authors on cell turnover (which had been postulated by Goodsir, chapter 3) and on cell function. When Hansemann began his career, the relationships of both these matters to the phenomena of mitosis (chapter 4) could be studied. Thus early histologists had seen the layers of cells in epithelium and they had guessed that the basal cells give rise constantly to the upper layers which are ultimately shed. However, not until (i) mitosis was established as the mechanism of cell reproduction and (ii) the location of mitoses was shown to occur almost exclusively in the lower layers of such tissues, could the whole concept of physiological turnover of cells be proven. For this reason, Hansemann's work (1891) on the distribution of mitoses in the normal human epidermis was significant. The current classification of tissues into "labile", "stable" and "permanent" was only promulgated in the mid 1890s (Bizzozero, 1894).

It is clearly an "altruistic" type of behaviour for a layer of cells (e.g. in the epidermis) to produce daughter cells which sacrifice themselves for the good of the organism just as much as it is for an entire cell type to serve the general good without sacrifice of cell life (e.g. adrenal cortical cells). Hansemann could easily have been led by his reading of Spencer's "biological altruism" (chapter 2) to "altruism" as a catch-all for both phenomena.

Thus it is possible that Hansemann may have simply modified Virchow's "philosophy of cell cooperation" by using the "updated" social concepts of Comte and Spencer to arrive at a "philosophy of cell altruism".

"Anaplasia", philosophically, may be another matter. In 1890 Hansemann invented this concept of cancer in a strictly rationalist/mechanist mode. His concepts were in accordance with contemporaneous and strictly scientifically-derived ideas of the functions of chromosomes in cells. After 1892, when the falsity of some of those ideas was exposed (i.e. Weismann revoking his – Weismann's – theory of chromosomal mechanisms of differentiation), Hansemann underwent a change in mode of contemplation (*Betrachtungsweise*). This change was not towards any "metaphysicalism" (which would have required an invoking of "forces" or "vitalism" or some similar concept) but was rather towards abstractionism. This path of advance seems to have been strongly modelled on Germanic philosophical traditions.

All this becomes clear by careful examination of Hansemann's "Studies ..." (1893c). A conventional rationalist/mechanist title of the book would have been "Mitoses in tumour cells: their possible morphological and physiological significance and consequences". However, Hansemann subdivided the overall discussion of tumour phenomena into three "conceptual niches" or abstract entities *viz*: – "Specificity", "Altruism" and "Anaplasia". These subsections contain the following material:

(i) "Specificity" of cells is expanded beyond ideas of embryonal development and lineage commitment (c.f. Bard, see chapter 3) to include concepts of specificity of mitotic appearances and location compatibility.

(ii) "Altruism" (derived from sociology – see above) was used by Hansemann to include not only simple interdependence in the functions of cells, but as well, wider functional effects which are now recognized as mechanisms in endocrinology. Ideas which now might be considered "autocrine" and/or "paracrine" or even endocrine are foreshadowed in this section.

(iii) "Anaplasia", in which Hansemann indicated the concept as an association of functional and morphological abnormalities. While this section seems to construct a kind of "cognitive niche", its drawing of attention to an association of biological phenomena in the one cell at the same time had some rationalist/mechanist basis. Scientifically-confirmed associations of events are not philosophical concepts, but on the contrary, are facts to be explained. Here, however, Hansemann stated that particular association of cellular abnormalities exist, and that some associations are cell-type-of-origin specific. These associations form the basis for interpretation of the histopathological features of malignant tumours, on which diagnoses can be made (see above).

In later works, Hansemann defended his idea of "Anaplasia" in the abstract mode of contemplation (*Betrachtungsweise*). Rarely did Hansemann return to specifically rational/mechanistic considerations of the possible biological basis for the association of abnormal phenomena in the cancer cell (chapter 12).

Only on "altruism" and "anaplasia" were Hansemann's thoughts overly abstract (by current standards). Hansemann's "The Microscopic Diagnosis ... " (1897o/1902h) is strictly rational and mechanistic. Even in works dealing with philosophical matters (Hansemann, 1909f, 1912f) he did not invent any new abstractions. Overall these works have a rational and modern general medical theoretical outlook.

Notes to chapter 5

1 See "Notes on the Works and Translations".

2 Hertwig (1890) gives an account of parthenogenesis as understood in Hansemann's time. The same work can be consulted for a discussion of the "differentiation" of the egg. The molecular biology of parthenogenesis is still not clearly understood (Parrington and Coward, 2003).

3 The American Type Culture Collection (ATCC) was established in 1925 as a non-profit organisation to establish and maintain a central collection of microorganisms that would serve scientists all over the world. It has also collected animal cell lines. Currently holds nearly 1,000 tumour cell lines, many of which are listed with their karyotypes.

   Reference: www.atcc.org

4 In point of fact Hansemann failed to find a suitable word for his speculative de-differentiation-associated process (*entdifferenzierungshaften Prozess*) which, unlike other de-differentiations but possibly modelled on oogenesis, leads to tumours. Initially, he meant that the fundamental process of tumour formation is normal oogenesis occurring in inappropriate cells; that is to say, non-egg precursors. Later, when the oogenic association became untenable, he may have thought it possible that the tumourigenic process is an abnormal oogenic process arising in non-egg-precursor cells. For that concept he could not use "caco-differentiation" because that would have been confusing since Lobstein had already used "cacoplasia" (chapter 4); it would have carried an insufficiently precise meaning anyway. Even "dysde-differentiation" would not convey the idea, and "dysanaplasia" would not be euphonious.

5 "Dolly", the name given to the first cloned mammal (a sheep) raised by Wilmut and co-workers (1997). The initiation of embryogenesis from a somatic cell nucleus requires (i) that the nucleus be inserted into a "ripe" ovum of the same species, and (ii) unphysiological stimuli, such as electric current, which perhaps act in some way similar to that of the stimuli required for the induction of parthenogenesis in animals such as frogs (note[2] above).

6 Alkylating agents are derived from mustard gases, and have cytotoxic, clastogenic, mutagenic and carcinogenic properties even in very low doses. As for carcinogens, the structure-effect relationships have not been established at the present time (see Bignold, 2006).

Chapter 6

Critics, reviewers, the forgetting of Hansemann, and what might have been

Introduction

Hansemann's theories tried to encompass a large number of different ideas which were then under consideration by biologists and pathologists concerning the nature of cancer. Foremost were ideas related to the details of the biological features which cancer cells exhibit: especially excessive and uncontrolled growth; loss of specialised activity; as well as invasion and metastasis etc. The second group of ideas concerned the conceptual role of embryological and other normal biological processes in cancer; particularly in relation to specificity of developmental cell lineages. In addition Hansemann was concerned with the significance of the abnormalities of mitotic figures and chromosomes in tumour cells.

Nevertheless the comprehensiveness of Hansemann's theory did not protect it from thorough critical review by other authors of the time. It was, after all, put forward within a culture which cultivated vigor of debate as well as of intellect and expression.

Some contemporaneous critics, however, vigorously attacked the detail of Hansemann's ideas, while others attempted to discount the main thrust, which was: altered chromosomes can cause altered cell morphology and function.

Ribbert and the theory of "control by connective tissue"

Hansemann's most constant critic was probably Ribbert (1855–1920)[1] who was the first into print, and perhaps the most persistent in the arguments which he advanced. Ribbert published his criticisms of Hansemann's ideas in three separate papers in 1890 (listed in Hansemann, 1892a), and in many subsequent articles. Quite early on, the dispute seems to have acquired a personal component. Nevertheless, in his book (1911) Ribbert was notably courteous in tone and relatively even-handed in his comments on Hansemann's ideas.

Ribbert's own theories (Bashford, 1905; Wolff, 1907; Ribbert, 1911; Beattie and Dickson, 1921) amounted to complicated variations on Virchow's theory of cancer which favoured a critical role for connective tissue cells in cancer formation. These versions became necessary when the lineage specificity of most types of tumours, especially carcinomas from epithelia and sarcomas from connective tissue cells, became irrefutable (see chapters 3 and 5). Perhaps Ribbert was attempting to preserve Virchow's discredited "connective tissue theory" of cancer by suggesting that the original cancerous change occurs in connective tissue cells, and that these cells then exert a "controlling influence" on the epithelial cells which are seen to be cancerous. Some residues of this idea are still published as "epithelio-mesenchymal interactions" (see Bignold 2003c), but are not widely popular today. Hansemann consistently expressed the currently most popular opinion which is that cancerous abnormality lies in the "parenchymal cell of the tumour", not in the "stromal cell of the tumour".

Lubarsch

Lubarsch[2] (1860–1933) was a notable writer on pathology, and produced many texts both for undergraduates and post-graduates. His theory that the basis of tumours is an "alloplasia" appears to have been substantially derived from Virchow's concepts of a role for metaplasia in cancer. In this way, he was perhaps a professional competitor of Hansemann. Considerable friction developed between them. The first dispute apparently began in 1895, and concerned the nature of kidney tumours (Lubarsch, 1902a). In the course of this article, Lubarsch (1902a) indicated that Hansemann (i) had attacked him unjustifiably, (ii) either had not read the works Lubarsch's works referred to, or had done so only sketchily, and (iii) had behaved in an ungentlemanly fashion.

Lubarsch (1902a) claimed that after September 1895 at the Nature Researchers' meeting in Lübeck, there was improper quoting and crediting of opinions concerning the nature of hypernephroid kidney tumours in relation to endotheliomas (Hansemann 1896b; 1897o; 1901b). A particular point was the distinction between myoliposarcoma and hypernephroid carcinoma of the kidney.

Lubarsch (1902a) wrote in the second paragraph: "Hansemann reproaches me because in respect of a personal demonstration and data which he had given me privately, that I had made this the object of quite unequivocal public criticism, and that therefore he has to regret ever having offered me such trust – a more incorrect representation is not easily possible".

Lubarsch (1902a) also objected to Hansemann's quotation of Lubarsch's views on significance of glycogen for this diagnosis of hypernephroid tumours. Hansemann apparently also ignored Lubarsch's work on new stains for glycogen in tumours, and did it in an insulting way.

> "In this kind of judgement of the relevant literature, it can come as no surprise that Mr von Hansemann, in his more pedagogic "Lecture on Tumours of the Kidney", does not mention a type of new formation which is not at all infrequent and which I myself described first of all in a much-cited work ... and he seems to have read Manasse's work supporting my view with the same thoroughness as he has read mine .... I do not need to remark further on Mr von Hansemann's use of the scientific works of other researchers for his pedagogic lectures".

Further friction between Hansemann and Lubarsch apparently flared at a meeting of the Committee for Cancer Research in March of 1902. The published report of the meeting (Anon, 1902) does not give details of the altercation which apparently took place. However, Lubarsch apparently particularly objected to any process (of which "anaplasia" was the example in question) which might begin in a histologically normal cell and give rise after some delay to actual, recognisable cancer cells (see chapter 5). He also believed that no cancer-related mitotic abnormalities occur at all. The section in Lubarsch (1902a) reads as follows:

> "And finally, Hansemann's theory of the anaplasia of cells could well use a cancer-arousing stimulus for completion, in that it would be this which makes the cells anaplastic. In a word, it could appear as if the parasite theory would open to us a deeper insight into the nature of malignant new formations than any other theory. Therefore, von Leyden also calls it a "biological theory" and opposes it to the "cellular" or "histogenetic" idea of Ribbert and von Hansemann. But in my opinion, unjustifiably. Specifically, Ribbert's and Hansemann's theories earn the name "biological", because just as much as Cohnheim's, they make the serious attempt to explain biologically the essence of malignant new formations too. They are at the very least pathogenetic, and decisively aetiological theories. Ribbert has always emphasised this, all his arguments reach their peak in explaining the phenomena of tumour formation from the normal laws of growth. If Hansemann repeatedly, and recently with particular reference to me, emphasises that his theory is only a histogenetic one, then I regret that he himself diminishes the great merits which he has gained for himself with his arguments concerning anaplasia. If his theory were really histogenetic, it would mean that every carcinoma is descended from an anaplastic epithelium, and then – from the histological standpoint – it would be scarcely discussable at all because it is quite unproved and unprovable that the epithelium, from which even a strongly anaplastic cancer proceeds, could be anaplastic. Anaplasia should make us understand the nature of destructive new formation; therewith the theory is at least already a patho- and not a histogenetic one."

In his "General Pathology" (1905) Lubarsch had a section "Phenomena of damage in self-dividing cells"/*Die Schädigungserscheinungen der Zelle beim Absterben*. Here, he discussed thickening and clumping of chromosomes, altered staining, and granularity, and then "Asymmetric mitoses"/*Die asymmetrischen Mitosen* (paragraph 5, p. 47 of the original):

> "Under this heading one understands those mitoses whose daughter stars do not have the same number of chromosomes (Hansemann), thus hypochromatic forms too can arise in this way. Asymmetric mitoses have hitherto been found in carcinomas and sarcomas (Fig. 12a) (Hansemann, Vitalis Müller, Stroebe, Lubarsch and many others), in adenomas (Lubarsch, Stroebe), in regenerative growth proliferations in the epidermis of skin (Stroebe), in regeneration of Salamander epithelia (if the regeneration proceeded under the influence of diluted anti-pyrin, cocaine and quinine solutions) (Galeotti, Figs 12 b and c). Finally Ranke has also observed them in Salamander larvae, when they were fully fed after a period of starvation (Fig. 13 a, b). In this, the CENTROSOMES too show deviations in that they are often of DISSIMILAR SIZE, so that Galeotti and Lustig assume inequality of the centrosomes to be the cause of the unequal distribution of the chromatic substance. Asymmetric mitosis is thus a not-infrequent finding which, in spite of its occurrence under virtually normal circumstances, must yet be regarded on the whole as an expression of cell damage, because:
>
> 1. Not infrequently other degenerative phenomena in the threads are associated with the asymmetry;

2. They appear above all when, simultaneously, disintegrative phenomena are present in the tissues. This is also the case, for example in Reinke's observations.

Hansemann has doubted Galeotti's observations and has explained the appearances pictured as being cut-off parts of normal mitoses; in my opinion, unjustifiably. I have convinced myself of the correctness of Galeotti's data and have also found asymmetric mitoses in surface preparations. That applies still more to Reinke's observations, whose preparations are exclusively surface preparations from the abdominal skin of the Salamander larvae."

In the next paragraph (6 of a section "Hyperchromatic and multi-parted mitoses"/*Die hyperchromatischen und mehrteiligen Mitosen*) Lubarsch (1905, p. 48) continued:

"By hyperchromatic mitoses we understand those which possess more chromosomes than normal. One can divide them into 2-PART AND MULTI-PART (PLURI-POLAR) mitoses. The former are large forms with many, up to 100 chromosomes, from which hyperchromatic cells arise "as the daughter cells contain exactly as many chromosomes as the mother cells possessed" (Hansemann). In the multipart mitoses on the contrary, where one finds three, four, six, or – according to Hansemann – even 12–20 poles with centrisomes and the spindles belonging to them, a reduction of the numerous chromosomes takes place, in that the cell divides into just as many parts as there are centrosomes present."

Thus Lubarsch differed with Hansemann concerning mainly (i) the possibility of a pre-tumourous abnormality of "normal-appearing" cells (i.e. pre-tumourous "anaplasia"), and (ii) the circumstances in abnormal nuclear division and their interpretation.

The argument concerning what is a "biological theory" and what is not may perhaps be seen as a dispute existing only at the level of over-abstraction of the issues; reminiscent of the Ancient Greeks and their philosophical descendants (chapter 2).

Lubarsch's other relevant opinion was to support Virchow's suggestion that metaplasia is a common phenomenon. He even reported that osteoblasts can turn into epithelial cells, which would have pleased Virchow (see chapter 4). He then introduced "alloplasia" for all metaplastic and related conditions, comprising "pseudo-metaplasia" (where the cells at the site change their form due to external conditions, previously called "adaptation" by Virchow, and "accommodation" by Hansemann) and "true metaplasias". Lubarsch used "true metaplasias" for the event in which the cells at a site undergo loss of differentiation ("metaplastic dedifferentiation") followed immediately by redifferentiation along a path which, although not usual at the site, is a normal path of differentiation at another site. An example of this is the squamous metaplasia which can occur in bronchial epithelium seen associated with chronic bronchitis.

Borst

Borst[4] was a prominent pathologist, but never worked in Berlin. In his book (1902) Borst pointed out that Hansemann's theory does not explain excessive growth. Borst discussed the aetiology of tumours (pp xii–xiii) under headings which include the following:

Older views (IRRITATIVE MOMENTS 79a; unique physical trauma. Other types of mechanical irritations 80; chemical damage. Inflammation, scar formation 80a. Tumour formation from hyperplasias …);

bacteria and parasites (including growth relationships and evidence against from studies of metastases) … congenital bases (Cohnheim's theories, hereditary factors, transplantation experiments etc) … and 'Inner Causes'.

In the last, Borst (1902) mentions congenital weakness or excessive strength of the tissues, local predisposition, abnormal idioplastic predispositions, Hansemann's and others' opinions, "blastomatosis", relation of the nervous system to growth, and "acquired disposition".

With respect to Hansemann's views Borst (1902) stated:

> "Most of the authors assume, as noted above, that in blastomatosis, a change in the whole nature of the cells appears (Hansemann, Hauser, Beneke, Lubarsch and many others). According to this the cells are supposed to gain quite new properties (greater capacity for independent existence, greater energy for proliferation, ability to exert a destructive effect on other tissues etc) and to lose other properties (reduction of specific differentiation, weakening or loss of functional capabilities, loss of formative influence etc). How this change in cell character ("anaplasia") is attained, has thereto received less attention.
>
> "With the word 'anaplasia' Hansemann wishes to say that morphologically and physiologically, the cells have become 'others'; he believes that perhaps asymmetric nuclear division leads to anaplasia; yet, as it seems, he does not attach any great value to this, as he says that it is a secondary question as to how 'anaplasia' comes about. Anaplasia as such, he thinks, has nothing to do with aetiology: anaplasia, he thinks, is the expression for the changes which the cells would have to undergo in order to possess malignant properties; in order, however, for a malignant tumour to arise, he believes, a further stimulation to proliferation must be added. If this latter stimulus hits a normal cell, then hyperplasia, in the widest sense of the word, arises; if it hits an anaplastic cell, then – he thinks – a malignant growth arises. According to this, the theory of anaplasia applies only to malignant tumours; specifically at this point, opposition, in my opinion, could begin."

In 1923, Borst contributed the chapter on tumours to the 6th edition of Aschoff's "Textbook of Pathology". On pp 655 of that book, Borst gives much credit to Boveri for a chromosomal theory of cancer. On pp 673 Borst continued:

> "In particular experimental tumour research shows us quite clearly that the special properties of tumour cells consist in a REDUCTION OF BIOCHEMICAL SENSITIVITY (lesser extent of differentiation) and in an intensification of the independent capacity for existence (see below, note 1). These are precisely the properties which Hansemann wanted to cover with his concept of Anaplasia; these peculiarities of tumour cells are also intended to be covered by expressions such as Hauser's "new races of cells", Beneke's "kataplasia", R. Hertwig's "return of the cells from the organotypical to the cytotypical growth". Whether an INCREASED AVIDITY OF THE TU-

MOUR CELLS FOR SPECIFIC NOURISHMENT OR GROWTH MATERIALS (EHRLICH) HAS TO BE ACCEPTED AS EHRLICH WISHED CAN BE HELD FOR LATER CONSIDERATION. The aforementioned specific properties of the tumour cells can now be comprehended as newly-acquired qualities; alternatively, one can more negatively assume that they become apparent by the falling away of certain inhibitions situated within or outside the cell. In each case, THE TUMOUR CELL HAS BECOME A DIFFERENT ONE VIS À VIS THE NORMAL BODY CELL, AND THIS CHANGE DOES NOT LIE ON THE NORMAL LINE OF PROGRESS, BUT REPRESENTS RATHER A DERAILMENT FROM THE NORMAL PATH. THEREFORE, COMPARISON OF TUMOUR CELLS WITH EMBRYONAL CELLS IS QUITE INAPPROPRIATE."

Thus Borst (1902, 1923) expressed Hansemann's position accurately, but without detailed or sympathetic analysis. Moreover, Borst failed to note Hansemann's priority in suggesting a chromosomal theory of cancer.

O. Israel

Oskar Israel (see chapter 1) was deputy director under Virchow at the Institute of Pathology. He wrote what was essentially a protest against a published comment by Hansemann. It was perhaps a little churlish for Hansemann to have attacked his ideas so vigorously. Perhaps the most important sentence in Israel's article (1902) is the enunciation of the view, which was to persist for 60 years, that chromosomal changes are only the effect, not the cause, of the neoplastic process. Israel apparently subscribed fully to Virchow's "chronic irritation" theory. He did not publish any theory of his own. Here is Israel's article in full.

Reluctance to become involved in personal polemics when scientific questions are involved is widespread and so deep seated, that fortunately it is only seldom set aside; and mostly only when an unusually personal and unjust attack has taken place. Herr von Hansemann can thank this circumstance for the fact that he has drawn upon himself such a complete rebuff as that which was administered to him recently by Lubarsch[1]. If now, in similar fashion I overcome my scruples in order to answer such an attack from von Hansemann, then what causes me to do this is the factually incorrect representation which von Hansemann gives of our controversy himself, and that the solution to it is not without scientific interest. Herr von Hansemann's tone is his affair and is at the very least dispensable for the factual proceedings; therefore, I do not intend to go into this any further.

Von Hansemann writes, among other utterances which on account of their lesser relevance I will not return to again here. In the second edition of his book "The Microscopic Diagnosis of Malignant Tumours" p. 187: "O. Israel denies (314) the concept of anaplasia wholly out of disinclination towards any theory. He asserts that he can give an explanation of tumours without theoretical considerations. Naturally one is very eager to know what he will bring forth. It then becomes apparent that he ceases his contemplations, as soon as the theory begins. That is naturally a very simple way of avoiding theories and if everybody were so sparing in this respect, as O. Israel we should find ourselves on the ideal foundation of pure facts. But would that satisfy everybody? Not me!"

The number 314 in this quotation refers to my essay which appeared among the centenary articles of the Berliner klin. Wschr. "On the pathology of disease-related tumours"[2], in part 3 of which I plead for a more consequential treatment of the tumour theory and as far as possible

---

[1] The diagnosis of adrenal kidney tumours. Remarks on Herr von Hansemann's essay "On kidney tumours". Zeitschr. f. klin. Med. vol. 44, pp 491 ff.

[2] Berl. klin. Wochenschr. 1900. Nos 28, 29 and 30.

---

with the methods of phylogenetic transformation. Earlier already von Hansemann referred to this passage in an essay "Concerning the concept and the essence of anaplasia"[1], in which he attacks the conclusions of Beneke[2].

He writes there: "Into similar error as Beneke, O. Israel falls, who in a recently published centenary article (Berl. klin. Wschr. 1900 No 28) expresses himself on the histogenesis of diseased tumours and touches on my hypothesis with the following words: 'An anaplasia in the sense of a cytogenetic atavism does not exist'. Thus, Israel too, like Beneke, presupposes that in anaplasia the cells return the same way as they took in a forward direction. I reserve the right to return on another occasion to the other differences of conceptualisation which exist between Israel and me."

These two citations contain, as far as my original utterances are confirmed, a series of errors which I must correct before I discuss what causes me to reject von Hansemann's anaplasia at all.

1. Von Hansemann reproaches me for "disinclination towards any theory" and says 2. that in spite of my assertion of being able to give "an explanation for tumours without theoretical considerations", I stop where theory begins.

The passage from which von Hansemann deduces my disinclination towards theories reads verbatim (*op cit*): "I prefer to show by one definite example how safely this mode of contemplation steers us around many a difficult rock which in this fashion I also avoid in the classroom when I am teaching, WITHOUT RESORTING TO HYPOTHESES AND CIRCUMLOCUTORY THEORIES[3]". My disinclination is only directed against hypotheses when I am teaching and against circumlocutory theories in general.

How far von Hansemann's view is justified, namely, that I cease my contemplations where theory begins, may be determined by those who have read Parts IV and V of the article in question, either in the original, or who will take the trouble to read up the theory given there on the histogenesis of carcinoma. I am of the opinion, however, that I have been successful in my presentation without hypotheses, and that that which I want to explain is not just simply a circumlocution.

I have not, however, in this explanation availed myself of von Hansemann's anaplasia for reasons which I will discuss further below. I have certainly used the word "anaplasia", which is in itself well formulated (*gutgebildet*), but with the express addition "in the sense of a CYTOGENETIC ATAVISM[3)]", which I reject, just as von Hansemann does, as the explanation

[1)] These Archives, vol. 162, p. 552.
[2)] These Archives, vol. 161, p. 70f.
[3)] Also emphasised in the original.

535 of malignant tumours. On the other hand, I agree with Beneke[1)] WHO REGARDS THE WORD "KATAPLASIA" AS MORE SUITABLE FOR WHAT VON HANSEMANN CALLS "ANAPLASIA". At various places in his publications, von Hansemann speaks of anaplasia as a theory as well as a hypothesis and, finally, for preference, as a concept. This absence of clarity in definition renders difficult *per se* to use "anaplasia" as an expression for conditions and processes which admit of precise denotation, and need such when it is a matter of clarification of a pathological process on the basis of proven conditions. There are two ideas which von Hansemann wishes to draw together: "THE CELLS HAVE LOST THEIR NORMAL AMOUNT OF DIFFERENTIATION AND HAVE INCREASED THEIR CAPABILITY FOR INDEPENDENT EXISTENCE" (CITATION ABOVE, P. 186) AND HE EMPHASISES EXPRESSLY "THAT ANAPLASIA DOES NOT EMBODY A PURELY MORPHOLOGICAL CONCEPT, BUT ALSO, SIMULTANEOUSLY HAS A PHYSIOLOGICAL MEANING".

Here, two things are coordinated which in my opinion do not stand equally to each other, and this is one of the reasons why von Hansemann's anaplasia has not offered us any means for explaining the origin of malignant tumours. As I discussed recently at the Congress of the German Society for Surgery[2)], the heightened reproductive capacity of the covering cells is the essential factor in the genesis of carcinomatous new formations, which is naturally not possible if the cells do not nourish themselves sufficiently. Thus both correspond approximately to what von Hansemann denotes as "increased capacity for independent existence", as the independence in carcinomas appears specifically in the descendant cells. The loss in morphological and physiological (functional) differentiation I regard correctly as secondary, as I think I have proved. It is the consequence of the – acquired by adaptation and increased in the course of the hereditary process – one-sided completely developed of the reproductive efficiency of the cells, whose other functions adapt themselves in similar fashion change, are changed and become partly or wholly lost. The morphological deviations in the cells – in a large part of their elements – are to be explained by the fact that they do not have any more function as covering cells. Absence of keratinisation and other phenomena of regular physiological development, changes in form, changes in the connections of cells between each other (especially evident in carcinomas arising from glands) etc; all those are circumstances which arise from the conditions in which the cancerous descendants of the cover cells arise and live. They form characteristics of the new formation, but offer no explanation for their origin. It is not because they are "anaplastic" that epithelial cells make carcinoma; what makes the cells anaplastic remains unexplained. Therefore, von Hansemann also emphasises

[1] cited before, p. 100.
[2] Verhandl. d. Deutsch. Ges. f. Chirurgie am 2.Sitzungstag, 1902.

that his theory is not an aetiological one. But histogenesis too cannot clarify von Hansemann's anaplasia; it only circumlocutes what we see in carcinoma; greater independence of the cells which have lost differentiation is indeed a brief and accurate characterisation but as discussed above, one which is not useful for the explanation of histogenesis, because it is an inappropriate pulling together of things which are not of equal rank.

As with anaplasia, when dealing with the essence of malignant tumours, von Hansemann tries through another word, "altruism", to surmount the difficulties of that relationship which was long since denoted as the correlation of the organs. Von Hansemann writes (citation above, p. 182):

"Here I would also like to remind ourselves of the particular connection between acromegaly and tumours of the hypophysis. In about 80 per cent of cases of this remarkable disease one finds tumours of the hypophysis. As far as these have been histologically examined, they are so made that one can conclude from them an over function of the organ. These data which I also provided earlier, were also confirmed by Benda. Marie has doubted whether the cases without hypophysial tumour are really acromegaly, and I completely agree with this. The case described by O. Israel is certainly not acromegaly, at least he has remained guiltless of any proof of this. To the increase in function in the hypophysial tumour, corresponds the altruistic growth of the rest of the body."

It is exaggerated to say that in 80 per cent of cases of acromegaly hypophysial tumours are found. Further there is no reason to conclude, for example, in a sarcoma of the hypophysis that there is an over function of the hypophysis. Thus, Sternberg[1] states that a sarcoma of the hypophysis was always found in cases of acromegaly which had taken an acute course; "He comes to the only logical conclusion that if there is a connection, the dissolution of the normal function of the hypophysis is the cause of the acromegaly, as on the other hand the sarcoma brings about the total annihilation of the organ, while von Hansemann postulates the opposite, over function. Because Marie doubts whether cases without hypophysial tumour are really acromegaly, and von Hansemann agrees completely with that, I am said to be guilty of not giving any proof that my case[2] was really acromegaly. Certainly no hypophysial tumour was found but otherwise all findings came together to justify the clinical diagnosis which *Geheimrat* Gerhardt had made with the patient. With the unproven increased function in the hypophysial tumour the "altruistic growth of the rest of the body" cannot have a better basis,

[1] Nothnagel's spec. Path. u. Ther., vol. 7, part II, Acromegaly. Wien, 1897, p. 78.
[2] These Archives vol. 164, p. 344.

537 than with the certain cessation of the unknown function of the hypophysis in those cases where the organ is reduced in size or completely destroyed by a "heterogeneous new formation, cysts and similar things"[1].

I am not, however, able to give a well-founded theory of acromegaly. Certainly I recently discussed an aetiological theory of carcinoma[2] namely that the most various and sufficiently-lengthy injuries, which lead to insignificant discontinuities of the covering cell layers, cause the neighbours of the injured cells to achieve a one-sided increase in their reproductive capacity as a result of their permanently-acquired replacing activity; this makes possible a temporally and spatially excessive number of descendant cells. If the regular resistance on the part of the connective tissue substance or if this resistance has been reduced by pathological processes (age, inflammatory and other processes) is unable to restrain new formation by the cover cells, then the new formation works in a destructive fashion and finds the possibility to spread itself under the given conditions throughout the whole body. The insults arising from the pushing out of place of the newly formed cells to the connective tissue and parenchymata of the organs, and just as much the losses of the newly formed parts themselves by regressive processes give the causes for the further triggering of cell divisions, for in this manner preparations of continuity arise in the epithelium (endothelium), as also in the connective tissue substance, which, just as they do this in the regenerative processes, hereto provoke cell divisions. Through its own effects the new formation is kept going: once the cells which have become particularly efficient in reproduction by adaptation and hereditary, once they have penetrated into the basement zone there exists a vicious circle which further intensifies the intensity and extent of the carcinomatous growth process, under certain circumstances until the death of the individual.

Through this histogenetic and aetiological theory the circumstances and processes are explained, which are drawn together by von Hansemann as anaplasia. Further research, however, will only be successful if it does not set as its object the discovery of cancer parasites in particular cancer-stimulating protozoa and the proof that carcinoma, sarcoma and so on are infectious diseases but on the contrary if it tries to clarify the mechanism of the biological processes, and in the individual case, where they have not been established with certainty, those moments which evoke pathological proliferation at the primary site. This is valid for all forms of proliferative tumours.

[1] Vgl. Sternberg, cited above.
[2] In press. Archiv f. klin. Chirurgie, vol. 67."

Other critics: Beneke, Wolff

Beneke[4] (1900) took up the debate on the precise nature of the abnormality of tumour cells, again arguing that "anaplasia", according to Hansemann's concept, in effect does not exist. He asserted that each mitosis represents a return of the cell to an "embryonal" state, and that in cancer subsequent specialisation is disordered with a displacement of functional activities by proliferation. He suggested "kataplasia" as a better descriptive word, but apparently did not discuss any chromosomal lesion as the basis of this change (Wolff, 1907).

Wolff's book (1907) has been the major source of reference for the history of the study of cancer, especially in Germany. We have already noted that this author did not record Hansemann in the "Index of Names". Hansemann was still alive when Wolff wrote his book. He is frequently referred to in the text, as though Wolff's readers did not need a guide to Hansemann's views. On pp 404 and 405 of his book, Wolff (1907) indicates that in "The Diagnosis of Malignant Tumours", Hansemann is uncertain of the significance of asymmetric mitoses in tumour formation (although the edition is not stated). But he does not mention Hansemann's idea of other mechanisms of chromosomal damage. Neither does he attempt any analysis of the issue of cellular heredity.

Boveri's ideas were similar to Hansemann's

Theodor Boveri[5] (1862–1915) has received considerable credit for espousing "the first" chromosomal theory of cancer. Boveri, who had made magnificent contributions to the biology of chromosomes in the 1880s, had been conducting experiments on embryos with a view to contributing to the major issue of "developmental mechanisms" (*Entwicklungsmechanik* – see below). His chosen method involved shaking embryos of sea urchins and studying the development of the resulting fragments. However, Boveri's ideas were not a significant advance on those of Hansemann. In fact, in many areas, they were simplifications of von Hansemann's fully-developed views (Bignold et al, 2006a, 2006b). The following is an extended account of the matter.

Boveri's first discussion of cancer came at the end of an article published in (Boveri, 1902, English translation 1974). He begins with the observation that sea urchin eggs penetrated by two spermatozoa ("dispermic eggs") undergo a tetrapolar mitosis with the formation of four blastomeres, beyond which no development takes place beyond formation of blastulae. Cells from the epithelial layers were seen to enter the interior, but their fate was unknown. Then Boveri eliminated the possibility that the dispermic eggs were abnormal before fertilisation, and showed that if the four blastomeres are separated (in calcium-free seawater), they develop often into gastrulae. He then discussed how mechanically shaken dispermic eggs (a method originally described by Morgan) can exhibit tripolar mitoses, resulting in three blastomeres, of which a considerable percentage develop into plutei, some of the latter being completely normal. Then he discusses these facts and comes to the conclusion that "These phenomena could only be explained on the basis of a process which itself is subject to corresponding variability and such a process is presented only in the manner of **distribution of the chromosomes**."

As point 6 in this paper Boveri (1902) addressed the question of whether the fate of the blastomeres depends on unequal quantitative distribution (of chromosomes) or on different qualities of the individual chromosomes. The simple quantitative model is disposed of quickly; the model of random assortments of chromosomes, each having specific qualities, is discussed. The conclusion is that "a definite combination of chromosomes" is essential for normal development, and that "the individual chromosomes must possess different qualities".

Following a discussion of the works of Driesch, Weismann, Hertwig and others concerning the nuclear-dependent features of embryogenesis, and considering on what basis the cells which wander into the interior of the abnormal blastulae might be thought of as "tumours", Boveri began to discuss "the possibility that multipolar mitosis might, under certain conditions, lead to the development of tumour-like formations". He considers that pressure, narcotics and abnormal temperatures might provoke the multipolar mitoses and "the entire causal sequence of certain tumours".

In Hansemann's terms, Boveri suggests tumours develop because multipolar mitosis occurs in somatic cells of mammals as an abnormality of histogenetic development. Boveri advances no evidence that multipolar mitosis can occur in the embryos of higher animals, let alone in their somatic cells, or that such changes might either occur commonly or uncommonly in such cells. In addition, Boveri does not mention how these changes could result in the development of cancer in such cells (i.e. the data discussed by pathologists in response to Hansemann's more general suggestions twelve years before).

Boveri's (1914) book presents an expansion of these basic ideas. In the first chapter he states that he believes a tumour cell to be one which has lost some qualities of normal tissue-cells. "In this view I follow entirely the idea which Hansemann characterised as Anaplasia". In chapter II ("Some Results of Experimental Cytology") Boveri reviews his own studies of the behaviour of chromosomes in eggs after dispermic fertilization. He refers to a 292-page account published in 1907. He mentions work by his student Baltzer supporting the "Theory of the differential value of chromosomes" (p. 21).

Chapter III ("Application to the Theory of Tumours") begins with discussion of the (possible) specific arrangement of hereditary factors in chromosomes, mentioning Mendel by name but without reference, and not mentioning Morgan at all. Boveri then speculates on "chromosomes which inhibit division" and others which might "promote" division, and how various assortments might cause "benign" and "malignant" features. Then he reasserts his conviction that tumours are formed from "an abnormal chromatin complex, however it arises" (failing

Boveri's ideas were similar to Hansemann's

to mention von Hansemann), but emphasising the possibility that multipolar mitosis might be the cause.

Chapter IV ("The Value of the Theory as an Explanation") discusses nineteen enumerated sections. These sections deal with (1) irreparability of tumourous cellular abnormality, (2) tumour uniformity (which is not always a correct observation) and proposes that the explanation is "because they too go back to common ancestors which also had the same abnormal constitution" (this is a travesty of all the theories of embryological derivation of tumour cells, see chapter 4). Boveri goes on to speculate (3) on the relevance of the metabolism of tumour cells, (4) the number of tumour types which can arise from a particular mother cell, (5) the differences between the tumours of men and animals, (6) multiplicity of tumours in one organ. Subsequent discussion concerns protoplasmic-nuclear interactions, sex chromosomes, (7) inheritance of tumours, (8) tumours composed of more than one type of cell, (9) the formation of metastases, (10) changes in the character of tumours, (11) differences between the cells of different tissues, which he suggests are "caused by certain diversities in the chromatin-complex" and then: "Rather the differences in question must have their cause in that in every tissue, certain parts of the chromosomes grow especially strong, while in other tissue, they fall into the background or disappear entirely". This is similar to von Hansemann's *Hauptplasmen* and *Nebenplasmen* without giving any attribution. In (12), Boveri mentions mechanical factors and chronic irritation as mechanisms of multipolar mitosis, without any evidence that it might ever occur. (13) deals with other aetiological factors, (14 and 15) with parasites, including Fibiger's work (unreferenced), (16) with transplantability, including Bashford's work (unreferenced), (17) organ-related frequencies of tumours, (18) capricious behaviour of malignant tumours, invoking embryological features (not referenced) and (19) increasing incidence with increasing age.

Nowhere does Boveri show that multipolar mitoses can be caused in mammalian cells, or that they are to be found more commonly than other types of asymmetric mitoses in tumours (they aren't – eds).

Chapter V ("Consideration of Some Objections") begins with a summary which includes the following "… it (the theory) maintains no more or less than that a multipolar or asymmetrical mitosis which appears in any cell normal up to that time may, though not necessarily, lead to the formation of a malignant tumour." Then there is an account of further growth of tumour cells "only by regular bipolar mitoses" and the incidence of atypical mitoses in tumours (no references, not Boveri's work, with no reference to Hansemann). Then Boveri discounts amitotic cell division, claiming that pathologists believe in this (which von Hansemann, as a leading pathologist, did not). Then there is further discussion of cytoplasmic-nuclear relationships. Boveri then describes his experiment on mitoses in regenerating corneal epithelium of a rabbit. He makes no mention of comparable studies as early as the 1880s (chapters 3 and 4). The four points of summing up in this chapter deal with amitotic division, not the objections.

Chapter VI ("Conclusions") introduces some observations on hybridizing cells (c f fecundation theories of cancer, chapter 4), but is otherwise a rambling collection of comments which repeat the ideas in the previous chapters.

It is difficult to see Boveri's book as anything but an attempt to argue some relevance of his observations on dispermic sea urchin eggs to mammalian cancer, using von Hansemann's and other pathologists' ideas almost entirely and without giving due credit. That Borst may have influenced Boveri in this has been speculated elsewhere (Bignold et al, 2006b).

Boveri's idea of "quadripolar mitosis" was not applicable to mammalian cells; his work with shaken embryos was flawed, as his biographer (p. 330 of Baltzer 1967) admitted. This should not obscure the fact that Boveri's early work on the role of chromosomes in cellular inheritance was the great contribution to biological science, as has long been recognised.

Hauser; Farmer, Moore and Walker; Bashford

Hauser[6] had published several articles on the pathology of carcinoma of the stomach and large bowel during the 1880s. These were summarised in a book (Hauser, 1890) in which he also illustrated multipolar mitoses in a carcinoma of the rectum and described the process as a "hyperplastic nuclear division".

Only in a later article (Hauser, 1903) did he propose that tumour cells represent a "new race" of cells. In this, he maintained that his views were different to those of von Hansemann. His theory did not include consideration of chromosomes, and the mechanism for the origin of the "new race" was unclear.

Ribbert thought that Hauser's theory was derived from Hansemann's (see Wolff, p. 405). The possible role of chromosomes was given little attention.

Farmer, Murray and Moore were English botanists who presented the idea the carcinomas arise via "fertilisation" of somatic cells by sperm (chapter 4). This was in the form of a short paper in the Proceedings of the Royal Society, London, in which a more detailed publication was promised in the future. Hansemann (1904q) complained that they had ignored his (Hansemann's) contributions to the field of "gametogenic concepts" in cancer. As noted in chapter 4, Bashford[7] initially (1905) supported these authors, but later withdrew this approval (1908). Farmer, Moore and Walker's idea was recorded by Beattie and Dickson (1921) as "unconfirmed and speculative". Their promised "long paper" never appeared.

Bashford (1905) in fact discussed the ideas of Thiersch and Waldeyer, Ribbert, Cohnheim, Farmer and Moore ("gametoid theory") as well as the parasitic theories (see above). Although he referred to von Hansemann's views of the later theories, Bashford did not mention any chromosomal theory in general nor Hansemann's in particular.

Other reviewers 1900–1919

Some attention was given to Hansemann's theory in the years after it was propounded. However, few authors explained in detail what the theory really was. The following summarises comments by various widely-read contemporaneous authors.

Bland-Sutton[8] (1906) mentioned **anaplasia** without noting its author, and then continued:

> "... and it is possible to express this structural alteration in the form of a law: **The degree of anaplasia exhibited by a tumour represents the degree of its malignancy.** This is a scholastic form for expressing a fact long recognised, **that the more a tumour diverges from the type of its matrix the greater the malignancy** (original emphasis)."

There is no mention of chromosomes in this work.

In an article (1907–8) James Ewing[9] discussed three "departments" of cancer research: the parasitic theory, the theory of cell autonomy; as well as the biological and biochemical study of tumours. Under the heading of "cell autonomy" Ewing discussed embryonal theories, the theory of tissue tension (which included a good discussion, of Ribbert) and chronic irritation. Hansemann was mentioned (p. 56 of this article) as the author of the concept of "altruism", but no specific reference to a work of Hansemann was given. Biological studies including transplantation studies and immunity were reviewed, but Hansemann is not further acknowledged. In his "Neoplastic Diseases" (4th edn, 1940) Ewing gave prominence to Cohnheim's theory of cell rests. Ewing may have been influenced in this by Borst and thus contributed to the later loss of interest in Hansemann's ideas (see "Why was Hansemann forgotten? – other factors", below).

In his "Principles of Pathology" (1908, pp 774) Adami[10] failed to distinguish undifferentiation from de-differentiation.

> "Von Hansemann regarded these as evidence of cell change, of the production of generations of cells which through altered distribution of nuclear matter do not so much undergo degeneration proper, but become incapable of attaining perfect structure and function. This modification he has termed **anaplasia**, cell races being formed possessing abnormal properties, one of which is that of increased vegetative activity".

In their popular student text (1921, p. 274) Beattie and Dickson confused anaplasia with embryonic reversion:

> "Now if, for any reason, the reproductive activity (the so-called "embryonic" character) of the cells should be re-established, the condition may be regarded as a reversion to the more primitive type of cell; and it is to this process of reversion, which appears to take place in the formation of neoplasms, that Hansemann has applied the term **anaplasia**, already referred to on (original) p. 260."

Whitman – overlooked insights

Whitman[11] (1919) attempted to discuss a possible Mendelian explanation for von Hansemann's concepts. While the article begins very well, its ending is disappointing. At the start, there is a good summary of von Hansemann's ideas in (1890a, 1891a, 1892a, 1893c, 1906c). There are some errors of detail. For example, the article refers to "hypochromatism due to a reduction in the amount of chromatin in the chromosomes …". Whitman also had difficulty with Hansemann's ideas of differentiation; he used the terms "undifferentiation" and "re-differentiation" rather than "de-differentiation.

However, Hansemann's main points were recognised: "Asymmetry of division which he regarded as analogous to the process by which he believes that differentiation …".

Moreover, Whitman (1919 p. 186) provides a good summary of the anaplastic cell:

> "The anaplastic cell then is one in which, through some unknown agency, a progressive disorganisation of the mitotic process occurs, which in turn results in the production of cells that are **un-differentiated** in the sense that those functions last to be acquired, most highly specialised, and perhaps most dependent for their continued functional efficiency on a continued altruistic relation to the other body cells, are **more** or **less** lost; but re-differentiated in the sense that the cancer cell is not at all an embryonic cell, but a new biological entity, differing from any cell present at any time in normal ontogenesis".

Whitman also makes the very perceptive statement (1919, p. 185):

> "In modern terminology it is, strictly and literally, a mutated cell. Since the process is, or at least may be, repeating itself from time to time, and here and there, in a tumor, it follows that the tumor cells are themselves by no means all alike in their biological properties; that on the contrary, an ever recurring process of mutation is taking place, with a tendency, however, to deviate more and more from the normal type. This explains why metastatic tumors, for example, are often more, but never less, malignant than the primary tumor, as well as other related phenomena of tumor growth".

Effectively Whitman suggests that "genetic instability" is present, and of a type which is not the result, but the cause of the chromosomal lesions of cancer. However, the remainder of the paper fails to consolidate this view. Whitman mentioned three other theories (Hauser's, Butlin's and Oertel's), as variants of Hansemann's, and does not mention Boveri at all. Then, Ribbert's and Ströbe's views are perceptively reviewed.

Then, beginning on p. 191, the work of Morgan and Bridges on mutations and chromosomes (including non-disjunction) of *Drosophila* is discussed. Whitman then argues against anaplasia having a chromosomal basis:

> "I incline strongly to the view that we are on safer ground in insisting, not on the loss of entire groups of chromosomes, and groups of chromosomes which anaplasia is said to produce, but rather upon the profound general disturbance of the mitotic process which is obviously

present, and the abundant opportunity for modification of factors, and the production of new factors, which is thus afforded".

Finally, Whitman discusses whether or not "somatic mutation" can occur. He (p. 197) notes the telling observation by Bridges that a mutation which might be lethal for embryos if it (the mutation) is in the germ line, might not be lethal to a somatic cell if the mutation arises as a somatic mutation. However, one's impression is that Whitman was disinclined, overall, to believe that somatic mutation can occur at all! There is no "general conclusion" to the paper.

This paper is regarded by the present authors as an opportunity missed.

Reviewers in the 1920s and after

Bauer[12] (1928) produced some remarkable insights into the possible role of mutation in a variety of human disorders, including cancer. Bignold et al. (2006a) have provided a translation of the section in this book which summarises these ideas. On Hansemann's idea of the role of abnormal mitoses and chromosomes in tumour formation, however, Bauer seems to have relied on Borst (1902, 1923, see above). He did not consider any of the detailed ideas (scattered as they were) in Hansemann's writings. Bauer was prone to generalisation and analogies, such as comparing the chromosome (of genes) with a battalion (of soldiers).

In his later work, "The Cancer Problem" (1949, 1963) Bauer gave fairly accurate, but still incomplete accounts of Hansemann's views. Bauer also made the statement that it was Boveri, not Hansemann, who contributed the first chromosomal theory of cancer (see Bignold et al, 2006b).

Levine (1931) gave an excellent review of chromosomal abnormalities in cancer and devoted nearly two pages to von Hansemann. Most of the statements concerning Hansemann were correct, but the oogenic concept in the original definition of anaplasia was not recorded. Levine's paper also reported studies of abnormalities of these in various human and animal tumours, as well as in crown gall on various plants. Levine drew several conclusions from this work. Most importantly he concluded that crown gall tissue represents a distinct pathological entity. It is the result of a protective reparative process of the plant against the invasion of the parasite. Cancer is a disease of the cell which manifests itself during cell division. The giant cells appear to play an important role in producing the substances which stimulate cell division. There appears to be no relation between polyploidy and the etiology of cancer. Polyploidy in crown gall tissue represents merely the products of nuclear division without cell division. In human cancer and animal tumors the polyploid mechanism is not altogether clear; it may represent stages in the development of chromatic substance necessary to stimulate cell proliferation.

Other authors have made little contribution to the understanding of Hansemann's ideas. Ludford (1925) mentioned Hansemann only briefly, and gave

Boveri credit for the chromosomal theory of cancer. Later Ludford (1930a) referred his readers to Whitman (1919). Ludford's other papers on chromosomes and the genetics of cancer cells (1930b, 1930c, 1934) mentioned Hansemann only in passing. Nicholson[13] (1933) in parts XI ("Causation: reaction and environment") and XIII ("Somatic development and tumour formation") of his "Studies of tumour formation" mentioned the work of Morgan and of Boveri, without mentioning Hansemann at all. Politzer (1934) catalogued the various opinions of previous German authors (above) and did not offer any new interpretation of Hansemann's views. Lockhart-Mummery[14] (1934) dealt with mutational bases of inherited predispositions to tumours. He mentioned mutation in adult cells, but without using the phrase "somatic mutation". He did not mention chromosomes, von Hansemann or Hansemann's theory at all. Cowdry (1940) reviewed the properties of cancer cells and recognised among these "a decrease in structural differentiation" without mentioning Hansemann's contributions. Willis[15] (1948) mentioned Hansemann by name as an author of a chromosomal theory, but with no further detail. He also strongly criticised mutational theories of cancer, singling out Lockhart-Mummery's theory as unsatisfactory. Oberling (1952) considered only three theories of cancer (chronic irritation, embryonal and parasitic), mentioned Boveri as first among those suggesting a somatic mutational theory of cancer, and did not cite von Hansemann at all. Wright (1954) mentioned anaplasia only in a descriptive passage "… at other times, especially in rapidly-growing tumours, the likeness may be slight or even absent, and the growth is termed an '*anaplastic*' one in consequence." Burdette (1955), in a long review of cancer which generally argued against a mutational basis for the disease, referred directly to some of von Hansemann's publications but missed the oogenic nature of the hypothesis.

> "He (Hansemann) believed that differentiation ordinarily occurs by asymmetrical division of the hereditary units, which he divided into Hauptplasmen and Nebenplasmen, so that successive generations of daughter cells become different in appearance and function. This process of differentiation was called prosoplasia, and the reverse process anaplasia."

In a valuable and detailed review of chromosomes in cancer, Koller (1957) referred to Hansemann's chromosomal theory, emphasising Hansemann's early suggestion that it is the "balance of chromosome numbers" in a cell which is the beginning of the cancerous growth. Koller also noted Boveri as having extended Hansemann's views by emphasising multipolar mitosis as the mechanism by which this begins. Koller (1957) did not address the concept of anaplasia, or the mechanisms of altered functional capacities of tumour cells.

Berenblum (1964) mentioned anaplasia only descriptively (and almost dismissively) as follows. "**Anaplasia** is difficult to define or describe because (*a*) it comprises a number of different qualities that do not necessarily appear together in every case, and (*b*) it represents an attempt to depict histologically what is, in fact, a clinical or functional concept – malignancy. The fact that the term has undergone frequent changes in meaning since it was introduced by Hansemann is irrelevant, since its value is essentially utilitarian: it represents those features which the histopathologist is able to diagnose as malignancy under the microscope."

Triolo (1965) discussed von Hansemann's concept at the end of a section on theories of cancer. Neither the oogenic analysis nor the question of increased capacity for independent existence is mentioned. However, von Hansemann's early association of changes of differentiation with changes of chromosomal numbers is mentioned, but not his later view (in Hansemann 1920a). Considerable space is given to von Hansemann's critics.

Foulds (1969/1975) gave a brief, although accurate account of von Hansemann's later statements on anaplasia, but ignored the earlier oogenic idea. In several long passages of histological analysis of neoplasms this author discussed "differentiation" at length, deciding that it, along with all tumourous phenomena, result from "differential utilization of the genome" (which he also referred to as "epigenetic"). By this, Foulds implied (as had Virchow) an inherently "natural-physiological" basis of tumours. On p. 383 of Foulds (1969) there is the remarkable (although completely inaccurate) analogy:

> "The relationship between embryonic cells and "anaplastic" neoplastic cells is much the same as that between a child and a senile old man in his second childhood; in the one potentialities are undeveloped and in the other, they are gone forever..."

Shimkin (1977) did not list Hansemann in the index of his book, but in the text mentioned Hansemann's contribution to grading of tumours. However, the reference was to Hansemann's 1890 article, in which grading was little mentioned. Elsewhere in his book Shimkin (1977) awarded originality for the idea of the "somatic mutation concept" to Boveri, although Boveri neither used this particular term nor deserved the credit for it (Bignold et al, 2006a, 2006b). Rather (1978) dealt with theories of cancer up to the 1890s and, although mentioning Bard (see chapter 3, Wolff, 1907) did not include theories produced in the 1890s or mention Hansemann. Cremer (1985) did not mention Hansemann, and Epstein (1986), in his chapter 14 entitled "Cancer", mentioned Boveri's (1914) book, but not Hansemann. Sandberg (1990) mentioned Hansemann briefly, but giving Makino (1975) as the reference. Harwood (1993) dealt with genetics and geneticists, but not tumour genetics. Harris (1995) believed that Hansemann's theory was "fundamentally incorrect" without offering any detail or reasons, and stated that Hansemann's opinion was "accepted by no one until it was taken up and developed with great virtuosity almost a quarter of a century later by Boveri (1914)". In a later book Harris (1999) did not mention Hansemann at all. Fitzgerald (2000) mentioned Hansemann only in a short description of "anaplasia". Lima-de-Faria (2003) did not mention Hansemann at all.

Subsequent developments in cancer research

Many of the biological phenomena which Hansemann discussed in relation to anaplasia have since been investigated and are fairly well understood. In particular the problem of endocellular sources to account for excessive growth are now understood in terms of "growth factors/oncogenes" and "tumour suppressor genes".

In relation to "increased capacity for independent existence" some issues are now reasonably clear. Thus Hansemann discussed the fact that normal tissue from one individual can rarely be grown in any tissue of another individual even of the same species (allo- or homograft[16]). On the other hand, tumour cells from one individual had been reported to survive as an allograft by Novinsky in 1875 and Hanau in 1889 (Shimkin, 1977). Progress thereafter was slow, although it was discovered that better "differentiated" tumours grow less readily after transplantation than the least differentiated ones. Loeb[17] (1945) considered that growth rate is the main factor in this, so that "poorly differentiated" cells grow faster; hence they have a better chance of growth.

However, it is now known that a major factor in survival of transplanted tumours is the degree to which the transplanted cell has lost those surface markers which enable the recipient animal to recognise it as foreign and reject it. Thus in the 1950s, it was shown that many tumour cells which are more highly metastatic have reduced expression of blood group antigens on their surfaces. More recently, expression of both "integrins" which control cell adhesion to connective tissue matrix structures, and "cadherins" which regulate cell-to-cell attachments, are reduced in more malignant tumours. Both these findings support a general concept of "immuno-identity-type" differentiation. Nevertheless the alternative possibility; i.e. that "local tissue-specific" growth-controlling circumstances (including interactions with local connective tissue and blood vessels) may play roles in growth of metastases has not been completely excluded. In some senses this implies that the "Cell Theory" in its extreme form of cells acting completely independently, excepting only under the influence of paracrine and endocrine factors is insufficient. It may also imply that cells behave physiologically in tissues as syncytia, perhaps communicating through intercellular gap junctions.

Finally, the problem of the nature of the genomic disturbance which might underlie anaplasia has not been solved. In fact, it has been little addressed. The aetiological characteristics of tumours, and the particular morphological features of "anaplasia" which Hansemann identified have still not been incorporated into any one, well-accepted single unified theory. Also unexplained are (i) the features of delay in appearance of tumour after application of carcinogen, (ii) invariable appearance of hyperchromatic cells (indicating aneuploidy) in many malignant tumour types, (iii) the fact of area-to-area variability of "differentiation" and (iv) the fact that "differentiation" may worsen and never improves.

Why was Hansemann forgotten? – more fruitful fields of research

In any complex scientific subject involving many individual researchers and issues there are usually many causes why good ideas can be lost. First of all, cancer research did not have the same priority in medicine which it has today. A century ago, infectious diseases were the major cause of death in all human populations. Second, it may be remembered that the period 1900–1920 saw the clarification in principle of many aetiological agents of cancer which are known today. Since aetiology is the key to prevention, these studies attracted more interest than investigations of theories of endocellular anomalies, especially because the methods for investigating the latter thoroughly were not yet available (Bignold et al, 2006a and see below).

Among these discoveries was that of the carcinogenic effects of ionizing radiations arising both from high voltage electrical apparatus (Becquerel, 1896) and radioactive isotopes. Initially there had been considerable unprotected handling of these agents by research workers, so that numerous cases of radiation-induced cancers resulted, including those of Marie Curie. With the advent of dosimeters the liability of the individual to tumours was found to be dose-dependent. Measures to limit exposure of individuals to non-therapeutic doses of agent were developed. Subsequently significant exposures to isotopes occurred only irregularly, for example those in the luminous watch-dial painters, who used their mouths to sharpened the points on the paint brushes which carried the thorium-containing luminous paint (Shimkin, 1977). After W. W. II, a second phase of interest in radiation carcinogenesis followed the development of nuclear weapons, and nuclear power for civil purposes.

Since the nineteenth century, chemical mixtures such as tar and paraffin had been recognised as responsible for a small number of tumour types in humans, but the identity of the carcinogenic chemicals in those preparations was unknown. Later in the same century, Hanau showed that arsenic is a carcinogen both in the skin of man and experimental animals. In 1895, aniline dyes were found to cause urinary tract tumours among exposed industrial workers, thus becoming the second pure chemical carcinogen identified as affecting man.

It was only when Hansemann's effective working life was drawing to a close that Yamagiwa and Ichikawa (1918) reported, in a European language, that epidermal tumours can develop in rabbits treated with coal tar. Not until the 1930s was any pure chemical carcinogen isolated from coal. Subsequently, many other chemicals, such as alkylating agents (Bignold, 2006) and nitrosamines, have become recognised chemical carcinogens.

Hansemann had not supported any infective theory of cancer, although such ideas had been in circulation since the seventeenth century. However, in 1911 Peyton Rous provided the first proof for the infectious cause of any tumour. This led to many additional infective agents being identified for various animal tumours, although research techniques for investigating the mechanism of these infectious tumours did not become available until the 1980s. Eventually it was established that the viral genome itself does not contain any carcinogenic gene, but rather that the virus takes up a normal fowl growth gene (cellular oncogene), and transmits it, either unchanged or in a mutant form, to other fowl cells. Thus the latter had the growth gene amplified by increased copy number. This, however, does not reduce the aetiological significance of the virus; hence the importance of such research work remains undiminished.

Why was Hansemann forgotten? – scientific faults of his work

Two of Hansemann's essential ideas were sound:

(i) that the essential quality (*Wesen*) of cancer is a disturbance in the genome of the somatic cell, such that the inheritable material of the cell is abnormal (leading to initial phenotypic abnormalities) and also subject to increasing abnormalities (leading to additional, and more severe phenotypic abnormalities).

(ii) that the resulting changes of phenotype (both chromosomal and cytoplasmic) can occur sometimes after a delay following application of carcinogens, and even then, at varying rates and in different intensities.

However, the ideas were lost. It must be conceded that the major reasons for the disappearance of Hansemann's name and ideas from the more recent literature may lie in the errors and complexity in his original exposition.

The specific scientific errors involving "oogenic de-differentiation" as a prototype of tumour cell biological abnormality; together with the uncertainty as to whether hyperchromatic or hypochromatic cells are tumourous, have been discussed above. Later, however, it was found that experimental tumours could occur without chromosomal lesions being detectable (Koller, 1955). Nevertheless, Hansemann had already anticipated this by suggesting that the chromosomal lesion might be too small to be identified by ordinary microscopic techniques (chapter 5); thus the experimentally-produced lesions may have been mainly "benign". Hansemann never claimed that his theory applied to such lesions. As a related issue, no constant chromosomal lesion could be associated with any particular tumour type. Apparently, the possibility that the nature of "anaplasia" could allow further chromosomal abnormalities (i.e. chromosomal and mitotic – type genetic instability) was not imagined.

More generally, we must address the charge that Hansemann was "too philosophical". In the late nineteenth century, most mechanistically-oriented scientists probably would have found Hansemann guilty of this fault. The most obvious incidence of inappropriate philosophising by Hansemann relates to "altruism", with its apparent roots in "biologistic sociology" (see "Hansemann's Philosophy" chapter 5). History has not been kind to this idea, especially because we now know that quite different cell biological mechanisms control the two different phenomena. Thus keratinisation occurs (we believe) by specific mechanisms of gene control in the epidermal cells, while the secretions of the adrenal cortical cells are controlled by hormones from elsewhere in the body (e.g. adrenocorticotrophic hormone from the pituitary gland). Hansemann down-played "altruism" in his book (1897o), but seems to have retained faith in the idea for many years afterwards (see Hansemann 1912d). Furthermore, it is difficult to understand his resistance to the evidence (provided by Banting and Best in 1902) that the anti-diabetogenic factor of the pancreas is in the Islets of Langerhans other than in terms of an adherence to a philosophical principle in the face of experimentally derived facts.

A milder form of over-philosophising may be identified in Hansemann's concepts of the possible mechanisms by which chromosomal abnormalities might have their effects. In its original exposition, Hansemann's chromosomal model was in the rationalist/mechanist tradition of Descartes – what ever **is** must have a cause, and that cause must **be** physical or chemical. Nevertheless, a semi-philosophical aspect is evident in Hansemann's approach to possible mechanisms by which abnormal chromosomes alter the essential qualities of a cell. Hansemann seems to have followed the approach which Virchow used in developing his (Virchow's) philosophy of "Cellular Pathology". This approach was: observe the cells in the lesions and then identify the "normal" physiological cell process which it most resembles. This was reasonable only in terms of Virchow's belief that cells change their appearances and functions often and easily. Hansemann identified "differentiation" as the "normal process" most likely to be abnormal in cancer cells. However, as shown above, this was soon found to have no basis in tumour cell biology: not then and not now in 2006, despite being used by histopathologists for descriptive purposes.

Hansemann's final tendency which may have contributed to his loss of popularity was that he insisted on considering "uncomfortable facts" of tumour cell morphology and behaviour. Thus the complexity of the histopathology of tumours – for example (i) the variability of cells within individual tumours, and (ii) the lack of consistent correlation between function and clinical aggressiveness – has made simple "germ line-like somatic mutations" unsatisfactory models for mechanisms of carcinogenesis (see Willis 1948, above). Since the 1960s, such a mutational type has been the major "paradigm" of cancer research, and only Loeb's idea of "mutator phenotype" has offered any explanation of increasing morphological and behavioural abnormalities in cells (see Bignold 2003a, 2003b, 2004).

Why was Hansemann forgotten? – other factors

A number of possible external factors may have favoured the forgetting of Hansemann. First is the "revolt against morphology". This aspect of the history of biomedical science has been emphasised by some authors in relation to embryology and genetics (Allen, 1978). However, another broader aspect of the same issue can be seen in the struggle which bacteriology and immunology underwent to obtain satisfactory status as laboratory medical sciences in the face of resistance from anatomical pathologists, especially Virchow. Generally no doubt, while researchers were assured of useful results simply from using microscopes with apochromatic lens in conjunction with new histological stains, more complex forms of laboratory work received less attention. In the late nineteenth century, at the Institute in Berlin, the anatomical pathologists had a well-documented dominance (Rather, 1962). This author discusses some aspects of the dispute concerning bacteriology at the Charité (chapter 3). In addition we note Hansemann's unsympathetic attitudes to bacteriological and immunological studies, particularly his ill-judged attacks on the concept of antibody-mediated immunity (chapter 12).

Yet another issue is the non-Mendelian focus of genetics in Germany after 1918.

German "Genetics" continued to be seen mainly as an issue of embryology, so that the latter questions received most attention. Mendelian genetics (after Boveri and Sutton, see Martins, 1999) was seen as able to answer only a few questions at the level of parent-to-child transmission of characteristics; nothing by way of answers was seen to be offered to the questions of the mechanisms for the controlled cellular changes which characterise both embryological development and normal histological function. The leading German "geneticist" of the period was Richard Goldschmidt[18](1878–1958), whose career initially involved study of embryological questions and only later those of Mendelian genetics.

Discovering mechanisms of embryological development was too difficult for the technology available at the time. Little progress was made. Currently it is considered that the mechanism of both embryological and histological "destined progressions of cell types" is that of cascades of gene activation. Even now, however, little is clearly understood. As a related issue, the relationships of development to evolution were neglected for many years; it is now under reconsideration as "Evo-Devo" (Hossfeld and Olsson, 2003). Nevertheless progress has been slow. Since the number of "genes" (defined as sequences of DNA transcribed into RNA and translated into protein) is smaller than was expected before the results of the human genome project became available, the basic concept of cascades of productions of active proteins may itself require modification.

Mayer (1952) detected a broader "holistic" trend in German pathology after 1900, based on advances in physiological chemistry. These factors may have led to a loss of understanding between the anatomical pathologists on the one hand, and the experimental pathologists and biologists on the other. Such a loss of understanding came to be entrenched in many medical school-hospital complexes when anatomical pathology became a diagnostic specialty of medical practice remote from the "academic" considerations of the nature of disease. Von Hansemann's attempts to include consideration of pathological phenomena in the debate concerning normal physiological processes were ignored.

Anti-Darwinism has been most public and prominent in the U.S.A. In the nineteenth century, the anti-evolutionary concepts of Agaziz (Lurie, 1960) did not help the acceptance of Darwin's theory in that country. In Britain, anti-Darwinism was expressed with greater subtlety, as suggested by Bowler (1983). In Germany since the 1920s, there has been little evidence of concern with Darwinism (as distinct from social Darwinism), so that the poor support for mutational theories of cancer was probably not related to any such considerations.

Could Virchow have contributed in some way to the forgetting of Hansemann? Virchow was obviously a courteous and tolerant man; he published all of Hansemann's important articles in his Archive. In an article of 1892, Virchow pointed out the potential for karyokinetic phenomena to alter pathological concepts, although there was no mention of this in Virchow's article of 1895. Virchow was philosophically inclined like Hansemann, and so probably would not have thought Hansemann unsound for this reason. Virchow was in a position to terminate Hansemann's employment at the institute whenever he wished, but never did. We have not been able to examine any material to suggest the kind of relationship which may have existed between Virchow and Hansemann. Certainly we have been unable to establish any basis for suggesting that Virchow was a negative factor on Hansemann's career.

Could Borst have had some negative role in the later appreciation of Hansemann? Borst was an academic competitor of Hansemann; his views (deriving from Cohnheim) were definitely in opposition to Hansemann's. Both Boveri and Bauer acknowledged Borst as a significant influence on their work. Moreover, Ewing may have been influenced by Borst (see above). In Germany and elsewhere, Boveri's and Bauer's works were more widely read than were Hansemann's. Thus it is possible that Borst's as well as Boveri's and Bauer's assessments of Hansemann's ideas may have been accepted without question.

Finally we ask, was Hansemann's personality a factor in the unpopularity of his views in Germany? There is evidence that he was argumentative, possibly unkind, and occasionally undiplomatic. He also freely published opinions which were contrary to the interests of bacteriology, serology, immunology, endocrinology and experimental tumour researchers. These issues do not seem to have much affected his career or his day-to-day relations with colleagues; he continued to hold positions of responsibility in the medical societies of which he was a member. However, the possibility remains that he was denied Virchow's chair (in 1902) because of his attitudes to bacteriology and other non-anatomical medical laboratory sciences (see above).

In general, however, even if personal factors did increase resistance to his opinions among some scientists in Germany, none of these issues would have influenced the assessments made by cancer workers in other countries of his scientific theories.

What might have been

Speculating on "lost opportunities" in science is of limited utility. However, a few points may be offered.

Hansemann was concerned particularly with chromosomal material, cellular heredity and cancer. At the end of the nineteenth century, Germany had a "scientific establishment" second to none. The German universities were well equipped; with the diligence and intelligence of their academics, they could have carried out the studies of Mendelism, for example, those on *Drosophila*, in a few years. Moreover, experimental X-ray laboratories were established in Germany, so that the work in the 1920s of H. J. Muller in the U.S.A. could probably have been carried out in Germany by 1910.

Furthermore: steps for identifying and enumerating human chromosomes using colchicine (purified in 1820 by Pelletier and Caventon) and metaphase plate preparations were also technically possible at Hansemann's time. Therefore, the correct number of human chromosomes could have been found had there been sufficient impetus to study them. Moreover, there might have been an earlier appreciation of the concept of genomic instability (see Whitman, chapter 5).

Nevertheless the critical step for the advancement of tumour genetics was the discovery of the structure of DNA. This depended on X-ray crystallography, which required high voltage electrical apparatus. Such apparatus was not available before W.W.I. Similarly, the processes of gel electrophoresis involving high voltage electricity applied to solutions for separation of proteins were not possible until the 1950s.

In all of this, it may be remembered that W.W.I caused an unprecedented break in the international scientific community. This applied right across the cultural-scientific spectrum; the waves of hostility in various directions meant that the broken links in both the sciences and the humanities could only be restored with great difficulty. Moreover, what seems in retrospect like a paradise-like era of freedom in Germany – 1919 to 1933 – was in fact problematic and fraught with difficulty. Certainly, the Weimar Republic in Germany saw a unique atmosphere of freedom and a corresponding flourishing of the intellect in many fields (Gay, 1968). But Hansemann had the double misfortune of dying not only at a relatively early age – 62 – but also at the very beginning of this epoch. His work was thus terminated and his reputation left with few if any to defend it.

Notes to chapter 6

1. Moritz Wilhelm Hugo Ribbert (1855–1920) b Hohenlimburg, studied in Bonn, Berlin and Strassburg, MD 1878 in Bonn, Professorial Assistant (*Assistent*) under Koester at Bonn, Dr habile 1880. In 1883 he was appointed *Professor Extraordinarius* in Bonn, and in 1892 was called to the Chair in Zurich. In 1900 he moved to Marburg to succeed Marchant; in 1903 to Göttingen to succeed Orth. In 1905 he returned to Bonn where he completed his professional career. As a person he was said to be "modesty itself", and did all his own technical and secretarial work.
   Wolff (1907) devoted 27 pages to Ribbert's theories; his exchanges with Hansemann are noted in the present text.

   References: Bashford (1905), Wolff (1907), Ribbert (1911), Dhom (2001).

2. Otto Lubarsch (1860–1933) b Berlin, studied in Leipzig, Heidelberg, Jena and Strassburg, State Examination (*Staatsexamen*) and M.D. 1884, Professorial Assistant (*Assistent*) at Giessen under Bostroem 1885. In 1886, he continued at Breslau under Ponfick, 1888 with Virchow in Berlin. After six months at the Zoological Station at Naples under Dorhn, he was from 1889–1891 *Assistent* under Klebs in Zurich. *Dr. habil* 1890, then 1891–1899 at Rostock under Tierfelder (and appointed *Professor Extraordinarius* in 1894). 1899–1904, leader of the Pathological-Anatomical division at the Institute of Hygiene in Posen. Other appointments were Prosector in Zwickau (1905–1907), Director of the Pathological Institute in Düsseldorf (1907–1913). After that he succeeded Heller as *Ordinarius* in Kiel (1913–1917). From 1917 to retirement in 1928 he occupied the Virchow Chair in Berlin.
   He was a prolific writer on pathology, was mainly an encyclopaedist, rather than an original researcher.

   Reference: Dhom (2001).

3. Maximilian Borst (1869–1946) b Würzburg, studied medicine in his home town, MD 1892, *Assistent* at the Pathological Institute under Rindfleisch as lecturer and first assistant at the University of Würzburg. Dr habile 1897. *Professor Extraordinarius* 1903. Called (to Professorial rank) at the Pathological Institute in Düsseldorf in 1904, and in 1905 to Göttingen, 1906 succeeded Rindfleisch at Würzburg. In 1910 he succeeded Bollinger at Munich. In W.W.I, military Prosector and Consultant Pathologist. His major works were "The Theory of Tumours and Microscopic Atlas" (1902, see main text), "Pathological Histology" in 1921, and "General Pathology of Malignant Tumours" in 1924.

   References: Shimkin, 1977; Dhom (2001).

4. Rudolph Beneke (1861–1946) was in Braunschweig (Lower Saxony) when this article was written. Dhom (2001) records only that he succeeded Eberth as *Ordinarius* at Halle in 1911. His father F.W. Beneke (1824–1882) was first *Ordinarius* in Pathology at Marburg; was less involved in microscopic pathological research than the Virchow School; and retained considerable interest in clinical disciplines (Dhom, 2001, p. 338).

5. Theodor Boveri (1862–1915), b Bamberg, studied at the *Realgymnasium* at Nürnberg, and then at the University of Munich and then worked under Richard Hertwig in the Department of Zoology there; appointed *Ordinarius* (Zoology) at Würzburg in 1893, holding that position until his death. Married Marcella O'Grady, an American student in his Department, in 1897. Marcella translated his 1914 book on tumours. Her English version was published in 1929. His scientific work was all within the field of embryology and genetics. His main achievement was recognition of the individuality of the chromosomes (in Cell Studies, 1888, see Baltzer, p. 66). His later work

using shaken embryos of sea urchins was in the vein of Roux' experimental embryology. It was methodologically flawed. Boveri had no medical or pathological training, and acknowledged Borst, Kretz and Schmidt as pathologists who provided "many a valuable suggestion".

Reference: Boveri (1914), Baltzer (1967), Bignold et al (2006a, 2006b).

6   Gustav Hauser (1856–1935) b Nördlingen, studied zoology (Ph D, on olfactory organs of insects), then medicine at Erlangen. He began studies of general pathology and pathological anatomy, with studies in Vienna and Leipzig, under Cohnheim and Leipzig. Appointed Professional Assistant (*Assistent*) at the Pathological Institute at Erlangen under von Zenker. Gained *Dr habil.* in 1883 in Erlangen, became *Professor Extraordinarius* in 1894 and succeeded Zenker as *Ordinarius* in 1895. He was at various times Dean of Medicine and Rector of the University. *Professor Emeritus* 1928.

Reference: Kirch (1937), Dhom (2001).

7   Ernest Francis Bashford (1873–1923). Research into cancer at that time was conducted partly under the auspices of the Imperial Cancer Research Fund in London. Bashford was the Director of Research (1902–1914); initially he supported Farmer and Moore in their idea of the "gametic"-fusion theory of the initiation of cancer. Hansemann noted that in one of their papers, these authors failed to quote his own work (see von Hansemann, 1904q). Hansemann (1906c) was a little sarcastic at the expense of their theory. He noted that, having sent their abstracts to the Lisbon meeting in the same year, they failed to appear.

Reference: Austoker (1988).

8   John Bland-Sutton (1855–1936) was surgeon to and member of the Cancer Investigation Committee of the Middlesex Hospital. He was interested mainly in the clinical manifestations and treatment of tumours. In a chapter entitled "Concerning the cause of cancer" (p290-300) in his book ("Tumours, Innocent and Malignant", 1906) he discussed "Embryologic", "Parasitic" and "Biologic" hypotheses. Bland-Sutton concludes the chapter by quoting from "Empedocles on Etna" (Matthew Arnold, 1833–1908)

> "The gods laugh in their sleeve
> To watch man doubt and fear,
> Who knows not what to believe
> Since he sees nothing clear,
> And dares stamp nothing false where he finds nothing sure."

Reference: Bland-Sutton (1906), Bett (1955).

9   James Ewing (1866–1943) b Pittsburgh, son of a judge, graduated Amherst College and subsequently MD from the College of Physicians and Surgeons New York. He was appointed Professor of Pathology at Cornell in 1899. Co-founded the American Cancer Society in 1913, first edition of "Neoplastic Diseases" published 1919. He described the cancer of bone known as "Ewing's tumour" in 1921, and was the only non-German contributor to the volume in Virchow's Archives marking the centenary of Rudoph Virchow's birth. In the 1920s and 1930s, Ewing was probably the most prominent oncologist in the United States. In 1940, he was named "Mr Cancer" by Time Magazine.

Reference: Virchow's Arch. for the year 1921; Huvos (1998).

10 John George Adami (1862–1926) studied natural science at Cambridge U.K., with post graduate work in Germany under Rudolf Peter Heinrich Heidenhain (1834–1897). He subsequently graduated in Medicine, was a Demonstrator in Pathology at Cambridge, and then from 1892, Professor of Pathology at McGill University, Montreal. In 1919, he was appointed Vice-Chancellor of the

Notes to chapter 6

University of Liverpool and died there in 1926. His text "Principles of Pathology" in its time had one of the best accounts, in English, of German theories of pathology, including neoplasia.

Reference: Anon (1927).

11 R.C. Whitman d 1937 (not to be confused with C.H. Whitman, Director of the Wood's Hole Marine Biological Institute, Maine), Professor of Pathology at the University of Colorado. The staff of the University has been unable to provide us with any further information.

12 Karl Heinrich Bauer (1890–1978) b Schwärzdorf, Upper Franconia, d Heidelberg. Studied medicine at Erlangen and Würzburg, served as a military surgeon 1914–1918; then worked with Aschoff at the Pathological-Anatomical Institute in Freiburg; published studies of osteogenesis imperfecta, haemophilia and ulcus ventriculi. In 1920 he began specialist surgical training at Göttingen under Stich; in 1923 gained *Dr habil*. He was appointed *Professor Extraordinarius* there in 1927; in 1933, he was appointed *Ordinarius* in Breslau, as successor to Küttner. In 1943 he succeeded Kirschner to the chair at Heidelberg. In 1945 Bauer was made first freely elected Dean of Medicine and Rector of the University. He was instrumental in the resuscitation of Heidelberg University after WWII. Retired in 1962 but continued active academic work, especially the foundation of the now-famous cancer research institute in Heidelberg in which he was actively involved until his death. Among many awards he received, in 1960, the Ernst von Bergmann Medal, of the German Society for Surgery.

Reference Schwaiger (1979).

13 Gilbert William de Pouton Nicholson (1878–1949) was Professor of Pathology at Guy's Hospital. These papers were among a total of 20 published between 1922 and 1938. The papers were summarised together as Nicholson (1950).

14 John Percy Lockhart-Mummery (1875 – 1957) was a surgeon at St Mark's Hospital, London. With Dukes he documented the family trees of patients with hereditary polyposis coli.

15 Rupert Allan Willis (1898–1980) originally from Melbourne, later Professor of Pathology at Leeds, was the leading British tumour pathologist of his time. He wrote several books (see Literature Cited under "Willis R.A."). In "Pathology of Tumours" (1948) he asked "what is wrong with the cancer cell" and gave his answer *Ignoramus* ("we do not know", see note[7] chapter 5).

References: Anon (1980), Attwood (1980).

16 "Autografts": from one site of an individual to another site on the same individual, "isografts" are between closely-related (inbred) individuals of the same species. "Allografts" (= "homografts") are between unrelated ("outbred") members of the same species; "heterografts" and "xenografts" are between members of different species.

Reference: Butterworth's Medical Dictionary, 2nd edn, 1978, London.

17 Leo Loeb (1869–1959), b and educated in Germany, worked with Ribbert in Zurich, but migrated to the U.S.A. in 1897. Most of his work concerned the behaviour of transplantable tumours and tumour cells grown in culture, apparently with stromal-tumour cell interactions as the "*raison de chercher*". He was a grandfather of Laurence Loeb, the originator of the "mutator phenotype" theory of cancer (Loeb 1996, 2001; see also Bignold, 2002, 2003b, 2004).

Reference: Loeb (1978), Witkowski (1983).

18 Richard Benedict Goldschmidt (1878–1958) b Frankfurt am Main, d Berkley, CA, began to study medicine in Heidelberg, but transferred to zoology under R. Hertwig in Munich. In 1912, appointed Director of the Department of Animal Genetics in the Kaiser-Wilhelm Institute for Biology in Berlin-Dahlem, but spent the years of W.W.I initially as a neutral and then as an interned alien in the U.S.A. In 1918 he returned to Berlin to further his embryological/genetic

studies, but was forced to leave in 1936. He held many unorthodox views (for which his reputation suffered) concerning the nature of mutation. In some publications he appears to have opposed the "beads-on-a-string" concept of the arrangement of genes on chromosomes.

References: Stern (1969), Harwood (1993).

Part II:

Translations

Chapter 7

On the asymmetrical division of cells in epithelial carcinomata and their biological importance

(Hansemann, 1890a)

Editors' Summary of Points

p. 299 no "cancer specific cell" exists; 300 mitosis generally; 301 mitotic abnormalities in tumour cells; 302 Klebs and Pfitzner on chromatin content of nuclei; 303 chromosomes generally – fertilisation theories; 304–306 Hansemann's first case of laryngeal carcinoma – many abnormalities including multipolar mitoses, hyperchromatic mitoses and chromatic connecting threads mentioned; 307–311 his thirteen cases of carcinomas – mitotic and chromosomal changes – hyper- and hypochromatic cells; 312 analogous appearance of some cells to the polar bodies; 313 histological methods; 314 no asymmetric mitoses in benign tumours (qualified, literature reviewed); 315–316 mechanisms of heredity – "idioplasms" "pangenes" and normal embryonic differentiation; 317 embryonic differentiation and "capacity for independent existence", egg as an example; 318 functions of cells determined by balanced factors for functions; 319 abilities of tissues to substitute for each other in autogenous transplantation experiments; 320 ideas of idioplasms need to be adjusted to accommodate this; 321 change from a somatic (ovarian germinal) epithelial cell to an egg cell is not an ordinary "forward differentiation" but a "backward de-differentiation" – "prosoplasia" and "anaplasia" for these respectively – balance of properties-related factors for this; 322 "differentiation" in embryos is not mechanical – begins summary; 323–325 relationship of all above to cancer.

Ever since initial microscopic examinations of cancer cells were carried out, we have been aware of the varying size and shape of these cells as well as of their nuclei. As early as Johannes Müller (On the finer structures of the pathological tumours) this particular attribute of the cells and their nuclei was demonstrated in characteristic fashion and illustrated in his Fig. 14 in Plate 1 and in Fig. 2 in Plate 2. It was specifically the polymorphic appearance of these structures that gave rise to intense debate, as to whether or not there is a specific cancer cell. It is well known that under Virchow's leadership (cf., also, from this period, Bruch, "Diagnosis of Malignant Tumours", Mainz 1847) this dispute was resolved in the sense that this was not the case, i.e., that it is not possible to deduce from the morphological appearance of a cell whether it comes from a cancerous tumour or not.

Although this agreement was reached, researchers have never ceased applying each newly-emerging method to the study of the morphology of cancer cells, still hoping to find a specific characteristic of these cells. Thus, for example, new staining methods provided fresh opportunities to test the chromatin content of the nuclei and its distribution within them. On the other hand, hitherto, it was precisely the absence of any consistent principle that proved to be the principle of cancer cells. In the same tumour, large and small nuclei were found, some with much, and some with little, chromatin. Some had their chromatin structured in fine

300 threads, others in multiple beads; often there are single large nucleoli in isolation, in other cells several small ones. In some, the nucleoli were absent altogether; in other cells they were so small that they could hardly be detected.

The major discovery of karyokinesis brought new impetus to these investigations, which promised to be all the more successful because here, along with characteristic distribution and ordering of important parts of the cytosol and nucleus, a new diagnostic element was added to mere morphology, namely that of movement. Under Arnold's leadership, a substantial body of literature accumulated on this topic. The first discovery was that tumour cells multiply by mitosis (Arnold, Observations on nuclear division in the cells of tumours. This Archive, vol. 78, p. 279), and it was established (same reference, p. 289), – "It was noted that in the cells of tumours during nuclear division, similar figures form as they do during cell divisions in plants, eggs of animals and in the embryonal development of plants and animal tissues as well as during inflammation and regeneration of epithelial, endothelial and connective tissues, although somewhat less in the latter". Arnold's words which follow on directly are so important that I quote them in full:

"It should be especially emphasised that in the cells of tumours, not just one or another form of nuclear division occurs, but that much more, during our investigations all the major forms were encountered which have so far been documented in different systems by other observers. However, these nuclear division processes are mostly similar to those in plant and animal eggs; so too similarly with those which prevail in the development of embryonal and pathological tissues, albeit, in some respects some minor differences may occur. The scientific finding of the most various types of mitotic figures in tumours generally, and in the various cells of the same tumour in particular, leads me to express doubt as to whether these differences are of any principal importance".

Specifically to investigate this last point further or in other words, to study to what extent these differences might be of principal significance for the formation of cancers, seems

301 to me to have been the aim of quite a few investigations on this point, which were carried out largely under Arnold's own direction. Thereto belongs first of all, proof of multiple divisions (1881) as they had been seen only in isolated cases during normal karyokinesis (W.A. Martin, The knowledge of indirect nuclear division. This Archive, vol. 86, p. 57). However, that this process is not at all so infrequent, in regenerative tissues, in tumour formation and even during lively (*lebhaftem*) growth generally, as one had in the beginning been in-

clined to assume, is proved by many publications of such findings by Martin, Rabl, Hegelmeier, Strassburger, Soltwedel, Mayzel, Waldstein amongst others. As sources of more references in this matter I might point to Martin (reference as above) and Schottländer (On nuclear and cell division processes in the endothelia of the inflamed cornea. Arch. f. mikr. Anat. vol. 31, p. 424). Particularly in this latter paper everything, which was published in regards to this matter by 1888, is carefully assembled. During further investigations, a number of smaller or larger deviations from the "normal" mitosis were found, to which, in each case dependent on the viewpoint of the respective researcher, more, or less importance was attached, so that, at the moment, in respect of karyokinetic processes in tumours, there seems to be a certain perceptible "confusion", which does not imply disagreement between the investigators themselves, but seems to reflect an apparently true jumbled-up (*durcheinander*) state of mitotic processes within the malignant epithelial tumours.

The original aim of the present work was to study these things more closely. Meanwhile, however, two factors have brought about a certain change in this work. The first, with reference to the content, yielded a rather surprising result. The second, in reference to the form of this work, was the appearance of Klebs' "General Pathological Morphology" (vol. 2, 1889, published by G. Fischer), in which a few of my findings were already touched on. For the moment, we do not need to go into all the new thoughts on tumour formation which Klebs sets in motion, but we will only emphasise that in Klebs' work, perhaps for the first time, the different amounts of chromatin were regarded as a particularly important factor for the

biological properties of the cancer cell. Klebs talks about a dwindling of the chromatinic core material, which is documented especially in "incomplete division", and can run independently of one another in the various parts*, to the extent that "not uncommonly we have found very chromatin-rich particles right next to chromatin-poor particles in the very same cell". Prior to Klebs, Pfitzner (this Archive, Volume 103, p. 281) emphasised the different chromatin content of tumour cells and thereby attempted to prove the embryonal character of the cancer cell, but he found the same relative paucity of chromatin in benign tumours as in simple regenerative processes after injuries ("under certain conditions"). Regarding the chromatin content Pfitzner put forwards two propositions: 1) The development of chromatin is a measure of the development stage of the cell. But, he then falls into the error of identifying "developmental stage" and age of the cells as one and the same thing, as his next sentence proves: "If namely we compare the cell nucleus in the same tissue in a young animal with one in a grown-up animal, we find throughout that the younger the animal is, the less chromatin the nucleus contains". 2) "Paucity of chromatin in the nucleus is a hallmark for the embryonal character of a cell". That this, however, is sometimes not correct has already been proved by Flemming (Arch. f. mikr. Anat. vol. 29);

furthermore, that the word EMBRYONAL in this context is completely out of place, I will return to later.

It is not difficult to convince ourselves of the fact that the cells within an epithelial tumour have different amounts of chromatin; the only question is, however; do these chromatin-rich cells arise by growth of their originally-present chromatin, or do they arise by uptake of new chromatin? Klebs believes that it is permissible to assume that at least in some situations the latter is true. But the pressing question arose, does the paucity of chromatin in individual tumour cells arise through a state of inanition, or by a loss of biological units of chromatin[1], i.e. is it a matter of pathological change in a single individual (cell) or of a process which entirely changes the character of a particular cell and its descendants? In these

[1] See further below.
* "of the cell" considered implied (eds).

questions, it is to be noted that the chromatin content of a cell can manifest itself in two ways: firstly, in the thickness and, secondly, in the number of nuclear thread segments. For the varying thickness of the segments (naturally it is always the same phases which are compared with each other) a different nutritional status may perhaps be sufficient, something which, by the way, I should not like to regard as always certain. For a different number of nuclear segments, one must exclude this with certainty. That the amount of chromatin is of supreme importance for the inheritance of specific cell properties and that it is precisely the number of segments to which high biological significance must be attributed, is proved by the constancy of this number in various tissues and kinds of animal. This was proved by the works of Flemming, van Beneden, Rabl, Strassburger, Platner, Boveri, Schewiakoff and others. Klebs (his figures indicate increase of segments) believes that he can attribute increase in chromatin to fertilisation by leukocytes. Virchow, too, on different occasions, has pointed to the possibility of this fertilisation from leukocytes (The nature of diseases and its origins. This Archive, vol. 79). I do not intend to discuss this much further here; but I should like to remark that uptake of leukocytes by epithelial cells alone does not, of itself, provide the proof that we are here dealing with some sort of fertilisation. Since the investigations of O. Hertwig, one has to demand that the association of two living nuclei results in a very specific way before one may speak of a fertilisation. However, there is no further biological necessity to demand, for the increase in segments, a new uptake of vital chromatin substance. Comparative ontogeny, and I should like to say specifically phylogeny, yields enough for such a process. Flemming too, has proved beyond doubt that the doubling of the segments in anaphase in the spermatocytes of salamanders occurs due to longitudinal splitting (Arch. f. Mikr. Anat. vol. 29). Finally, one can doubt whether the nuclei of leukocytes truly contain the vital substance in the sense of a fertilising body. Now, however, concerning the reduction of the

number of segments, it is unthinkable, given the already-mentioned high biological importance appropriate to them, that this change should arise by a simple diminution, almost as unthinkable as it is impossible to make a rat into a mouse through starving.

    Elucidation of these questions was most easily achieved by considering an epithelial cancer, whose nuclei showed the widest possible extremes of chromatin content. For one such sample I have to thank Professor Krause who removed a part of a tumour from the larynx for anatomical diagnosis and sent it to me in alcohol for examination. Despite fixation in alcohol, the mitoses were most splendidly preserved and thus the examination was most particularly straightforward, as I was dealing here with an extraordinarily large-celled cancer. How different form, size and chromatin content of the nuclei were, is shown in Figs 1, 2, 3, 5, 6 and 7, all of which were drawn with the same magnification (Zeiss Apochromatic Immersion 2.0 ocular 8). Most of the nuclei, as in Fig. 7, are not lobulated, whereas others, even little ones, show lots of indentations (Fig. 5), which seem to have a special relationship with their nucleoli, in such as way that almost every small lobe of the nucleus contains at least one nucleolus. In Fig. 2 one sees literally one really giant nucleus. The more sharply–delineated parts reveal the horizontal cuts in the optical plane of individual cell projections. The main mass of the nucleus shimmers through as a dark body.

    Every slide is rife with karyokinetic figures. Most of them correspond completely to the normal type, only that their individual loops cannot be counted properly because of their high number, as is often the case with mitoses of higher order animals. I omitted illustrations of those because I did not believe they would add anything new to what has long been familiar. All phases are encountered, from the very first "ball of tangled threads" shape (*Knäuelform*), through to separated daughter cells. The achromatic figures are in places very clear, but often quite invisible. There were no polar bodies to be seen anywhere.

    Along with the normal mitoses, there is next found a large number of triple and multifold divisions which in like manner agree with familiar forms. Only one deviant form

is to be found. It is depicted in Fig. 12. The loops are somewhat baked together (*zusammengebacken*), the figure however, is in the stage of the daughter stars, perhaps in transition to the daughter chromosome balls (*Tochterknäuel*). The two main stars are joined to each other by finest threads, otherwise nothing is visible of an achromatic figure. On the one star, there is in addition an appendix, which clearly represents another complete star. The figure thus forms a triaster with an irregular position of the third part. We will discuss the presumed emergence of this figure later on.

Then there are found many two-fold divisions which are still connected with a thread of chromatin (see also Schottländer, Flemming and others as above) and also star-like figures in which the chromatin loops are rather short and thick, similar to those which Flemming illustrated (see above, Plate 25, Figs 45 to 47). Lastly, there is a significant number of other individual deviations, which need not be discussed here, but which, however, according to the opinion of others, do not represent anything of pathological significance.

Further there are found numerous hyperchromatic mitoses, which are easily interpreted as early stages of giant nuclei with large nucleoli and masses of chromatin threads and dots. Then, however, one sees on the other hand an abundance of chromatin-poor mitoses, the origin and fates of which remain for the moment obscure. And in point of fact, this paucity of chromatin was not only based in the thinness of the threads and loops, but on their number. One extreme example of such a figure is depicted in Fig. 14. This is a monaster with nine clear loops; a number which will certainly not otherwise be observed in higher animals. The cell measured 18 micron by 16 micron. Thus the question arose, where do such chromatin-poor cells come from, and how do they arise?

During exacting scrutiny of the slides, the cell depicted in Fig. 11 was accidentally noted. Here one sees two groups of loops, one group clearly contains five segments, the other one eight or nine. In the drawing there are eight, as this appeared to be to me most probable. On the other hand, one area in section (at "a") was not entirely clear, so it could also be nine segments. It is to be noted that the loops lay not exactly in one plane as Fig. 11 represents it, but to see them all, the micrometer screw had to be adjusted a little. Between the segments, which point to each other with the open side of their angle and which are of different thicknesses, one can see fine achromatic joining threads. No spindle or pole radiation is to be seen. The interpretation of the mitosis, to my mind, is beyond doubt. The figure is at the beginning of anaphase. That metakinesis has already finished is evidenced by the position of the shafts with the tips pointing away from each other, with open angles turned towards each other. For this reason, a confusion is not possible, and also not with the deviant metaphase of its so-called homotypical form as illustrated by Flemming (above, Figs 38–40) and described in the text. But the number of loops in these two parts is not the same. So thus, we have a process here which clearly contravenes the commonly accepted law of van Beneden, Rabl, Heuser, Roux and others, namely that the chromatic nuclear substance has to be divided with mathematical regularity into two similar halves. As far as I am aware, this is the first definite proof of such an occurrence, with the exception of a finding of Boveri's, to be mentioned later. What remains unclear is whether not all of these segments split or whether the split segments embark on an asymmetrical movement. Neither here, nor in the forms to be described later, was there any reason at all to assume any perishing

(*Untergang*) of individual chromatin loops. All these loops were absolutely intact, stained very well and showed no signs of disintegration[1].

[1] There would still be the possibility that a piece of the cell had been cut off by the microtome knife, something which does happen sometimes. Such cut-through cells are always recognisable as such and never form such a closed-off body as the cells under discussion.

Once I had discovered this cell and convinced myself that this was not an artefact, I began searching for similar figures in other epithelial cancers and other epithelial tumours and hyperplasias and soon discovered a large number of such mitoses, which I will go on to describe in the sequence of mitotic phases.

Thirteen epithelial cancers were examined, the diagnoses of which had been proven absolutely by the microscope, and in some cases also through the clinical outcome. There were five cancers of the vocal cords, one rodent ulcer of the right temple of a 55-year-old man, one cancer of the seborrhoeic skin gland (v. Volkmann), a breast cancer, a cylindrical cell cancer of the descending colon of a 45-year-old man, a lip cancer of a 73-year-old man, a carcinoma of the cheek of a 60-year-old woman, a skin cancer of the nose of a 70-year-old man and one liver metastasis of a cancer of the stomach. In addition, the following were control tissue for comparison: a tuberculous pachyderma verrucosa of the posterior laryngeal wall; a wart of the posterior aspect of the uvula; a naevus pylorus of a 2 year-old child; a wart from the tip of the uvula; two warts from vocal cords and a corneum cutaneum of the nose of a four-year-old girl; a typical skin wart; a leukoplakia of the vocal cord; a similar one in the vicinity of a cancer; and papillary condyloma of the penis. THE FINDINGS COMMUNICATED IN THE FOLLOWING WERE ALL FOUND IN THE 11 (*sic*) MALIGNANT TUMOURS, WHEREAS THE OTHER TUMOURS AND OTHER SKIN CONDITIONS AND HYPERPLASIA DID NOT ALLOW US TO RECOGNISE ANY HINT OF ANY SUCH SIMILAR CONDITIONS.

During the anaphase, there is nothing to be discovered of any, in principle, important irregularity. It seemed to me to be of importance to determine at which time the longitudinal splitting may have happened; given the small size of the objects, however, this could be achieved with any clarity only in a few of the tumours and even then in only a few mitotic figures. The most certain findings on this question were found in the same tumour, from which Fig. 11 originates. Here, I was often able to confirm adjacent chromatin loops with parallel shafts lying closely beside each other, both in the monaster phase as well as

in metakinesis. It is thus certainly possible that a delay in the longitudinal splitting has, in parts, taken place.

An asymmetrical division of the segments naturally becomes visible in the anaphase. Next, I should like to report a case from the early stage of this phase, where the asymmetrical division was clearly evident by counting. The figure is taken from a rodent ulcer and is shown in Fig. 21, meaning that in the style of Fig. 11, the segments appear all in one plane. This figure is of unusual clarity as one can see from the achromatic joining threads and spindles, which made interpretation very easy and virtually ruled out any error. Moreover, fixation had taken place in Flemming's solution and hardening in a most meticulous way in a Schultz' dialysator. The segments differ only a little in thickness, they are arranged in two groups and the open sides of their angles turn towards each other. The one group contains 11 loops and the other 16. Here, again, an odd number in the sum of the segments is striking, which by the way was not entirely clear in Fig. 11, but only probable. Should this prove to be a more frequent or even a regular finding in the presence of asymmetrical mitosis, this would indicate very strongly that we are dealing here with a missing longitudinal splitting of individual segments. This would immediately mean that in the one half, material would be retained that should belong to the other half. Nothing on this point can be concluded from the differing thickness of the loops, because the segments often undergo irregular and uneven shortening and thickening in the anaphase (see also Flemming as above). Thus, for the moment, these two observations do not yet allow any certain pronouncement on the reason for such asymmetrical divisions. Unfortunately I cannot report on any further mitoses in which the data of asymmetry can be given in terms of numbers. Such observations must naturally be placed among the extreme rarities. First of all, one must find mitoses with very few segments; secondly, however these must all be in a very narrowly limited stage of mitosis. For if the

309 anaphase has only progressed a little more, it is no longer possible to count even a low number of segments. As they lie closely alongside each other, then also, under the influence of reagents, (they) will much more easily fuse with each other. Finally, these figures must have a favourable position *vis à vis* the optical plane. The coinciding of these three factors, to which still many chance factors associate themselves, and given that asymmetrical mitoses are already rather rare, means that such mitoses are extremely uncommonly seen.

 The further fates (*Schicksale*) of the asymmetrical karyokineses are, however, so clear from other figures that one can be in no doubt at all as to what one is dealing with once one is aware of it, even if the exact number of the segments can no longer be counted. Such figures are not at all rare. That is to say, one should not expect to find them at every step. Often, discovery of these requires a considerable amount of time and tenacity, but so far I have never missed one in any single epithelial cancer I examined, whereas I have never found one hitherto in benign epithelial tumours or in simple hyperplasias.

 Here perhaps belongs Fig. 12, already described, because it seems to me that one is dealing here with an asymmetrical division into two, in which, in the larger part, a second asymmetrical division has occurred, thus resulting in an asymmetrical tristar. Further, Fig. 8 certainly belongs in this category. It is hard to interpret and it cannot be said how much here is artefact and how much is nature. Only one thing seems to be clear and firm, namely that in a cell which does not yet show any evidence of division, two chromatin figures, each of very different mass (in tangled ball form – *Knäuelform*- eds), are situated.

It should be mentioned further, in order to complete the examples of unclear forms, that Figs 13 and 23 represent diasters whose asymmetry is indeed very slight, but which according to our knowledge of other findings is not to be doubted. On the other hand, I will not attach any particular value to these figures and will not throw a stone at anyone who doubts that they are actually asymmetrical, based on the drawings alone, because in judging

divisions with only a small amount of asymmetry, the thickness of the nuclear figure which cannot be reproduced in the drawing, plays a great part.

It is very different with other figures, however, of which examples will be given here in Figs 10, 15, 16 and 24. Fig. 10 is taken of a young cancer of the right vocal cord of a 48-year-old man. In the surrounding of the cancer there was found ordinary leukoplakia, against which, however, the cancer was clearly demarcated, so that there was only a narrow zone at most of tissue where one could have doubts as to whether one was dealing with cells of the cancer or of the leukoplakia. This specimen, which was obtained by laryngotomy, is of special interest precisely because it allows one to recognise very clearly the contrast between the karyokineses in the area of leukoplakia and those of the cancer. Thus Fig. 10 shows a cell of moderate size ($22:16\,\mu$)*; it contains two daughter stars, one of which is more than twice the size of the other. Both stars are joined by achromatic threads, the peripheral ones being slightly bent outwards. In the larger star a clear spindle can be recognised, which appears to me extraordinarily sharply angled. Fig. 24 is taken from a carcinoma of the lip and follows directly on this figure. The same is in anaphase but progressed a little further than the one in Fig. 10. One notices already in the cytoplasm a slight creasing which allows us to suspect an impending division of the cell into a larger and smaller part. Fig. 15 is taken from an ordinary breast cancer. Here the indentation is well advanced, so far that a small part of the cell is already detaching itself from an approximately four-fold (by surface) larger part. Both parts lay obliquely to the plane of cutting so that the smaller part lay higher than the larger part, so that the connecting stalk, which should still be present at this stage, was covered over. Thus in reality both cells could not be focused in one optical plane. But the evidence for them to be still joined, however, is proved beyond doubt from the clearly visible achromatic joining threads and by the fact that the transverse division of the cytoplasm was complete at high and deep focussing, but at middle focussing was clearly interrupted, as is

* it is unclear whether Hansemann means a ratio or a range (eds).

illustrated in the drawing. The figure is apparently/obviously (*offenbar*) just at the end of the diaster phase, shortly before the dispirem. Fig. 16, finally, comes from a sebaceous gland cancer. The difference in the number of loops in the various other mitoses of this tumour is extraordinary. Fig. 16 itself represents an analogue to Fig. 15, but it is much clearer because both parts lay in the same optical plane.

These individual examples may be enough, seeming to me, as they do, to prove that an asymmetrical karyokinesis occurs, and I believe further that I may be allowed to propose the assertion that the mitoses with a lesser number of segments are derived from those with more segments specifically by asymmetrical division*. In consequence of this, these cells containing** fewer segments must be viewed as the aftermath of the processes described above and must be considered valid proofs of the occurrence of asymmetric divisions, even if these latter are not to be found. In this, however, it is to be noted that here one may consider only the absolutely hypochromatic cells *vis à vis* the hyperchromatic cells and not the relatively hypochromatic cells. In this way one derives three forms, hyper-, normo- and hypo- chromatic cells for which, however, no exact measure can be given at this point, so that the borders between the forms become indistinct and only the extremes can be adduced as proof.

If one now seeks to investigate further what becomes of these things, we have, as I believe to distinguish between the larger part pieces (*Theilstücken*) and smaller part pieces of such cells. If we first deal with the latter, it is indubitable, according to available findings, that cells with a small number of loops are still capable of further division, to be precise, following the usual scheme of karyokinesis with little deviations which do not exceed the extent of the physiological deviations. Thus Fig. 14, already mentioned, demonstrates a monostar with nine loops and Fig. 22 such a one with only eight loops, of which one is slightly displaced (see also Flemming above). In both cells the polar (*polständige*) localisation of the loops is striking. But then, really frequently, figures are found whose interpretation causes considerable difficulty.

*this point, even with what follows in this paragraph, caused confusion among contemporaneous authors – see chapter 4 (eds).
** *enthaltenen* thought to be a misprint for *enthaltenden* (eds)

312   I give examples with 19 loops in Fig. 9 and with 18 loops in Fig. 19 (in both figures the loops have been projected into one plane). Both, with a little trouble, can be recognised as being at the beginning of the metaphase. In such cases there was never anything more to be discovered of achromatic threads. Now, however, thirdly, one finds forms which are entirely uninterpretable and for which Klebs' term "disorder" (*Unordnung*) seems particularly appropriate. As examples I cite Fig. 4a (carcinoma of the larynx), Figs 17 and 18 (cancer of the sebaceous skin gland). Especially the latter two, as far as their position in the sequence (*Reihe*) of mitosis is concerned, are quite incomprehensible, and Fig. 18 is then the example of a further phenomenon, in which the individual chromatin pieces take up the dye only badly, and their borders appeared somewhat blurred, as if they were in

the state of initial dissolution in the cytoplasm which, of course, would mean the ruination (*Untergang*) of the cell. This question, whether one would be entitled to place these three forms into a relationship of interdependency, I do believe one can affirm by reason of the analogy with other observed facts in living cells. I mean the expulsion of polar bodies (*Richtungskörperchen*) from the egg. Certainly, in general, nothing is known here of a numerical difference in the nuclear thread pieces. Only twice did Boveri observe (Jenaische Zeitschrift, vol. 22) that the direction body in the worm *Ascaris megalocephala* contained only one rodlet, whereas the egg contained one extra loop. During the expulsion of the direction body, by a typical karyokinesis, a part – which is very unequal to the egg – is expelled, which either immediately perishes or beforehand divides one or several times mitotically. When in our cells the process of ruination follows on, it is obviously not tied to a specific number of nuclear thread pieces.*

What happens to the larger segments is perhaps more difficult to tell. There is in any case nothing to discourage us from assuming that they re-form themselves into the resting nuclei of the cancer cells proper, whose chromatin content depends essentially on the number of segments. The size of these nuclei is not solely connected with this process,

* whether the "our cells" refers to tumour cells, or human cells in general is not clear (eds).

for one finds small nuclei which contain unequivocally more chromatin than some large nuclei. These cells now may perhaps divide symmetrically for a long time, or also soon again yield asymmetric part pieces. Nothing definite can be said about this.

I wish to comment only briefly on the methods of investigation used. The best results were obtained as usual by fixation in Flemming's solution or sublimate. Individual good successes were also obtained with 100 per cent alcohol which, however, I never applied deliberately. Numerous colleagues, in the most charming manner, sent much material in 100 per cent alcohol, but only 10 per cent of these samples were suitable for the detailed study of the mitotic figures. Therefore, I recommend 100 per cent alcohol usage only if, for external reasons, the more complicated method is not appropriate. The sections were embedded in paraffin according to protocol and after being glued on to the glass slides, were then stained with haematoxylin and eosin or saffron and nigracin. Staining *en bloc* of the pieces beforehand was less successful.

It should be noted again that asymmetrical cell divisions and their probable resulting phenomena were found in 13 epithelial cancers whereas in 11 "benign" tumours and hyperplastic states nothing of this nature was discovered. On the contrary, apart from regular mitoses, only a few triple and multi-divisions were shown. Now, however, I must expressly emphasise that I am not trying to say that asymmetrical mitosis only occurs in epithelial cancers. The material examined is not remotely extensive enough for such a statement and apart from this, there are four reports in the literature, albeit doubtful, concerning asymmetrical divisions in non-cancerous tissue. 1) Mayzel reports in a Festschrift for Hoyer (this document is in Polish and I therefore cite Schottländer) on a quadripartite division in a connective tissue cell of an axolotl larva which, while he observed it directly, was carried through into four in such a fashion, that from the one cell, three small connected cells were formed with tiny nuclei, together with one large cell with a large nucleus. 2) Rabl (Morph. Jahrb. vol. 10. 1884) observed in a kidney epithelial cell of *Proteus,* two daughter stars of unequal size, one approximately half the size of the other. He interpreted this to mean that originally three poles existed, two of which had joined together. 3) There is a figure of Schottländer's (see above, Fig. 12) which I find suspicious. The figure clearly shows an asymmetrical division but nothing is said about this in the text, so it is not obvious from this whether perhaps some loops were still situated under the plane of optics and are not depicted in the drawing 4) Fig. 50, p. 528, in Klebs' book, points to similar processes with the corresponding explanations and text which I have already cited above. The figure is meant to depict a papilloma of the bulbar conjunctiva, very likely the same that he has mentioned in Fortschritten der Medicin (1888, p. 906, "On the formation of nuclear chromatin"), the malignancy of which, however, as Klebs says himself, cannot be excluded without doubt. Although these four findings described above may be interpreted in different ways, they do not yet provide the negative proof for the exclusive occurrence of asymmetrical mitoses in cancers. However, one can probably maintain that no epithelial cancer occurs without asymmetrical mitoses. And I believe that I can support this assertion: firstly, through my own findings described above; secondly, through the data of Pfitzner and Klebs concerning the different number of nuclear thread pieces and cancers; thirdly, by the different shape and size of the nuclei in cancer cells which have always been a generally-recognised and much emphasised characteristic feature of tumours and, as I believe that I have shown now, have their origin in asymmetrical division.

In the general law of the symmetry of karyokinesis, an exception to this law must be given greater weight especially when it is repeatedly found in a particular class of pathological structures, this being cancers of the epithelia. In addition, there is the significance which in recent times has been attached by all researchers to the number of nuclear thread segments for the biological attributes of the cell. Asymmetrical division seems to be

particularly critical from the point of view of panmerism which means, as is well known, that certain biological properties of a cell are intrinsically linked to definite formed elements of the cell. These formed elements consist of more than one molecule, and by growth and division, pass on from mother cell to daughter cell. Whether now one collects all these properties together, and with Nägeli ("Mechanical-physiological Theory of Heredity". Munich and Leipzig 1884) and Weismann (On Inheritance, Jena 1883 and "The Continuity of Germinal Plasma as the Basis of a Theory of Inheritance". Jena 1885 and so on) calls them "idioplasmata", or whether, with Hugo de Vries ("Intracellular Pangenesis", Jena 1889) one identifies them individually as "pangenes", I still believe that I must maintain that the parts characterising the cell, even if mainly from the nucleus, are not exclusively – as many would like to maintain – in the chromatic substance of the nucleus, but are also to be sought in the cytoplasm. The facts which speak for this have been recently assembled by H. de Vries (as quoted above) and he, as a botanist, draws his examples mainly from plant biology. I believe there are sufficient analogous examples from cell theory of the animal kingdom. Unfortunately I must refrain from going into the details of these interesting studies and should just like to mention in advance that the following considerations are all built up on the basic idea of Panmerism in the sense already indicated.

From this standpoint, one will find numerous asymmetrical cell divisions in each embryogenesis, in the sense that the daughter cells are not equal to each other in value, and taken together represent up to the potential worth of the mother cell. The qualitatively unequal cell division alternates in ontogenetic development with qualitatively equal ones, so that, in tracing out cell pedigrees, one can identify certain steps or "generational stages". It is not difficult to find examples for this in the field of comparative embryology. Already the first cleavage of the egg is in many cases a qualitatively uneven one. A classic example of this

process is the paper of Weismann (Contributions to anatomy and embryology, Festschrift for Henle, Bonn 1882, p. 80) on the development of *Rhodites Rosea*. One divided piece of the first nucleus migrates to the posterior and the other one to the anterior pole of the egg. The posterior one divides first, forming the "blastoderm". Only then does the anterior one divide and there arise the so-called inner germ cells which form the wall of the mid gut and then also move into the mesoblast.

Similar communications are given by Grabben (Arch. f. Mikr. Anat. vol. 14) and Dohrn (Zeitschrift f. wissensch. Zool. vol. 26). In other cases, on the other hand, the very first division of the egg signifies no qualitative- but a quantitatively different division, in the sense that the "first plane of division of the egg represents already the median plane for the future embryo, so that it divides the material of the right body half from that of the left body half" (Roux). This was found by Roux (this Archive, vol. 114) and by Pflüger (On the influence of gravity on the division of cells. Arch. f. d. ges. Physiologie vol. 31, 1883) for the frog egg; van Beneden and Ch. Julin (Segmentation in the *Ascidia* and their relationships to the organisation of the larvae. Arch. de Biologie 5. 1884) for the *Ascidia;* Kowalewsky (Zeitschrift f. wissensch. Zool. 1886) for *Carassius auratus* (bony fish). In many other cases the same things may occur, and the qualitative work division must only begin later. Only the cells of the *Homoplastidia* (described by Götte) would, during the entire development stage, proceed solely by quantitative work division.

If we could monitor these processes during the entire period of ontogenesis right into their details, then we would have reached the ideal as Virchow in his "Cellular Pathology" (p. 82, 4th edition) says: "A more detailed knowledge of the pedigrees of tissues will solve many a still-remaining riddle." But we are far distant from this in the case of the highly differentiated tissues*. For plants, already since Mohl's time, we have begun with this, and for many plants, the pedigrees are virtually complete (for example, for *Equisetum*. K. Goebel, "Basic features of Systematics and of Special Plant Morphology" 1882, pp 286-304). Weismann has begun to lay the ground work, especially for the germ lines of some animals

* here von Hansemann uses differentiation in relation to comparative studies: i.e. the phylogenetic meaning, chapter 3 (eds).

(Concerning the question of the immortality of uni-cellular organisms. Biol. Centralbl. vol. 4, nos 21 and 22; "The origin of sexual cells in the Hydro-medusae". Jena, 1883, and elsewhere). In higher order animals it is granted to us to begin only at single points in the cell pedigrees and to have the ability only to follow them through for a short while. From these studies, two pivotal statements can be derived:

1) WITH EVERY FURTHER QUALITATIVE WORK DIVISION, THE CELLS LOSE THE CAPABILITY TO EXIST AUTONOMOUSLY.

2) WITH EVERY NEW GENERATIONAL PHASE A CHANGED GROWTH ENERGY ["NUTRITIONAL, FORMATIVE, AND FUNCTIONAL ACTIVITY" (VIRCHOW)] TAKES PLACE WHICH OFTEN MANIFESTS ITSELF IN A CHANGE IN DIRECTION OF GROWTH.

Concerning 1) The least differentiated cell is the mature egg cell. It contains potentially the sum of all cellular properties of the future body. In contrast, the cell also possesses the largest degree of autonomy because it detaches itself from the body of the mother animal in order to embark on long wanderings, and finally, with or without fertilisation, to form the basis for a new individual. This property of the autonomy of the egg cell is so prominent that it caused Rolph ("Biological Problems", Leipzig 1884) to attribute equal importance to the egg cell compared to the whole of the rest of the body in the sense that there is a generational change between the sexually differentiated egg cell and the sexually not differentiated multicellular parent organism (pseudosexual main generation)*. If the mature egg cell divides and if the part products of division are of unequal measure, then a certain altruism arises between both daughter cells, that is to say, one cell takes on a sum (*Summe*) of the kinds of functions of the now two-celled individual, and its activity is also of benefit to the other cell which has taken over the rest of the functions, and thus for its existence has become dependent on the other and vice versa. In other words, one of these daughter cells cannot exist without the other. The same takes place at each further generational stage, only that now, by divisions which are often of equal value, single cells are substituted by large groups of cells.

* this refers to asexual versus sexual proliferation in fungi etc (eds).

Hereto, the same altruism exists between different groups of cells; for example, protective epithelia, secretory cells and phagocytes (*Resorptionszellen*) and so on. If only one of these kinds of tissues is removed, then the sum of everything else goes to ruin. Also the findings by Roux (as noted above), that one cleavage sphere of the frog egg develops into a hemi-embryo, if one destroys the other sphere, speak completely in favour of these views even if they also present a negative proof, because the same researcher has shown that the first division of the egg in frogs is a qualitatively equal one, and thus not compromising the autonomy of each half.

The division of functions between two unequal sister cells is, on the other hand, certainly not so complete as, according to all this, one would have to assume, and has also in fact been maintained by some researchers. For example, let us imagine a cell which essentially has two functions which, however, maintain balance and as a result of this are latent. Such a cell, for example an embryonal epidermal cell from which glands later develop, could be represented by the following scheme: _ _ _ _ _ _ _ _ . . . . The dashes should represent the later epidermal properties, the dots, the gland-cell properties. Then, in further differentiation, the division cannot possibly proceed in such a way that the two daughter cells would look as follows: one, _ _ _ _ _ _ and one, ... If that were the case it would be inexplicable how superficial epithelium could be developed from glands, eg, as found in the puerperal uterus (see also Friedländer "Physiological and anatomical investigations of the uterus" Arch. f. Gyn. vol. 9, p. 22). Probably here too belongs Heiberg's attempt, (Centralbl. f. d. med. Wiss. 1872, No 12) who, by transplanting a piece of tissue from the wall of an atheroma* cyst, that is to say derivatives of glandular cells, created normal epidermis on a wound. (Heiberg himself on the other hand interpreted his own experiment in the opposite sense, concluding that atheromata must have been generated by invaginated epidermis). This substitution of related tissues seems, however, to take place only when the common ancestral cell lies only a few generational stages back. For example, it is not possible to substitute cells of the ectoderm by enterodermal cells and vice versa. The

* thought to mean the lesion known as "epidermoid" or "epidermal" or "sebaceous" cyst (eds)

surgeons know the persistence capability of the epidermis and not infrequently it causes them difficulties, for example, for the plastic covering of large defects in the urinary bladder. It is well known that keratinisations in gut lining cells are not rare, particularly pachydermia of the larynx has recently often been an object of research. Similar situations have been described concerning the bronchi of the stomach* of low order mammals, the renal pelvis, the uterus, etc (see also the recently published work of Posner in this Archive, vol. 118, p. 391). I retain a preparation of a congenital everted Meckel's diverticulum, the outer epithelial layers of which, although not exactly keratinised, are nonetheless multilayered and flattened in the upper part. However, all these examples, to my mind, do not seem to prove that these tissues have become external epidermis with identical properties to skin, but only that the cells of the gut gland lining and so on, given certain circumstances, have the ability to keratinise. There are reports alleging that even frog skin transplanted on to human wounds has led to the healing of those wounds (Baratoux and Dubousquet-Labordie, Animal grafting with the skin of the frog in losses of cutaneous and mucous substance. *Progrès med.* 1887, No 15). The same is reported of transplantations of small pieces of cornea taken from rabbits into human beings (Chisolm, Maryland Medical Journal, 1888, June 30, and New York Medical Records XXXV, 1. Jan. 1889. Also, Williams, St. Louis Medical and Surgical Journal, vol. XXXV). Here there can be no further question at all of a real substitution, but only a certain stimulation of neighbouring tissues to elicit renewed growth activity caused by those transplanted pieces. The significance of those transplantation experiments in regard to these questions has already been elaborated by Virchow (this Archive, vol. 79). Even in lower animals such a substitution of endoderm by ectoderm and vice versa is not possible as Nussbaum has proven (second essay on the divisibility of living material, Arch. f. mikrosk. Anat. vol. 29). Thus the opinion of O. Hertwig (Development of the Mesoblast (*mittleren Keimblattes*), Jenaer Zeitschr. 1883) that "the protoplasma of a cell conceals within itself various capabilities in order to be able to differentiate in this or that direction; and it

* "bronchi of the stomach" probably means the "pits" of the gastric mucosa through which the secretions of the glands-proper of the mucosa empty (eds).

depends only on the specific demands which are made of the cells occupying a specific position in the body, so that they develop this or that property in a special way, and thus can function better according to the object in each case" – is only correct under certain conditions, that is to say, only for closely related cell types, but not, however, for those whose common ancestor cell lies many generational stages back, or perhaps is only to be sought in the egg.

Kölliker (Zeitschrift f. wissensch. Zool. vol. 40, 1884) and Fol (Rev. med. de la Suisse romande, 1884) as well as Haeckel (Jena Scientific Journal 1884) are of the same opinion, up to a point, as Hertwig. Thus, I have come to the conclusion that the division of idioplasmas is never a completely pure one, so that in every cell main and subsidiary plasmas are present, of which the main plasmata form the actual idioplasma of the cell, whereas, on further differentiation, the lesser plasmata disappear more and more and, finally, are no longer noticeable at all.* However, there seems to be evidence that even these last unsuspected remains of lesser plasmata can achieve a certain mastery under special opportunistic circumstances. The interesting experiments of M. W. Beyrink show that under the influence of cells, the *Poa nemoralis* can develop roots at a place where this normally never happens ("The gall of the *Cecidomyia Poa*". Botan. Zeitung, 1885, no. 2) and causes roots to grow forth from the actual galls of *Salix purpura*, which were totally identical with young roots of the same species of willow (On the cecidium of *Nematus Capreae*. Botan. Zeitung, 1888, no. 1). Here we seem to be dealing with the re-emergence of germinal plasma in an otherwise purely somatic (*somatischen*) cell line.

To come back to our initial scheme, a division of this embryonal epithelial cell could look like this: _ _ _ _ _ . and so _ _ _ _ . .

So far we have only been talking about a steadily increasing rate of differentiation with asymmetrical division. This assumption, however, is only applicable to the so-called

* This presages the "obligatory-" and "facultative-" genomes of Foulds (1968; 1975) and the "specialisation" genes of current cell biological terminology.

maximally undifferentiated cell, the unfertilised mature egg. Thus, at some stage there has to be a dedifferentiating process as opposed to differentiating ones, because it is beyond doubt that at certain times, the immature egg cell represents a fully characterised somatic epithelial cell. [Were one to give names to these processes, the differentiating and the dedifferentiating one, then "prosoplasia" (from $\pi\rho\delta\sigma\omega$ forward) should be chosen for one and "anaplasia" (ν "backwards") for the other]. Whether this is the significance of the first polar body as Weismann claims (On the number of polar bodies. Jena 1887* and earlier papers by the same author cited there) or whether this happens beforehand, in some way or other, in any case I cannot see how this process can be interpreted in any other way than in the sense of the expulsion of all parts bringing about the overweighting of individual plasmas, so that those remaining behind maintain their balance once more. If thus I may use a simplified scheme again, where the germinal cell, as long as it is still a somatic cell, may be depicted with _ _ _ _ _ . ., then, following completed maturity, it should assume _ _ _ _ ., meaning that _ _ have to vanish from it. One can see that my theory is very much similar to Weismann's views, and I would only like for the moment to leave indefinite whether in this process, it really is the first polar body or the latter** alone that is responsible.

Concerning 2) When I said, "with each new generational phase there is a different energy of growth which manifests itself in a change of direction of growth", one has to explain that this has often been interpreted exactly the other way round in the sense that mechanical circumstances change the direction of growth and, therefore, cells would assume a new meaning. This may actually happen in several instances, for example, when the originally cubical epithelial cells of the Malpighian body of the kidney develop into the covering epithelial cells of the fully-grown glomeruli and their capsules. This has on occasions led people to call them endothelia because of their flat nature.

* English translation on pp 337–384 of Weismann (1889) (eds).
** meaning the loss of excess chromosomes before the expulsion of the first polar body (see previous sentence) (eds).

If, however, Hertwig states recently in his textbook (pp 59 and 60), concerning glands and the central nervous system that these only arise by the formation of folds, then it seems questionable to me that he will be able to maintain this for long, especially in the light of him recognising differentiation (sharing of work) as a second fundamental principle of development (p. 63). Specifically, in the two processes that Hertwig describes as examples, the invagination of the folds occurs in the direction of higher resistance, and is thus, for the moment, not mechanically explicable, something which has already been pointed out by Boll ("The Principle of Growth", Berlin, 1876). One must therefore ascribe to the relevant cells [which, by the way, are usually very well-differentiated morphologically before invagination, as, for example, the animal stage of the vegetative organism before the formation of the gastrula of Amphioxus (Hatschek, Studies of the development of *Amphioxus*, Arb. aus d. Zool. Instit. zu Wien u. Trieste. vol. 4, 1881), or also, specifically, the cells of the medullary plate], already before their invagination, their ability to effect precisely this invagination, i.e. the differentiation precedes the change in direction of growth.

I am very conscious of the fact that in the above deliberations I have dealt with a very broad and complex topic only in rough outline, and very incompletely. A detailed working over of the matter would require space far exceeding the framework of a mere essay. Touching on this theme may, however, be excused by the fact that in so far as I wished to draw conclusions from my findings of epithelial cancers, I had to take up a position with respect to a number of biological questions.

If, now, from the standpoint of these biological questions, we summarise the results gained from observation of asymmetrical karyokinesis in epithelial cancers, we have the following results:

In cancers one finds alongside the usual asymmetrical* mitoses such which lead, immediately or only after a few divisions, to cells with extraordinary few nuclear thread

* it is unclear whether Hansemann meant "symmetrical" here (eds)

pieces. These asymmetrical divisions do not follow any rules as far as the number of segments is concerned, that is to say, in this process, in one and the same tumour, cells containing different numbers of loops are split off. This leads to an ever self-repeating metaplasia of the tissue. It may well be that this occasionally represents a so-called prosoplasia (which can neither be proven nor disproven). It is likely that in most cases we are dealing with an anaplasia because one result of cancer formation is epithelial cells with an heightened degree of autonomy compared to their mother tissue. Those cells can often develop in the body far away from the site of origin and lead there to ancestral cells of a new tumour of exactly the same kind. This can even happen if cancer cells from one animal are implanted into another. This fact, the possibility of which was doubted for a long time because the corresponding experiments (see Virchow's "Tumours", vol. 1, p. 87; further Novinsky Centralbl. d. Med. Wiss. 1876; and Ware, Deutscher Chirurgencongress 1888 and 1889) were not quite perfect, has recently been placed completely beyond doubt by Hanau's success in rats (Fortschr. d. Med. No 9, 1889). Nothing similar has ever been observed of a normal epithelial cell. For all such experiments have hitherto led to the result that normal epithelial cells, placed in a foreign location, will perhaps grow for a little while, but will soon after be reabsorbed (compare Kaufmann, On the Eukatarraphie of epithelial cells. Dissertation. Bonn 1884 – Zahn, Congrès period Internat. Geneva, 1887 – von Dooremal, Arch. d. Ophthalmol. vol. 19, p. 359 – Schweninger, Centralbl. f. d. med. Wiss. 1881, no. 10 and Goldzieher, Arch. f. exp. Path. II, p. 387 and many others, in particular, Klebs on Embolisms of the liver cells in his book in 1889, p. 120).

Each asymmetrical division of the cell means a change in its differentiation; it is thus to be placed in parallel with a new stage of ontogenetic development. According to this, the asymmetrical division must in every case be associated with a change in growth energy and growth direction.

In epithelial cancers one has to distinguish two different types of cell which can hitherto only be recognised by the type of their karyokinesis: firstly, those with consistently lesser numbers of segments which either immediately or after a few more divisions, but in

any case soon, die a physiological cell death. Secondly, there are those which divide symmetrically and somewhat regularly and thus contribute to the enlargement and spread of the tumour. The latter are the real tumour cells, the former might just be waste products. The main cells can keratinise and perhaps also undergo fatty metamorphosis, and then die a physiological death sooner or later, like the epithelial cells from which they originally developed (epidermis, sebaceous glands, milk glands). A large number of these tumour cells, as is well known, do not perish in a physiological way, but in contrast, in the pathological way.

I have called many cells, perhaps all major cells of epithelial cancers, "anaplastic", i.e. they have passed from a higher state of differentiation to a lesser one. The question now is: is one justified, as happens on many sides, in calling these cells embryonal? Here, I do not wish to adduce all the reasons which have been advanced against this with complete justification. Only a few refutations of this terminology should be mentioned here. Embryonal epithelial cells are those which have not reached the highest possible degree of differentiation, in which, however, the capacity lies to reach this degree of differentiation. Specifically this latter ability is extraordinarily constant in all embryonal cells, and they do not abandon it even in relatively unfavourable circumstances. For example, if one implants in the anterior chamber of the eye of a rabbit a tiny piece of skin of a rabbit embryo just before the hairs have developed, from day 14 to 18 of embryonal development, this piece of skin will heal without problems but the epidermis keeps developing and forming hair follicles which can be clearly seen with a magnifying glass through the cornea. This development of hairs is only a little retarded, despite this great change in circumstances and can be seen with the naked eye in 14- to 18-day embryos, about 11 to 15 days after the

operation. I have carried out such experiments several times with constant results. Once the circumstances were still more unfavourable. Five days after the operation, the iris prolapsed, through which the already fixated fragment managed to get out. Even despite a heavily purulent conjunctivitis which developed afterwards, 16 days after the operation the greatly enlarged skin fragment was covered by long hairs. After the pieces of skin have grown for a while, the hairs fall out and the whole tissue is resorbed. Based on this I believe it is rather unlikely, after such successes, that any piece of epithelium which is not "differentiated out" (un-*aus*-differentiated) can persist anywhere in the body*. Thus, as far as anaplastic cells are concerned, they must not be confused with embryonal ones, in fact, there is a clear contrast between the two and the embryonal cells begin where the anaplasia ends, with the egg.

* "persist" here seems to mean "persist in an embryonal state". Such an opinion would be in opposition to Cohnheim's theory of "cell rests" (see chapter 4 – eds).

Plate

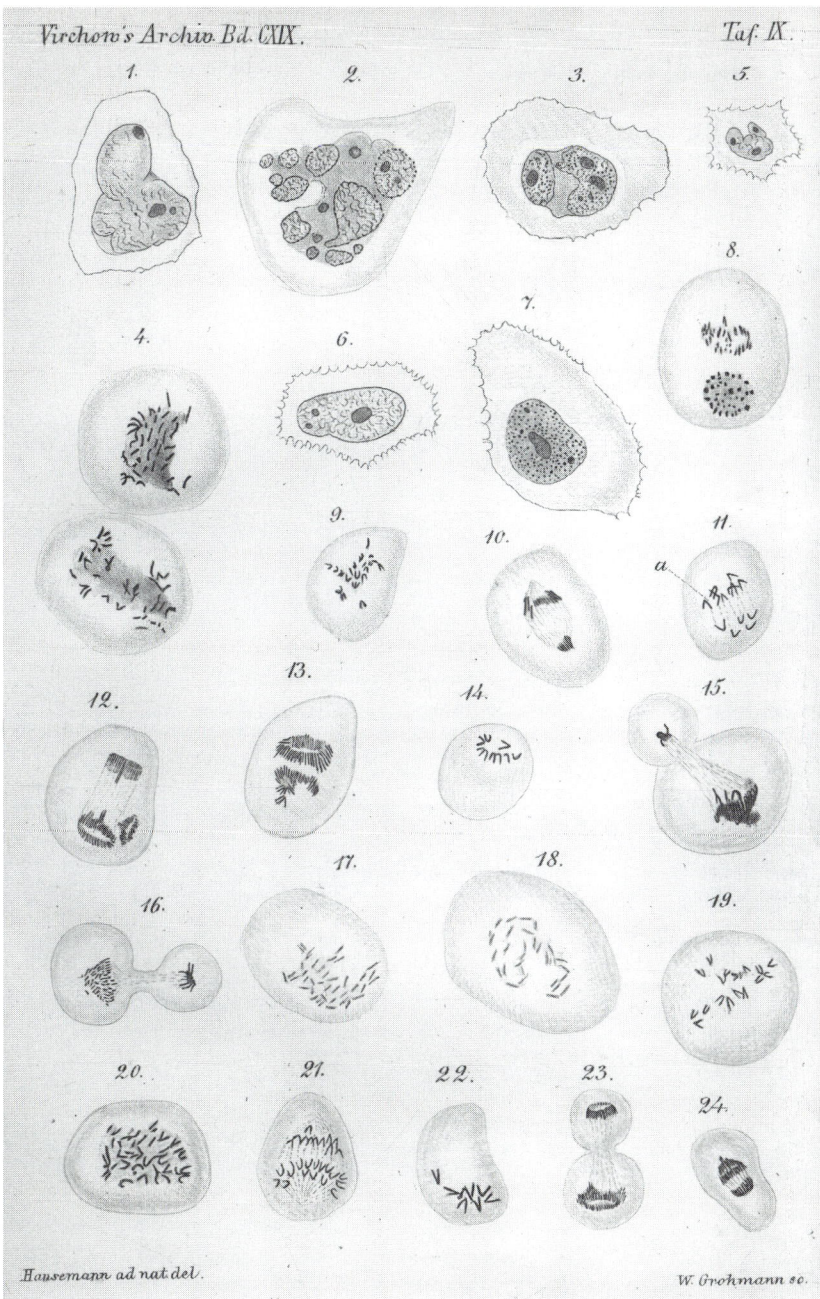

Plate IX

Explanations of the diagrams: plate IX

All figures are drawn with Zeiss apochromatic 2,0 oil immersion. Ocular 8. Only Fig. 16. with Ocular 4.

In Figs 9, 11, 14, 18, 19, 21, and 22 the thread pieces are laid in plane; in the remainder, the thread pieces of other planes appear as a diffuse shadow, as they are in reality seen through. As a general principle, the figures are presented in the most realistic way possible.

Figs 1, 2, 3, 5, 6, 7, resting cells from a cancer of the larynx.

Fig. 4. Two cells lying alongside each other with different numbers of loops from another throat cancer. a. scattered thread pieces and loops; the stage cannot be interpreted. b. somewhat unordered monaster in transition to metaphase.

Fig. 8. Asymmetric diaster from the cancer in Fig. 1

Fig. 9. Hypochromatic cell from the cancer of Fig. 4.

Fig. 10. Asymmetric diaster from the same tumour.

Fig. 11. Asymmetric diaster from the beginning of anaphase with countable loops from the cancer in Fig. 1.

Fig. 12. Asymmetric diaster from the cancer in Fig. 1.

Fig. 13. Probably asymmetric diaster from the cancer in Fig. 1.

Fig. 14. Hypochromatic cell from the cancer of Fig. 1.

Fig. 15. Asymmetric dispirem from a carcinoma of the breast.

Fig. 16. Asymmetric dispirem from a skin cancer.

Fig. 17. Unclear monaster (?) hypochromatic cell from the same cancer.

Fig. 18. Hypochromatic cell with disorder in the thread pieces and initial dissolution (?) of the same, from the same cancer.

Fig. 19. Hypochromatic cell, monaster, from the same cancer.

Fig. 20. Somewhat disordered monaster from the same cancer, normal chromatin content or hyperchromatic.

Fig. 21. Beginning of the anaphase, with countable loops from a rodent ulcer.

Fig. 22. Hypochromatic monaster from the same rodent ulcer.

Fig. 23. Asymmetric diaster from a carcinoma of the sigmoid colon.

Fig. 24. Asymmetric diaster, earlier stage than in Fig. 23, from a cancer of the lip.

Detailed descriptions are to be found in the text.

Chapter 8

On pathological mitoses

(Hansemann, 1891a)

Editors' Summary of Points

p. 356 methods, significance of early fixation – disagrees with Ribbert on this point, uses sublimate; 357- more on methods; 358 mentions Klebs' work as supporting his own – mentions Hauser disparagingly; 359 reports studies of mitoses in more cases – finds none in sarcomas or non-tumourous conditions- discusses hypochromatic, normochromatic and hyperchromatic cells in detail; 360 these terms refer to the number of chromosomes per nucleus – difficulty of counting human chromosomes; 361 continues discussion of nuclear chromaticity; 362 abortive forms in hypochromatic cells – loss of individual chromosomes from the spindle as a mechanism of altered chromatin numbers; 363 normochromatic nuclei can also show many pathological deviations – shortness and thickness of chromosomes – not in normal human organs – delay in longitudinal splitting of chromosomes; 364 "chromatic connecting threads" (now understood as chromosomal stickiness – eds) – polar bodies not seen in normal humans but are seen in human tumours – division of the cell body occuring too late after division of the cell nucleus being a cause of binucleate cells; 365 spindles and their fibres – resistance of these to destruction; 366 cells with two or more nuclei in division – pluripolar mitoses; 367 pluripolar mitoses are pathological forms – hyperchromatic cells in sarcomas; 368 Schottländer's account of pluripolar mitoses – hyperchromatic cells show most aborted forms; 369 clumpings of chromatin – variable chromaticity of nuclei may be a diagnostic feature of malignancy.

In February 1890 I reported in Virchow's Archive on a pathological form of mitosis, which until then I had only had the opportunity to see in carcinomata. This phenomenon has been reported on several occasions since and I personally have observed more of such pathological mitoses in cancers as well as in numerous other normal and pathological human tissues. Thus I was able to form a certain conclusive judgment on their significance.

Most of the tissue material was given to me courtesy of Prof Küster, currently Director of the Augusta Hospital and by *Geheimrat* von Bergmann and many other dear colleagues, to all of whom I am grateful for the friendly donation of fresh material to me. I might explain at this stage that it is necessary to have the best tissue preparations in order to study pathological mitosis, meaning those which have been transferred straight from the living body into fixation fluid warmed to body temperature. Incidentally, on this matter I do not quite agree with Ribbert (Centralblatt für Pathol. Anat. vol. 1, p. 667) in that I demand any further tissue preparation should be omitted in order to get the earliest possible fixation. This is best achieved with concentrated aqueous sublimate solution. The way I do it is that I dissolve sublimate in excess in boiling water and let it

356

crystallise when it gets cold. If kept in a dark bottle the solution lasts a very long time. In this solution I place my pieces of

357 organs, the pieces as small as possible and they remain in the fluid for anything between 10 and 60 minutes depending on their size. If there is a necessity to fix larger pieces, fixation of which would take longer than one hour, I recommend choosing an alternative method. This is because if organs are fixed in sublimate any longer than that, most tissues, especially smooth muscle and epidermis, become so solid that the blade of the knife will break on them.

Directly from the sublimate, small pieces are transferred into diluted methylated spirit without a washing step. From there they will be transferred into 100 per cent alcohol in Schulze's dialysator and finally embedded in paraffin according to standard protocol.

In order to see karyokinetic figures I never stain pieces first, having had several bad experiences with that method. I prefer to glue the slices on to the slide and then stain them while vertical in a tall vessel. This way precipitates are kept to a minimum, especially when one stains with haematoxylin, as I usually do. The dye should be as dilute as possible and the staining process should last 15 to 24 hours. The reason for this is that the chromosomes look more slender, which is of some importance given the small size of the karyokinetic figures. All aniline dyes create precipitations on the chromosomes, which I find extremely awkward, the only exception being the safranin method of Flemming. However, this staining method gives the chromosomes a strong shine, which blurs their borders. High-contrast staining of diluted Böhmer's haematoxylin, after 20 hours of incubation, delivers the best results for human mitoses.

The slices should not be too thin, otherwise it may happen quite often that cells get cut in half. The best safeguard is that one only estimates the amount of chromatin, or the numbers of chromosomes, in such cells in which one can definitely see the upper and lower border and as well, the upper and lower borders of the neighbouring cells. This insures us against evaluating cells which have been cut through. Even in perfect preparations one must not evaluate any suspicious cells. Otherwise one might find oneself in the same situation as Schütz

358 ("Microscopic Findings in Carcinomas", Frankfurt a.M., 1890), namely being accused of having evaluated lots of artefacts. This accusation has recently been refuted by Alberts as far as asymmetrical karyokinesis is concerned (Deutsche Medicinalzeitung, 1890, vol. 93, p. 1043).

Klebs, and quite recently Hauser ("Cylindrical Carcinoma of the Epithelium", Jena, G. Fischer 1890, p. 72), have confirmed my findings. Klebs says (Deutsche med. Wochenschr. 1890, vol. 24): "Whilst in place of the normal secretory activity of the epithelia, or of activity generally directed to the production of specific products of metabolism, excessive and irregular growth appears with irregular karyokinesis, as was especially described by me in my book, and recently announced by Hansemann as confirmed, the assumption of a deep-seated change in function seems quite specifically to be a postulate whose real existence, on the other hand, remains to be proved." I would like to remark that in his book Klebs has only spoken of the following "... that it is not uncommon to find very chromatin-rich parts right next to chromatin-depleted ones in the same cell...", while true asymmetrical cell division, as far as I know, has been described first of all by me. I see that this might well be more than mere confirmation of Klebs' findings.

Hauser must have been oblivious of my findings as well as those of Klebs since he fails to mention them. As far as the asymmetrical karyokinesis is concerned Hauser limits himself to the sentence "... that not infrequently the mother stars disintegrate into daughter stars of consistently unequal size."

As far now as asymmetrical mitosis is confirmed I would like to say in advance that I found these phenomena, since February 1890, in 20 further carcinomata (and in all which I examined when they were fresh enough), sometimes more frequently and sometimes less commonly. Some examples are shown in Figs 1–8. Here, of especial interest are two cells from the same case (cancer of the lip in a 69-year-old man) but from different cuts, no. 7 and 8. no. 7 is characterised by an extreme asymmetry and in no. 8 the asymmetry is

present in a tripartite division (cf. my treatise, this Archive, vol. 109, Plate 9, Fig. 12). 359

In no other tumour, not in sarcomata, in no hyperplasia, in no inflammation, nor in state of regeneration in any normal tissue could even a hint of asymmetrical divisions be found[1]. One is thus confirmed in the view that asymmetrical mitosis is likely to be characteristic of carcinomata. However, I have pronounced the theoretical possibility (see above) that they could be found during normal development at the interfaces of generational stages.

In contrast, in almost all pathological tissues other forms of nuclear divisions can be found, which will be the subject of systematic discussion in more detail here. The latter can be classified in two ways; first, according to the number of the chromosomes and, secondly, according to the physiological valence of the cells. If one combines those two principles the following order will be revealed:

I Hypochromatic cells (with fewer chromosomes than the tissue in question usually reveals, thus the hypochromasia is always a relative one).
   a) Bipartite partitions
   b) Multiple partitions
   c) Aborted forms

II Cells with normal chromatin content
   a) Altered chromosomes
   b) Altered centrioles
   c) Altered cellular division

III Hyperchromatic cells
   a) Two component giant cells
   b) Multipart giant cells
   c) Aborted forms

As far as the assessment of the amount of chromatin goes, this is never possible in a "resting"* cell, just as little does it depend on the thickness or fineness of

[1] In total, I have at my disposal the most exact examinations of more than ninety perfectly-fixed specimens.
* interphase (eds)

chromosomes, but only their number is important. And if in the following text the terms hyper- or hypo-chromatic are used, then that refers only to the number of chromosomes. Now it is indeed correct that only in most rare cases is one truly able to count the number of chromosomes. Hauser reports (his abovementioned publication on p. 72) that the number of chromosomes in cancers of the stomach might vary between eight and 12. That is certainly based on an error. In normal human tissue I have never been able to count the chromosomes with absolute certainty given their great number. In one case, I was convinced I had 18 chromosomes, in another case that I had 24; however, without having any guarantee for the certainty of these numbers. In a third case [of loose tangles (*Knäuel*) within a normal endothelial cell without longitudinal splitting of the chromosomes] there were with certainty more than 40 chromosomes. I have shown (cited above) that in carcinomas, hypochromatic figures with seven chromosomes occur; however, these are decided rarities and are, as I have said, probably a so-called 'aborted form'. As until now, in most cases, it is impossible to determine the number of chromosomes; one has to hold on to extreme values as is also the case with asymmetrical figures.

I. The hypochromatic forms are probably only found in carcinomata. One can assume in general that each cell whose chromosomes can be counted in the state of the monaster, must be hypochromatic. Where this is not applicable, one must determine the average size of all mitoses found in one specific phase and according to this, judge their chromatin content. Thus, for example, in Fig. 9, cell "a" is in a monaster (diastole), from which I have formed the opinion that its chromatin content is to be regarded as the norm for cells of a cancer of this type (breast cancer of a 60-year-old woman). Cell "b" of the same Figure in the same phase thus represents a hypochromatic figure (this latter cell was in the same optical plane as cell "a").

One might perhaps object that research based so much on such subjective opinions rests on very weak feet (*schwachen Füssen)*, and I have to recognise the awkward situation in which I find myself because of the lack of any absolute measure for the chromatin content. However, everyone who has ever concerned himself thoroughly with these questions, will admit that one can readily gain the necessary experience to judge chromatin content with some certainty. After all, in the case of other investigations, one very often speaks of increased numbers of cells, of enlargement of an organ and so on, without being able to give numerical data and without the need to demand these data, but supported solely by an individual's experience. From this standpoint, I should like, in the same manner, to explain Fig. 11 (from same cancer as Fig. 9) as being hypochromatic. In the same way, Fig. 10 (from the same cancer as Fig. 7 and 8) belongs here, and one can compare this one with Fig. 14 (from the same cancer), the latter picturing a hyperchromatic form. Now the hypochromatic form doubtless occurs also in multiple divisions, which is all the more striking, in that one must regard the multiple division as a process which reduces this enlarged number of chromosomes back to the normal measure (*Masse*)*. Fig. 13 represents such a hypochromatic multipolar cell, which, quite by chance, was not cut through, although it was large in size. Here we are dealing with a metakinesis (same cancer as Figs 9 and 11) with six spindles, of which spindle "a" contains a sufficient number of chromosomes, whereas in spindles "b" and "d" too few are found, and spindle "c" has hardly any, with two double chromosomes on the left side only. The only explanation for a cell like this is that it was generated by over-production of chromatin in a hypochromatic cell.

Incidentally, this figure is instructive in another sense. It clearly shows the achromatic spindles; often, however, these are less clearly seen or even completely invisible. If one follows on with the idea of achromatic spindles, and looks at the chromosomes only, they form a seemingly disorganized picture, especially when one imagines that they are all in different planes, and in the drawing they have all been transferred into one plane for illustration purposes. One can see from this example that to understand any mitotic figure, the achromatic spindles are always necessary. This must always

* here the noun "measure" has the sense of overall amount (eds)

be taken into account in all those seemingly incomprehensible (*unverständlichen*) mitoses*, such as are found very frequently, specifically in carcinomata.

As I have shown earlier (see above), abortive forms occur commonly amongst the hypochromatic cells. Usually they present (compare also the diagrams there – previous article) as pale, indistinct structures, the mitotic phase of which cannot be clearly determined, whose chromosomes show irregular shapes and often have blurred borders, such as are also found for example in Fig. 15. In many cases one would be inclined to view these cells as being cut through**. However, they are distinguishable by their clearly-delineated cell border, which can be confirmed above all by the fact that above and below them still further cells lie in the same cut.

When I first saw these hypochromatic figures in conjunction with asymmetrical mitoses I believed that they could only come about through asymmetrical division. Meanwhile, I have seen figures such as those in Nos. 16-22. Common to all of these is that beside the ordered chromosomes and the monaster, a few single additional ones are found, seemingly lost. All these figures originate from carcinomata, with one exception – and this is really notable: – the one in Fig. 20, taken from a sarcoma; in the latter, it was the only cell of its kind. Fig. 16 is perhaps less reliable because the material had been taken from a corpse, whereas all the others were taken from a living body and have been fixed without delay. In these cells now, it is possible that the lost chromosomes somehow participate in mitosis later on; because some of them show a clear longitudinal splitting, eg, Fig. 21 and Fig. 22. But it is also conceivable that these chromosomes permanently exclude themselves from the interior of the nucleus, and that in this way a hypochromatic cell would come into existence. I was strengthened in this view by a statement of Boveri's (Studies of Cells, Jena, 1890, booklet 13, p. 63), which describes a similar occurrence and places it in relationship with the reduction of chromosomes in gametes. Schottländer has also described similar figures (Arch. f. mikr. Anat. vol. 31, p. 457) as "lost loops" in the process of regeneration

* currently often referred to as "mitotic catastrophe" (eds)
** by the microtome (eds).

of Descemet's membrane in the frog. In his case it seems likely that these lost loops can regain a relationship with the nucleus figure later on, which is a scenario not totally excluded from my figures either.

II. The pathological deviations in the division of cells with normal chromatin content are very manifold. They occur in part also in hypo- and hyperchromatic elements. Some of these are so minor that one is tempted to classify them within the framework of the physiological area; as they are typically found, however, as a rule only in mitoses which occur in unusual places, eg, in the high strata of the Malpighian layers of warts, this seems to justify placing them among the pathological processes.

The changes in the chromosomes consist mainly in the fact that they are strikingly short and thick. Flemming (Arch. für mikr. Anat. vol. 29) has described something similar in the testes of salamanders, and one can find them there very commonly, usually in clusters. Apart from that I have found changes in chromosomes in primordial eggs in the ovaries of newborn and embryonal rabbits as illustrated in Fig. 28. In normal human organs, however, I have never seen such structures, but I certainly have in pathological formations. Figs 9a, 13, 17, 22 and 23 give examples of this. With the exception of Fig. 23 all the Figs come from carcinomata. Fig. 23 is taken from the highest layer of the rete Malpighii of pointed (*spitzen*) condylomas. It seems that certain conditions, which cannot be more closely defined, lead to the creation of such forms; in many cases none of them are found; where, however, they are found they are usually abundant, often in one optical field.

Already earlier (as cited above) I have proposed the idea that a delay occurs in the longitudinal splitting of chromosomes. More recently, as well, I was able frequently to find many mitotic figures in the monaster phase, which made this seem very probable to me. However, up to now it has not been possible in this respect, to achieve certainty.

Chromatic connecting threads have previously been explained and well illustrated as pathological phenomena, especially by Schottländer (as cited above). I do not regard them as pathological since they are also found in quite normal human tissues.

The polar bodies (*Polkörperchen*)* in human beings are usually at the limit of what is visible at all, and in most mitoses they cannot be seen at all. In strong proliferations and especially in certain carcinomata, they attain, however, a considerable size. They stain intensively with eosin and are usually weakly shiny (in the fixed and stained state). They have a round or slightly oval shape; in the latter case, the long dimension is always perpendicular to the axis of division of the cells. The polar bodies are well visualised in Figs 9b, 12, 13, 24 and especially so in 25 (metakinesis in a lip cancer).

That the division of the cell sometimes lags considerably behind the division of the nucleus has been described by Flemming in pigmented cells of the salamander larvae (Arch. für mikr. Anat. vol. 35), and Zimmermann showed and proved subsequently that this process is only present in those larvae (same Archive, vol. 36), which have been deficient in nutrition, and postulated that this process might be pathological. In pathological conditions in humans, I should like to regard the same phenomenon as a very frequent occurrence. In all possible pathological growths of any considerable kind one finds cells in which the daughter nuclei have already built a membrane, yet a constriction of the cell membrane is not to be noted. In addition, cells with two nuclei are relatively common as I have seen for myself in many cases. Finally, there is no shortage of shapes where the constriction only starts after daughter nuclei have been well formed previously. A very nice example was delivered by a polypoid condyloma in its epithelial cells.

Sometimes cells can be found in the anaphase, which were not divided by constriction, but by the formation of a dividing wall as in plant cells, see also Figs 26 and 27, but only apparently however. In the case of Fig. 26, one can see with certainty a break in the middle of the so-called 'wall' by exact focusing, and in the case of Fig. 27 the constriction of the chromatic connecting threads, allows one to recognise easily the true situation.

* Hansemann may have meant centrioles, not the polar bodies of oogenesis (eds).

365 Such behaviour is shown in Fig. 18, Table XXII in Schottländer's work (Arch. für mikr. Anat. vol. 31).

The spindles and achromatic connecting threads, which are best demonstrated after long exposure to diluted aqueous eosin, show remarkable constancy. I have never seen a deviation from normal in them worth mentioning. That one can sometimes see the achromatic structures, as also the polar radiation very clearly, whereas in other situations they are hardly perceptible, seems to depend on some chance factors, the nature of which has not yet been elucidated. But only one thing is very striking here, namely that the spindles are most obvious in material from corpses, which has been fixed at least 24 hours or longer post mortem, as opposed to organs fixed when they still had body temperature*. If one looks at Figs 31–34 with this in mind, it is easy to see that the chromatic figures can be already completely destroyed (Fig. 34), whereas the spindles have lost none of their clarity. However, central bodies (*Centralkörperchen*)** have not been identified in these specimens.

III. Hyperchromatic cells are abundant in any state of pathological cell proliferation and in point of fact, are the more common the more stormy the proliferation. It is therefore probably explicable that they are found much more often in cancers than in other proliferative states, but sometimes in very rapidly growing cancers they only occur sparsely. In others, on the other hand, they are so common that one finds several in every visual field with the usual magnifications of 500 to 600. If now, it is beyond doubt that most hyperchromatic cells lead to multiple divisions, it is also still quite certain that bipartite giant cells do also. Examples for this are Fig. 14 (from a cancer of the lip), which one should compare with Fig. 10 from the same tumour, and also with Fig. 37, taken from a sarcoma of the thumb, the usual cell size of which is depicted in Fig. 36; finally, there is Fig. 39 from a common wart, in which the remaining cells were of the size of cells to be found in Fig. 38.

Of greater interest than the bipolar giant cells are the giant cells with multiple poles. Here, we have to differentiate between two sorts:

* this suggests an autolytic phenomenon revealing the stainable structures (eds)
** thought to be centrosomes (eds)

366 Firstly, there are cells with several nuclei in the process of division. Their mitotic figures can be in the same or in different phases of mitosis. Such forms are depicted in Flemming's publication in the Arch. f. mikr. Anat. vol. 18, Plate VII, Fig. 16 and Plate IX, Figs 49a to 52. Furthermore, similar phenomena are described in plant cells. Whether this form occurs in human beings as well I am unable to say with certainty. The best object on which to study it might be the giant cells of sarcomata. Klebs has described pathological mitoses in such giant cells ("Pathological Morphology", vol. 2, p. 730); these cells were however, pluripolar[1] as he very kindly told me personally.

Baumgarten too (Zeitschrift für klin. Med., vols 9 and 10), describes nuclear division figures in a tuberculous giant cell (p. 253 vol. 9); however, these were not so clear that he could dare to produce a drawing*. Finally, the data given by Fütterer (Report of the Meeting of the Würzburg Phys. – Medical Society, 1887, 4 June) are not very satisfying either. Namely, Fütterer says, "As far now as the finding of giant cells (in a sarcoma of a mandible) are concerned, no clear mitotic figures were visible, as appears to be necessary to assume karyokinetic processes; yet, according to what we have seen we don't doubt that they must be present". My own experiments have not fared any better, only one single figure in a sarcoma, in the absence of any better interpretation of its appearance, could be regarded as mitotic.

[1] It should be mentioned incidentally that Klebs' pronouncement (same Archive, p. 721) "I have to draw attention to the fact that nuclear divisions of cells labelled "karyomitoses", so far as they originate in human tissues (especially sarcomas), hardly justify this appelation. In part they are darkish linear structures which proceed from the surface of the cell membrane, and divide the nuclear substance into two or more segments; in part they are those incomplete divisions as described by Arnold etc..." may well be in error. In every sarcoma I have examined so far, I have seen beautiful and mostly typical mitoses, so that in this respect I agree entirely with Siegenbeek van Heukelom (this Archive, vol. 107). I find these mitoses even more clear than they are depicted in his illustrations. Fragmentations as Arnold describes I have never observed in sarcomas.
*this is not sarcastic in the original German (eds).

However, that is by no means certain, and if a picture is given here, then this happens only because, perhaps, a chance finding in a more suitable specimen could shed more light on this controversy some time later on.

Secondly, one observes the oft-described pluripolar mitotic figures (Figs 8, 12, 13, 24, 29-35, 41 and 42). Here, one could dispute, whether these are to be understood as pathological phenomena or not. I have never found these phenomena in normal human or animal tissue; as far as I know, they have been described, in not provenly pathological circumstances, only in the testes of salamanders (Flemming, Arch. f. Mikr. Anat. vol. 29). Flemming is inclined there to place them among pathological forms; as far as humans are concerned, I would like to associate myself with this unconditionally, because here, under pathological circumstances, they are found very commonly. I saw the most beautiful and most regular forms in an atypical epithelial proliferation (Friedländer) on the edge of bad granulations (Figs 29 and 30), here however, they were not numerous. In carcinomata they are very common, and sometimes so common that they outnumber dual divisions. Of the correctness of these observations of Martin (this Archive, vol. 86), Tizzoni and Poggi (Rivista Clinica di Bologna) and others, I have had various opportunities to convince myself on many occasions. When Klebs states (as above, p. 529) that hyperchromatic nuclei are the rule in sarcomata, this can only be admitted for a selected few sarcomata. By far the majority of sarcomata, especially lymphosarcomata and the slowly-growing osteosarcomata, feature only very tiny mitotic figures. Only in large-celled rapidly-growing sarcomata and in spindle cell sarcomata can one sometimes find hyperchromatic structures. It should not be denied that one may occasionally find a sarcoma for which Klebs' statement is correct, but it is only the generalisation of this finding that I must energetically resist. It was striking for me that I never found pluripolar mitotic figures in proliferating connective tissue, here they must either be very infrequent, or proceed so rapidly that one does not easily catch them in the act (*in flagranti*).

Nauwerck ("On the Regeneration of Muscle", Jena, 1890, p. 11) was able to prove these figures in the connective tissue of rabbits.

In most detailed way Schottländer concerned himself with pluripolar mitoses in a very beautiful experimental work (Arch. f. mikr. Anat. vol. 31). It may well be difficult to pronounce anything specific about the significance of these mitoses. For the most part, I would like to reiterate the abovementioned explanation, which is that through these multiple mitoses, the immoderately accumulated substance of chromatin is reduced back to its normal amount*. However, we see from the fate of these mitoses that perhaps this still succeeds in tripartite or perhaps also in quadripartite divisions, but that later a sure cell division after the nuclear division was not observed, so that here the urge to restore the *status quo ante* may still be present, but the result is inadequate. I myself have only ever observed a constriction of the cell membrane with tripartite divisions (Figs 31, 41 and 42), but never found them in quadruple and higher order divisions.** Martin (source as above) produces a drawing of a quadruple division with a constriction of the cytoplasm and Schottländer also describes this quite expressly for a quadruple division. In cancers where multiple divisions are so dominantly common, I have never seen the subsequent divisions of the cytoplasm. On the contrary, I have always observed that an extraordinarily high number of epithelial giant cells with many nuclei was revealed, especially in a breast cancer as depicted in Figs 12, 13 and 14.

Nowhere are aborted forms so frequent as in hyperchromatic cells, and nowhere are their forms so manifold. They are distinguished by the fact that the chromosomes – if one wants to still call them chromosomes at all – take the most bizarre shapes. In Fig. 15 I give a typical example originating from a cancer of the lip. Proof that this is indeed a mitosis is provided by the light zone which occupies the inner part of this cell. No achromatic figures are to be noticed. The cell is of an unusual size. I consider it improbable that this is an artefact caused by reagents because, specifically, all slides of this cancer were faultless and, particularly, all the parts around the cell seem perfectly fixed. In such abortive forms I was never able to identify a division of the cell body proper.

* is he suggesting that this is a physiological cell rectification process? (eds)
** his notion is that if there are no constrictions, there are no subsequent cell divisions. (eds)

I have often seen aggregations of chromatin and coalescence of the latter in homogeneous drops, not only in cancers but also in other perfectly fixed tumours and in proliferations of inflammatory nature. But I have not been able to convince myself here that these are actually mitotic figures. On the other hand, I believe that some of those bodies so frequently described in recent times as 'parasites in cancers' belong here; these have no further significance than as a form of necrobiosis of single cells.

I should not like, for the moment, to draw any more conclusions from the data presented here. It follows from the latter that all pathological forms, except the asymmetric cell division and the hypochromatic forms, are not found exclusively in carcinomata. However, their frequent occurrence in tumours and their predominance, compared with normal mitotic figures in some carcinomata, may well, as emphasised by Klebs (source as above) and also by Schütz (source as above), provide support for the anatomic diagnosis of carcinoma.

More detailed communication on this point, I will reserve until another occasion.

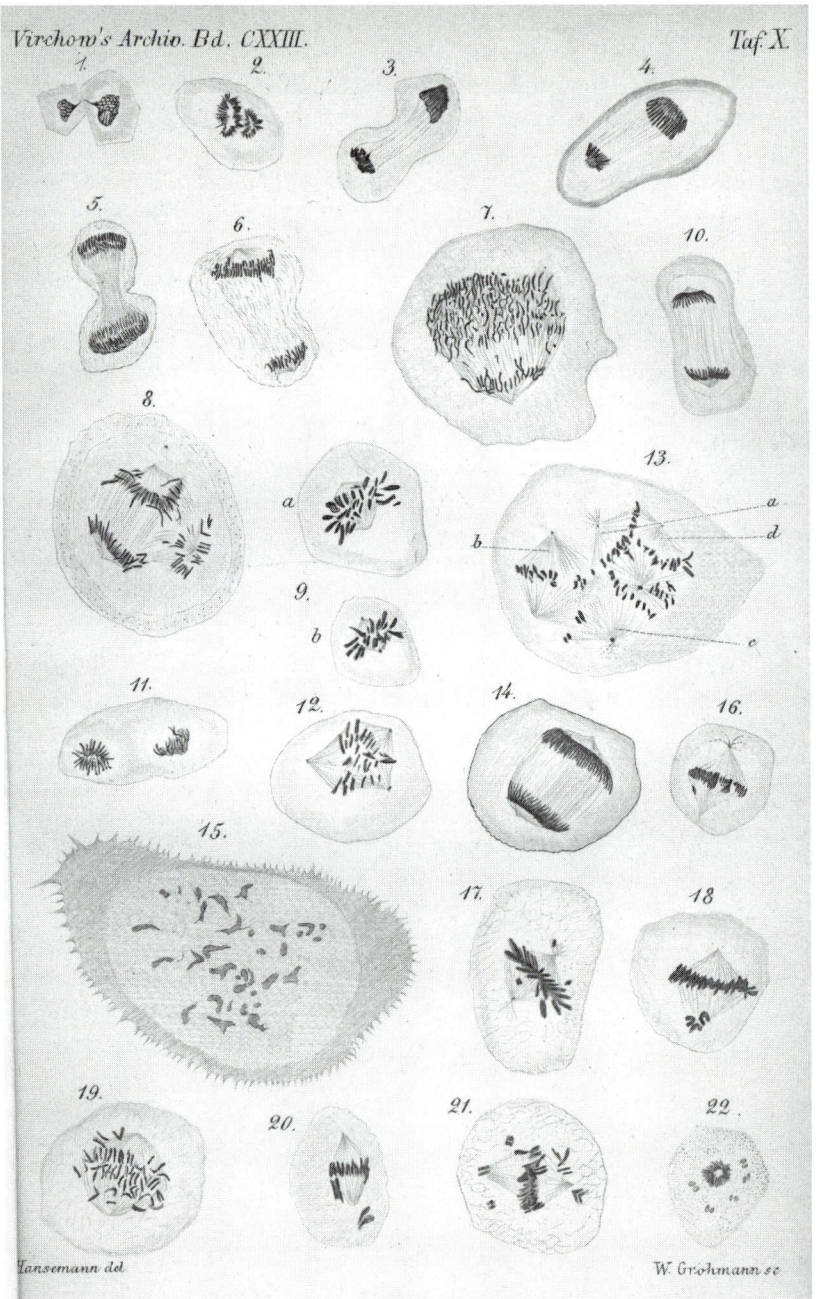

Plate X

Plates

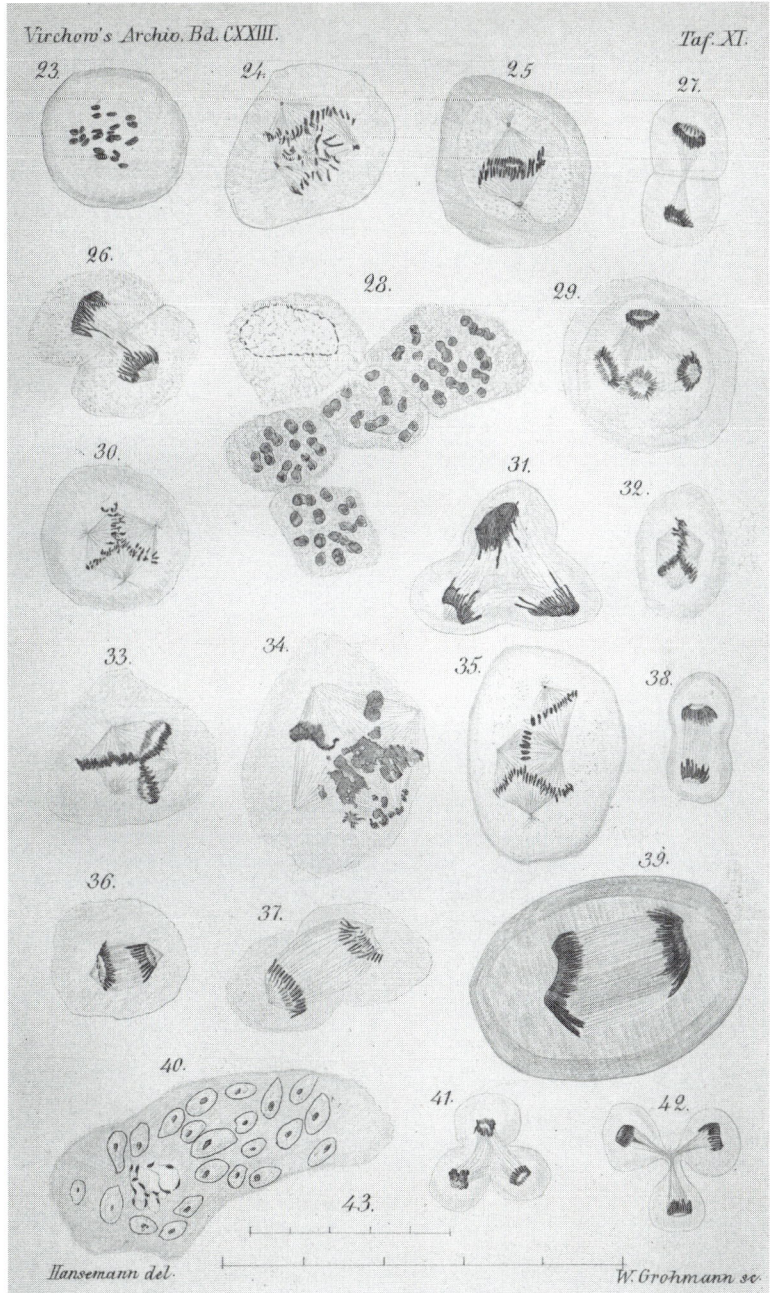

Plate XI

Explanation of the illustrations: plates X and XI

The Figures are wholly prepared with Abbe's drawing apparatus. The enlargements were presented via the Zeiss apochromatic oil immersion, with aperture of 1.30, tube not drawn out, and the apochromatic compensations oculars 4 (Figs 40–42), 8 (Figs 1–27 and 29–39) and 12 (Fig. 28). For this, the drawing table was situated at the height of the object table. As a measuring rod, a fragment a millimetre long and divided into 10 parts with the ocular 4 and 8 is reproduced under the same conditions.

Figs 1–8 asymmetric figures: 1 from a laryngeal cancer, 2 from a gut cancer, 3 from an epithelium of the cheek, 4 from a lip cancer, 5 from a cancer of the digestive tract, 6 from the same, 7 from the same lip cancer as Figs 4, 8 from the same, tripolar.

Figs 9a and b. Two mother stars from a breast cancer situated closely alongside each other.

Figs 10 and 11. Hypochromatic cells from cancers.

Figs 12 and 13. Multipolar, hypochromatic (relatively) cells from cancers.

Fig. 14. Cell from a cancer (hyperchromatic).

Fig. 15. Abortive form from a cancer (hyperchromatic).

Figs 16–22. Mitoses with errant chromosomes wholly from cancers. Only Fig. 22 from a sarcoma.

Fig. 16. From cadaveric material.

Fig. 23. Cell with short chromosomes from a condyloma.

Figs 24 and 25. From cancers with clear polar bodies.

Figs 26 and 27. Apparent squamous cell formation.

Fig. 28. From the ovary of a new-born rabbit. The resting cell strikingly poor in chromatin.

Figs 29 and 30. Multipolar mitoses from atypical epithelial proliferation associated with granulations.

Figs 31–34. Multipolar cells from cadaveric material.

Fig. 35. Multipolar mitosis from a breast cancer in a male.

Figs 38 and 39. Normal and giant mitosis from a common wart.

Fig. 36 and 37. The same from a sarcoma.

Fig. 40. A doubtful mitosis from a sarcoma giant cell.

Figs 41 and 42. Multipolar mitoses with cell division.

Chapter 9

Karyokinesis and "Cellular Pathology"

(Hansemann 1891c)

Editors' Summary of Points

p. 1039 General, positive comments on the Cellular Pathology and Virchow's role – bacteriology seen as an attack to be repelled – specific antibacterial factors in serum discounted; 1040 early studies of cell division and nuclear division reviewed – incidence of mitoses in general – mitoses can be abnormal as part of injury to a cell – concerning forms of mitoses, there are differences between different tissues; 1041 pathological mitoses different in regeneration and malignant tumours – concerning the number of mitoses, various factors, resistance to lack of cell nutrients, effects of poisons; 1042 increases of mitoses need time to develop – increases not only in malignancy – concerning the place where they are found – different capacities of different tissues to regenerate – peroration on role of cellular pathology as a medical science, the pre-eminence of which has not been eroded.

When the "Cellular Pathology" appeared summarised as a book in 1858, the struggle surrounding its theory was not then concluded, but was already decided in its favour. The present generation scarcely thinks about what struggles it cost to make valid those scientific fundamental principles which are now so familiar to every young doctor; and they can scarcely understand that all these concepts which appear today as natural as one's mother tongue, once did not exist, and had first of all to be defended step by step against sharpest opposition. If those who were not themselves in the struggle wish to understand it correctly, they must study the first thirty to forty volumes of Virchow's Archive; thereby they will be able to gain an idea as to what courage and strength were required to fight this struggle through, since at that time Virchow stood almost wholly isolated on the one side. Then it will be clear how his party gradually won more supporters, until finally no serious voice dared to raise itself against it[1].

Although Virchow's teachings have now been transformed into flesh and blood, so that now no research in the area of the morphology and biology of plants and animals can be undertaken without proceeding from his teachings and building on them; nonetheless, twice in recent times, "Cellular Pathology" has still been under attack. The first attack was fended off by Virchow himself in his essay "On the nature and causes of diseases" (his Archive vol. 79, p. 185). The second attack originated recently from the bacteriological side. Whilst some of the researchers (Metchnikoff, Arnold, Leber, Hertwig etc) see in infectious diseases a struggle of the cells against bacteria; the other researchers (Bucher, Charrin and Roger, Behring) appear to place the chemical side of the processes in the foreground to such an extent that they believe themselves compelled

1039

to reach back – for some processes – to humoural pathology. As one example among many, Landerer may be cited here, who probably expresses himself most unambiguously ("Directions and Aims of the Newer Surgery", Leipzig, 1891) thus: "One thing we can already say now, is that the days of exclusive 'cellular pathology' are numbered. We only want to hope, if the presumed dead 'humoural pathology' should suddenly arise from its grave, that we may not be thrown from one extreme to the other, and that we will be successful in joining the old 'cellular pathology' with the demands of 'humoural pathology', free of irrelevant outgrowths, in one permanent building". Here, as with many other authors, it is a matter of a clear misunderstanding of cellular concepts being obvious, so that Buchner – from whose ground-breaking works these and similar conclusions are usually drawn – will scarcely wish to take the responsibility for this on himself. That blood serum in the body, with its disinfecting properties, is a constantly changing product of cells, will probably not be denied by anyone. Thus I do not see how one can hold anything responsible, in the last resort, for everything that proceeds through the blood serum, other than the cells which produce the blood serum – just as as one makes the micro-organisms responsible for the poisonous metabolic products which derive from them. And these latter are themselves nothing other than cells. Just as metabolic products of bacteria can kill animal cells, so metabolic products of animals cells can kill certain bacteria. That, however, is not "humoural pathology", but the most excellent "cellular pathology" in its purest form. Thus Orth states, with reference to the views cited above (Keynote Address given 4th June 1891, Göttingen, p. 25): "The newly gained recognition that blood and lymph, in particular possess properties hostile to bacteria, independent of their cellular elements, could arouse the idea that thereby the significance of cells had been reduced. Absolutely wrong. Whence, then, do the body fluids receive their chemical components? What does not come directly from outside, comes from the body tissues; which comes from the tissue metabolism; which comes from the tissue cells; which rule and guide metabolism. And what arises in the blood itself certainly does not arise without the collaboration of new cells, both the white and red blood corpuscles. Thus here too it is cells which in all dispositions play the essential and main role."

[1] A perhaps little-known but really significant episode occurred in 1847 at the Conference of the Natural Researchers in Aachen in the first session (20th September) of the second section (for Medicine, Surgery and Midwifery). Virchow spoke about the parenchymatous inflammation, particularly of the kidneys, the liver, the muscles, and thereby argued his observations on cellular processes. After twenty minutes he was interrupted by the chairman, *Geheimrat* Dr Harless (Professor in Bonn), as his time for speaking had now run out. Only after energetic calls from the younger doctors: "Carry on!" was Virchow able to conclude his lecture. (personal report of *Geheimrat*-Health G. Mayer, in Aachen). Harless added to the lecture the hardly encouraging remark that Virchow had indeed exactly described microscopic processes in inflammation but the chemical part had remained very much in the background. (Official Report of the 25th Conference in Aachen, p. 106. Aachen, 1849.)

Whilst on the one hand, we can certainly say "Cellular Pathology" has experienced unjustified attacks, on the other, research in the area of cells has experienced the greatest triumphs. By this I mean the more exact recognition of cell division by Schneider, Eberth, Strassburger, Mayzel, Flemming etc. I won't speak here of the great significance of this process for the understanding of biological processes, particularly those of fertilization (Hertwig, Boveri, van Beneden etc) and heredity, but rather of the influence of these things on the recognition of pathological processes. After Flemming developed the methods of investigation (*kennengelernt*), the pathologists took possession of these things – Arnold in the vanguard, and under the leadership of Flemming, Arnold, Ziegler, Marchand and others – a rich literature on karyokinesis in regeneration, hyperplasia and inflammation soon developed. What importance is attached to these researches today is proved by the position which has been accorded to them in new text books, and also by the innumerable works on them which appear continually. I myself have been concerned with these studies for years, and can scarcely imagine more interesting and rewarding microscopic work.

In this, a sequence of viewpoints has come to me which could have particular significance for the recognition of pathological processes. They are:

1. The incidence of mitoses in general;
2. Their form;
3. Their number;
4. The place where they are found.

Concerning 1. We know that the cells of all tissues without exception increase by karyokinesis at the time of development and growth. In their full-grown condition, however, a substantial part of the tissues no longer shows mitoses, whilst in others, a permanent regeneration for replacement of the discarded or died-off cells takes place. In the first group belong the connective tissues, the musculature, the central and peripheral nervous tissue, true glands such as liver, kidneys, mucous, salivary, and sweat glands, the peritoneum and the endothelia of the vessels. In the second category belong the covering epithelia of the outer skin, and of the mucous membranes, the gland excretory passages, further the lymph glands, the spleen, bone marrow, Lieberkühn's crypts of the gut, sebaceous glands, and probably bones too. Intermittent mitosis is seen in the cells of the breast gland (namely only during pregnancy) and the testicular epithelia.

The absence of mitoses in the first group is *inter alia* important, in so far as we learn from this fact that in the glands, secretion does not cause perishing of the cells, as has been widely assumed. Bizzozero and Vasale (Virchow's Arch. vol. 110), first pointed to the fact that in most glands, cell division figures are absent. These two researchers and also Heidenhain (cf. Schmidt, "Concerning Nuclear Changes in the Secretory Cells". J. D.* Breslau) then recognised that mitoses, wherever they occur, are not related to secretion. Altmann too ("Elementary Organisms", Leipzig, 1890) reached the same result via a different route. The only apparent exception in human beings is in the sebaceous glands. Looked at more closely, however, one will find that here we are not dealing with real glands at all, but that the sebaceous follicles – which is a better way of putting it – are equivalent formations to the hair roots. With the same justification one could regard the hair as a secretion of the hair roots, just as hitherto one has understood sebum as a secretion of the sebaceous glands. The distinction lies only in the fact that in the one case the cells perish by peculiar keratinisation, in the other case by a peculiar fat metamorphosis. In the concepts of perishing and of secretion / *Secerniren*** there is already a certain distinction; the one is a passive and the other is an active process.

If now mitoses appear in the tissue of the first group, one must deduce a pathological process (of inflammation, regeneration or hyperplasia).

The cells of the second group are not in principle distinguished from those of the first group by permanent mitosis. The difference consists only in the fact that processes which occur only exceptionally in the first group, are completed regularly in the latter, and these we are accustomed to including amongst the physiological processes, although strictly speaking, they are pathological in nature.*** This is most clearly apparent in covering epithelia, for example in the epidermis, (cf. Concerning cell division in the epidermis. In: "Festschrift for Virchow by his Assistants", Reimer, 1891), where, in the keratinisation we observe a continuing death and expulsion of cells – caused by external stimuli – which (i.e. the cells) regenerate themselves by mitosis of the remaining viable cells. It is rather more difficult to gain a comprehensive view of the process in lymph glands and in the organs of blood formation. Here, a continuous loss of cells at the periphery takes place, partly on the surface of the body, partly in certain organs, which then have to be regenerated in the central places – the germinal centres.

In this second group too, given particularly occurring pathological stimuli, the formation of mitoses can increase considerably, whereby the individual organs can undergo significant changes in their entire configuration.

Concerning 2. The form of mitoses in the human being coincides on the whole with that propounded by Flemming and others. In the individual case, however, there are characteristic deviations for every type of tissue which are so perceptible that, with some practice, one can easily distinguish the cells of individual tissues by the form of their mitosis. That applies particularly to tissue types which are very distant from each other, for example, the lymph glands, the epidermal cells and the endothelia.

*   a name of a publisher may be missing (eds)
** lit. "separation" or "secretion" – thought to mean apocrine and/or holocrine secretion (eds)
*** The distinction is between a mitosis in a pathological condition of the whole cell, and a mitosis which deviates in its own form and successful outcome from normal mitoses without the involvement of damage to the rest of the cell. (eds)

But also in some closely related cells, for example the epidermis and hair root cells, such a difference is clearly perceptible; likewise in the endothelia and connective tissue cells (reticulum cells). Some cell types, however, have not hitherto been distinguishable by their mitosic form, for example those of the salivary glands and of the kidney. This, however, is almost certainly because of the smallness of human cells in general and our deficient knowledge of characteristic points. Fortunately this mostly concerns cells which – on account of their other properties and their separate position in the body – do not easily cause confusion between themselves. In the formation of granulations, however, and in the proliferative growth of the lymph glands, one can distinguish by the form of mitosis whether, in the individual case, we are dealing with a reticulum cell (connective tissue cell), an endothelial cell or a lymph cell. The same applies to most other combinations of tissue. Differences between individual cell types extend to all hitherto well-recognised cell parts and stages of mitosis; either to individual parts or simultaneously to several. The differences concern the form and shape of whole mitotic figures, of individual chromosomes, connecting threads, attraction spheres, the duration of the individual phases, and finally the cytoplasm.

Under pathological conditions the mitoses can either retain their characteristic form, or change so considerably that they can no longer be recognised as belonging together. The former takes place mainly during regeneration, the latter in malignant tumours. In between, however, there are all possible transitional forms. The slightest deviation from the norm is to be seen in tripartite and multipartite division. Then come the giant forms; finally the asymmetrical karyokineses, which hitherto have been found only in cancers*. All these forms have biological significance. In addition to these, however, there are abortive forms, which overall lead to a dissolution of the cell.**

These particular properties of the individual cell types are especially important for the processes of regeneration because through them we recognise without any doubt that every cell can only be regenerated from a cell of the same type as itself: muscle cells only from muscle cells, connective tissue only from connective tissue, endothelia from endothelia, epithelia from epithelia and so on. A transition from one form into the other can indeed be deduced from resting cells lying along side each other; every cell passes on unchanged to its descendants the properties it acquired at embryonal differentiation. The only exception is caused by the asymmetric division. Here, daughter cells with unequal properties arise which therefore, in their external appearances and in their mitoses, are not necessarily any longer similar to the mother cells. Thus the origin of the carcinoma cells in the individual case is not to be deduced from the form of the mitoses alone.

Concerning 3. From the number of mitoses one can generally judge the degree of the process; in this, however, we have to take into account that mitoses almost always appear in groups – thus the degree should never be assessed in one section alone. Furthermore, the larger the number of mitoses which is visible, the shorter is the resting phase in comparison with the duration of division. The duration of division appears to be quite constant for the individual tissues; the resting phases, however, can vary because of different factors, for example by the degree of nourishment flowing in. In order to draw a conclusion as to pathological conditions, it is important to know approximately the number of mitoses normally occurring in a tissue. In the epidermis, for example, this number varies in each case according to the site; and similarly, external*** damage uncovers more exposed points, so that particularly the most freely exposed body parts demonstrate more mitoses than the protected parts. Lieberkühn's crypts show extraordinarily numerous mitoses; at least eight to ten times as many as the human skin. The mucous membranes, too, have a greater rate of cell increase than the epidermis. Quite markedly numerous, however, are the mitoses in the lymph glands, where in their germinal centres they are not less in number than in the rapidly growing tumours.

Under pathological conditions the number of mitoses can increase or decrease. The decrease is not automatically connected with lack of nutrition, for Morpugo (Archivo med. XII, no. 22, 1888) has shown that even in starvation, the karyokinesis proceeds almost unchanged. In spite of this, one will not be able to deny the influence of nutrition for the mitosis. Thus in sclerosis of the skin, one finds the mitoses in the epidermis extraordinarily reduced in number. In the lymph glands in fibrous degeneration, a significant reduction of mitosis is apparent. That, however, can also proceed without a new formation of fibrous tissue in the lymph glands, as when these glands are transformed into small bodies, in which Flemming's germinal centres lose their characteristic shape or form. The cause for the inactivity of the cells has not been explained in this case****. More understandable on the other hand is the reduction in mitoses by the effect of poison. If the tissue is in a state of phlegmony, or is flooded with leukocytes, mitoses disappear completely – a circumstance which was first recognised by Baumgarten in tuberculosis, but which probably has general validity. This can be related mainly to a poisonous effect of the simultaneously-present bacteria. Thus Baumgarten (Mycology vol. 1, p. 315) saw no mitoses in sites of pus which had been brought about by *Staphylococcus pyogenes aureus*. Perhaps, however, the excessive number of the leukocytes themselves or the serous insudation of the tissue can also play a role here, because I observed the same process where I was not able to prove the presence of bacteria.

*   Hansemann is not quite right here, – see chapter 6 of this volume (eds)
**   the modern word is "karyolysis" (eds)
***   "äusseren" is considered a misprint for "äussere" (eds)
**** The irony is that the lymphocytes, which he notes as multiplying so much in a way which cannot be explained, are the source of the antibodies (of Behring) which earlier in the article Hansemann has discounted (eds).

On the whole, the reductions of mitoses by pathological processes are less frequent than increases. The latter, however, do not follow on pathological stimulus, but need a certain period of time before they appear – the "incubation period"; between three hours (Garré: Chirurgische Beiträge von Bruns, IV 1889) and 3 days (v. Büngner: Regeneration of the nerves, Ziegler's Beiträge vol. 10, p. 321) – in each case according to tissue and process. One finds the most numerous mitoses in new formations; these, however, do not therefore always have to be malignant, as Schütz ("Carcinoma Findings", Frankfurt, 1890) believes. IN AND FOR ITSELF, MALIGNANCY HAS NOTHING TO DO WITH THE RAPIDITY OF GROWTH AND THE NUMBER OF MITOSES OBSERVED.

Concerning 4. It has been shown that regeneration of most tissues, particularly physiological regeneration, does not occur just anywhere. Flemming was the first to indicate that a layer – the germinal layer – exists in the skin, in which mitoses are found exclusively. In the same way he described the germinal centres in the lymph glands. A similar matrix, we know, through Kraft's work (Ziegler's Beiträge vol. 1. p. 85) is present in the periosteum for bone formation; for cartilage growth we have long since recognised the epiphyseal plate as the place for cell division. Under pathological conditions these germinal places can become more extensive – such as in the skin, the cartilage, and the periosteum, – or they may become completely indistinct as in the lymph glands. They may disappear completely or almost completely by the reduction of the mitoses. By this change the whole tissue acquires a definite stamp, which is characteristic for any condition.

In those tissues which normally contain no mitoses, we know of no such germinal centres or layers, even in pathological changes. The division figures appear, furthermore, at the most various points; mostly apparently without cause, sometimes, however, localised by a recognisable cause. Thus for example, they occur in liver cells in closest proximity to loci of interstitial inflammation.

In the above I have only hurried over a large area which, in part, is still only in a state of development (*Werden**). I have picked out only single examples from the wealth of material available, in order to show what significant contribution the understanding of karyokinesis has made to the recognition of pathological conditions, and is still able to make. From this, the conclusion may be drawn that Virchow's teaching of cell physiology and pathology, brought to victory under such difficult circumstances, has no limitations, as some believe; but that on the contrary, we can still expect many important things from it, and that in it, the master of pathology has raised an imperishable monument, on which the most stormy advances of science have left no signs of erosion.

* The usage of the word echoes Luther "*Nun steht es mit uns aber so: wir sind's nicht, wir werden's aber.*" ("Now this is how things stand with us: We are not, but we are becoming." – eds).

Chapter 10

On the anaplasia of tumour cells and asymmetric mitosis

(Hansemann 1892a)

Editors' summary of points

p. 436 no cancer-specific cell – no carcinoma-specific karyokinetic processes either – carcinomas of the various epithelia behave differently; 437 carcinomas show variable specialised functional features – anaplastic means "less differentiated" than mother cells and possessing relatively greater capacity to exist independently – anaplasia does not exist to the same degree in all circumstances; 438 Ribbert's and Ströbe's attacks on role of "polar bodies"; 439 Weismann has retracted ideas on polar bodies – but egg-type dedifferentiation and cancer cell behaviour might still be related – Noeggerath makes similar error – other misquotations of Hansemann; 440 anaplasia can exist in different degrees in the same tumour – often more in metastases; 441 returns to processes of cell and nuclear division – these are most different from normal in carcinomas – cell type-specific differences in karyokinesis; 442 these differences in shape, number of chromosomes etc – it is possible to identify a cell type by the appearances of its mitosis – but not to identify types of carcinomas; 443 Ribbert disagrees with Hansemann's theory of anaplasia, because of changes in metastases – semantic problem of "epithelial character"; 444 counting of human chromosomes – perishing versus wandering of individual chromosomes – Ribbert's views; 445 literature review of errant chromosomes – Ribbert's view discussed; 446 Ströbe's objections – Ströbe's methodological errors; 447 Ströbe has probably not avoided the "incomplete mitosis" artefact through cutting sections too thin – and made further incorrect interpretations; 448 Karg has objected to Hansemann's findings without good reason – reports finding an asymmetric mitosis in a sarcoma cell; 449 Ströbe's error on frequency of asymmetrical mitosis – case of carcinoma of urinary tract diagnosed by asymmetric mitoses in fragments in urine – difficulties of diagnosing asymmetric mitoses when chromosome counts cannot be done.

When one first began to analyse tumours in a histologically more detailed way, many investigators pursued the goal of discovering the histological *specificum* for carcinomata, and for a while it was believed that in the tailed cells (*geschwänzten Zellen*) in specific carcinoma cells this criterion had been identified. However, soon it was realised that such specific histological criteria do not exist; just as little as caseation and giant cells are characteristic of tuberculosis, no specific cell serves as the characteristic feature of carcinomas.

Then, recently, it was proposed that one could see certain karyokinetic processes as specific features in carcinomas (Schütz, "Microscopic Findings in Carcinoma", Frankfurt a. M. 1890). When I described asymmetric division of cells a few years ago, and reported that I had found it only in carcinomata in man – and that it was a rare exception in the rest of the animal kingdom – the widespread view developed that this form of cell division was absolutely characteristic of carcinomata. Nevertheless, I had always stated the theoretical possibility, or even

436

indeed the probability, of the existence of this process in other situations (this Archive vol. 119).

Now in almost all papers that are concerned with the process of cell division in carcinomata – from work carried out with the declared aim to find the histological *specificum* for carcinomata – the talk is always about carcinomata in general. However, it has been known for a long time that carcinomata of the stomach, for example, or of the gut, the epidermis, of the liver or oesophagus etc, behave completely differently; thus as we must assume – from all more recent investigations – that carcinomata

develop from the specific parenchyma and the stroma of each organ, so one would have to conclude that the carcinomata compared to each other should themselves really behave just as differently as the organs (are different) from each other.

But not even the carcinomata of one and the same organ are identical as far as their configuration and the physiological capacities of their cells are concerned. Thus, for example, there are carcinomata of the epidermis – the cells of which behave in a very similar way to normal epidermal cells – which form clear squamous cells (*Riffzellen*) and which perish with the same regularity after keratinisation as the squamous cells do. Carcinomata which consist of such cells do not form ulcers but only form an epidermoidal organ which is vaguely reminiscent macroscopically of scar tissue or scleroderma. In contrast, the cells of other epidermal carcinomata only incompletely keratinise and do not transform themselves into a protective cover: these can lead to eczematous or ulcerating proliferations. Yet other epidermal carcinomata lack any hint of any keratinisation; it is those which often produce extensive ulcerations. Similar differences can be brought forward for the carcinomata of almost every other organ. Thus, for example, there are colon carcinomata with lovely cylindrical and goblet cells which look very similar to simple polyps when looked at superficially histologically; there are others, however, where the cylindrical form of the cells and the formation of gland-like tubular structures can hardly be recognised; in others again, the structure does not even remotely resemble that of the original tissue.

When I was developing a histogenetic theory of carcinomata (this Archive vol. 119 pp 314 ff) I introduced the word "anaplastic" to describe their cells and meant to express by that, that the cells of the carcinomata are less differentiated than the cells of the mother tissue and that they possess a relatively greater ability to exist independently. One can see from the examples above that anaplasia of tumours does not reach the same degree in all situations. To return to the extraordinarily characteristic example of the epidermis, I suggest that there is a lesser degree of anaplasia in carcinomata with strong keratinisation than in those lacking keratinisation.

Or, in gut cancers, those cells which still contain tubular structures with cylindrical cells or even allow us to recognise goblet cells preserved, show a lesser degree of anaplasia than gut carcinomata with polymorphic transitional cells.

Ribbert has reviewed my work (this Archive vol. 119), in the Deutsch. Med. Wochenschr. 1890 and in the Centralblatt für pathologische Anat. (1890, p. 362) as well as in discussion (D. med. W. 13 October 1891, p. 1183, no. 42) and has dragged exclusively into the foreground the comparison used by me of the expulsion of the polar body in the case of the egg. Ströbe too (Ziegler's Beiträge vol. XI, pp 10 and 11) seems to have interpreted this the same way, as if my theory of anaplasia of tumour cells was only built on the comparison with the polar body. My comments in that respect (see p. 321 as above) are as follows:

"Whether or not the significance of the first polar body is as Weismann says, or if this (namely the de-differentiation/*Entdifferenzirung*) has already happened beforehand in some way or another"

and further below that:

"One can see that my theory is very much similar to Weismann's view; however, I want to leave it aside for the moment whether this whole process can be attributed to the first polar body alone."

Here you can see, as from the entire development of my theory on anaplasia, that they did nothing more than just use the comparison, and never attempted to explain the process of anaplasia by the expulsion of the first polar body. Neither is my theory built on the theory of expulsion of the polar body as Ribbert and Ströbe seem to think. This is more than evident from the sentence I coined earlier: "Every asymmetrical division of a cell means changes in degree of differentiation. It thus has to be seen in parallel with a new generational stage of oncogenetic development. Therefore, asymmetrical division each time it occurs, has to be linked to a change in the energy of growth and direction of growth". Where here is anything about the polar body? And yet it is precisely in this sentence that the essence of my theory of anaplasia is very clearly declared. But it seems to me

that the analogy with the polar bodies was so blinding that everything else disappeared, and therefore I really regret that I ever made this comparison at all. One can see from this that I strayed onto the polar body only because of the significance which Weismann attributed to it. Weismann himself has now himself given up this theory ("Amphimitis" Jena 1891) and it does not occur to me to defend a theory against its originator. Therewith my comparison with the polar body falls down, but not the matter itself. I still would like to maintain that the development of the mature egg from the somatic cell, just as much as is the development of a carcinoma cell from the mother tissue, happens through anaplasia, that is, by dedifferentiation and increased capability for independent existence. Even if the polar body has nothing to do with anaplasia of the egg, it has no relationship to asymmetrical cell division either, which does not change anything of the matter at all, as Ribbert and Ströbe seem to think.

But matters did not end with these expressions of opinion by these two authors; the representation that Ribbert had given to my theory has had further consequences. Noeggerath namely, on p. 31 of his monograph ("Essays on the Structure and Development of the Carcinoma", Wiesbaden, 1892) copies Ribbert's lowermost paragraph verbatim (up to the omission of the word "Figures" after the word "asymmetric" and the addition of the word "first" in front of the word "polar bodies" in lines one and four of the paragraph) from the work (Deutsche med. W. 13 Oct 1891, separate print, p. 12, lines 25–36) without citing him. Naturally, all the erroneous views of Ribbert are therefore also repeated here. But that is not all, for Hauser has reviewed the work of Noeggerath (Münchener med. Wochenschr. 1892, 7 June, p. 411) and said there that Noeggerath has refuted my "hypothesis based on wrong premises", in which I "bring into parallel the asymmetrical nuclear division as observed in carcinomata with the expulsion of the first polar body of the egg" and so on and so on.

Now, however, the relevant sentence by Ribbert (as above, p. 12, lines 25-36), contains two further erroneous statements about my theory which I have never expressed, namely that the carcinoma cells "lose their property of being epithelial cells and thereby become indifferent and particularly capable of proliferation." Ribbert has placed "indifferent" where I said "less differentiated (*weniger differenzirt*)" and "capable of proliferation" where I used "greater ability to exist independently". But these are words are not synonymous and cannot be interchanged at will.

440   After all, "less differentiated" does not mean "quite de-differentiated" which only then would mean "indifferent"; and a greater ability to exist independently is a long way from involving an increased ability to proliferate. Every healthy animal cell is capable of proliferation, but the daughters of the metazoa are dependent on each other, and it is this dependency which, in my opinion, is reduced in carcinoma cells but not totally abolished.

The term "capable of proliferation" indeed means something completely different. It creates the impression that I had composed a theory of the aetiology of carcinomata which indeed is believed by Noeggerath and also, it seems, by Hauser. Likewise Alberts (Deutsche Medicinalzeitung, 1891, no. 34), and Ströbe seem to be of the same opinion too. However, according to my entire deliberations which naturally I cannot reiterate here in full, I am only proposing a histogenetic theory which does not touch upon the question of aetiology at all.

If now a certain degree of anaplasia applies to every carcinoma it would be of interest whether this degree can be changed in the very same cancer. Probably not every carcinoma can provide such information, but only those which display a certain degree of anaplasia, have metastases, and originate from an organ with cells which possess well characterised physiological properties. Such organs, for example, are epidermis, oesophagus, trachea and the colon. I have found by study of a large number of such carcinomata with little anaplasia – and their metastases – that the degree of anaplasia does not always change; however commonly it increases, and in a manner such that in the first regional lymph node group, the degree of anaplasia changes only little; but with each subsequent group of lymph nodes it increases more. Never have I observed the step backward to normal which would represent prosoplasia; in all this, however, I cannot state with confidence that this might not occur occasionally.

For example, I was studying a cancroid of the oesophagus with squamous cell formation and characteristic keratinisation. In bronchial lymph nodes which were situated very close to the primary cancer, keratinisation was less clear and found to a lesser degree with only a few scattered spinous cells being present here and there. Further metastases were present in the mesenteric lymph nodes, and in the liver. Those did not display any keratinisation

apart from scanty evidence of it occasionally and spinous cells were altogether absent. Thus, these cells are able to change their character; they depart in their nature ever further from the mother cells and the result is different each time. The whole histological picture in extreme cases can be so different in the metastases compared to the primary tumour, that* one might be led to believe one was looking at a completely different cancer if one did not have the different transitional stages in all the lymph nodes as evidence.

If after this, I return to the processes of cell and nuclear division, then what comes out of all of this is that one may not contemplate nuclear division processes in carcinomata in isolation, but should always compare them with what goes on in the mother tissues. In this, it is generally established that the mitotic processes in the stroma are not necessarily different from simple regeneration or inflammatory proliferation, whilst the karyokineses of the "carcinoma parenchyma" are often substantially different from those of the mother tissue.

It is only natural that until now one struggled to trace all forms of karyokinesis back to the common scheme; through the careful investigations of many researchers, agreement has been achieved concerning such a scheme in most tissues. There are only a few indications in the literature pointing to the fact that here and there some authors found specific deviations from this scheme in individual types of tissue (for example, Grawitz, Verhandlungen d. X intern. Congresses, Berlin, vol. II, chapter III, p. 9; Müller, On the question of leukaemia, Deutsches Arch. f. kl. Med., vol. 48, p. 51. Also Flemming and others).

In an abbreviated form, I pointed out last autumn (Karyokinesis and the Cellular Pathology, Berl. klin. Wochenschrift, 13 October 1891) that with sufficient training one can differentiate the mitotic figures of different tissues from each other and specify the characteristics of them; on that occasion, I mentioned that these differences might be extended to all parts of the process, or also only to individual parts of them. The differences

* "se" is considered a misprint for "so" (eds)

are in regard to the shape, perhaps to the number of chromosomes, to centrosomes, to the achromatic spindles, and to the area of the divisional zone or to the size of the entire mitotic figures; furthermore, there are differences in terms of duration of the phases and the situation of the mitoses within the tissue. Here unfortunately, I must restrain myself from presenting the proofs of these assertions of mine because the reproduction of all of these would clearly be beyond the scope of this particular journal. The differences are so characteristic that they can be easily demonstrated by the means of photography. During the Surgical Congress in Berlin in 1892, I exhibited a large number of such photographs which I was thus able to demonstrate to a large number of colleagues. These pictures will soon be published in another place. The typical figures recur in the individual tissues with extraordinary regularity again and again, and if one has seen a large number of them, one becomes so used to the differences in shapes, that one can determine the type of tissue from the individual mitosis.

In the parenchyma of carcinomata, however, this changes significantly and in fact the mitoses are the more different from the mother tissue the more strongly the cancer is anaplastic. This finding is repeated everywhere with the utmost regularity: the mitoses of slightly anaplastic tumours are very similar to those of the mother tissue; the ones of strongly anaplastic tumours, however, bear little or no resemblance any more to those of the mother tissue. In addition, mitoses become extraordinarily different from each other, so that sometimes one cannot speak any more of a specific type at all. In these cases, dwarf or giant forms and excesses of the most general kind most often are found; and it is in these tissues that one finds the clearest asymmetrical mitoses – a process by which normal cells give rise to cells with fewer than a normal number of chromosomes; which I believe has an intimate relationship to the anaplasia of tumours.

Against this theory of mine Ribbert argues (Deutsche med. Wochenschr., 13 October 1891, separate print, p. 13)

with the words: "If one now adds the fact that there can scarcely be talk of the presumed dedifferentiation of epithelial cells in so far as the cells maintain their epithelial character even in the latest metastases, then it becomes questionable to some extent whether the interpretation of asymmetrical mitoses which Hansemann attempted, will be sustainable". From this it is not clear whether "original" refers to mother tissue or to the first beginnings of the carcinoma. In reference to the first, it is well known that carcinoma cells maintain neither the morphological nor functional characteristics of the mother cells to the same extent. If it is possible that cancers with transitional cell characteristics can develop from cylindrical epithelium – or that cancroids can develop from ciliated epithelium – one can hardly any more call this the maintenance of the original "epithelial character"; the more so in view of the countless finer differences which can be recognised between the respective resting cells; and particularly in those undergoing the process of dividing. Above I deliberated on the different degrees of anaplasia and made clear that the very definition of this is based on the varyingly strong degree of deviation of the carcinoma cells from the mother tissue.

As far as the second possibility is concerned, namely, that Ribbert with the word "original" was referring to the early stages of the carcinoma formation: I have shown before and proven through numerous slides that in many cases the metastases contain cells with deviations which are different in principle from those of the primary tumour, morphologically as well as especially functionally: this can be defined as the degree of anaplasia increasing in the metastases. Thus in this case too, I have to contradict Ribbert's view.

Finally, however, I have great reservations about the term "epithelial characters" in general. Indeed, one reads this term in many places, but by this everyone imagines something different. It would lead too far here, if I were to go into the meaning and the history of the term, and its enlivening admixture of theories of germinal layers. At the moment the circumstances have not been clarified at all, and it certainly is not in vain that in Kölliker's masterly "Handbook of Histology", 6th edn, 1889, there is no mention of epithelium anywhere in the classification. Here, where we are talking of morphological things in the fully grown body, one can certainly not make the definitions other than morphologically; and accordingly "epithelial" signifies only a location. However, as one comprehends the definition, it is always the LOCATION which thrusts itself into the foreground, with emphasis on the covering of surfaces and the lining of hollow spaces with the orientation towards an upper surface. The word "character" demands that one regards the cell in and for itself, dissociated from its environment. Here it has always been incomprehensible to me how one can speak of an epithelial character in general; on the contrary, the history of normal and pathological histology has taught me that much confusion has been caused by this. One can speak of the character of a renal, a liver, an epidermal cell, and so on,

or of a cubical, cylindrical, ciliated or goblet cell; but it is not possible for me to establish a morphologically common character for all these cells. However, often too, in the literature, there is talk of "epithelial character", even of an "epithelioid" one. I have nowhere been able to find a really satisfying definition of this character, and now, indeed, the "originally epithelial character" in carcinomas is supposed to be retained in cells which arrive at a different location with every new* lesion and which are often so different both amongst themselves and from the mother cells. To sum up, it may perhaps be more correct to drop the word "epithelium" completely for a type of tissue, and to apply it only where the matter has to do with cells in particular locations as moreover, is done by Disse ("Basics of Histology", Stuttgart 1892).

Human chromosomes usually cannot be counted; one must estimate them and that poses major difficulties. In carcinomata one finds cells which are clearly not cut through (because there are layers of cells above as well as below) and in which it is very easily possible to count the chromosomes, and in which one also finds occasionally a rather surprisingly low number of them. Such cells are generated, as I believe I have proven (this Archive vol. 119 and 123) in two different ways which are not different in principle from each other. Firstly, through the perishing of individual chromosomes (not to be confused with errant chromosomes) and secondly due to asymmetrical cell division. Now Ribbert says (same separate printing as above p. 12): "I should like to set against the view (namely, the view in "On the meaning of asymmetrical mitosis") that I (Ribbert) failed to establish any clear distinction between asymmetrical mitosis and pathological nuclear division figures[1]. It seems to me as though the asymmetry and displacement of single or small groups of chromosomes simply resemble different degrees of the same abnormality. And if a cell division can follow there, then, given the relatively slight deviations, there is really nothing striking here". Ribbert simply states here what I have said myself already (vol. 123, p. 362, this Archive). Such errant chromosomes, to my knowledge, were first described by Retzius

[1] That should probably be: "the REMAINING pathological nucleus division figures" because after all it is not to be doubted too that the asymmetric division figures are pathological ones.
* metastatic implied – eds

(Biological Researches. 1881, no. 9) as "peripherally situated loops" and were depicted in Tab. 12, Figs 11, 14 and 26. Schottländer subsequently (Arch. f. mikr. Anat. vol. 31, p. 457), has declared these to be pathological and has introduced the name "displaced loops". Flemming has proved their frequent occurrence in the lungs of salamander larva and demonstrated this at the Anatomical Congress in 1891 (in Munich). I have convinced myself of this latter fact with numerous preparations. These errant chromosomes usually lie in the region of one of the poles at the stage of the monaster, and they are not only found in the lungs of salamander larva, but also in the gill plates, in the mylo-hyoid plate, in the pulmonary mesentery and in the peritoneum. They are just as sharp and clear as all the other chromosomes and I do not have any doubts that these later enter the mitotic figure. I base this on the fact that in later stages such irregularities cannot be proved. Such figures, which are not infrequently found in humans as well, thus cannot be considered pathological.

Now, however, there are figures which I have published, for example, in Tab. 10, Fig. 22 (this Archive vol. 123). There the chromosomes lie completely outside the mitotic figure – not only outside the spindle, which can happen normally – but also outside the entire divisional zone. They stain less intensively and are not as well delineated, so that they give the impression that they are in the process of dissolving in the protoplasm. These forms of errant chromosomes are, in my opinion, about to perish, while the rest of the mitotic figure looks completely intact and leads, as I discussed above, to hypochromatism. Thus Ribbert is in complete agreement with me as far as he refers to this second form of errant chromosomes, as he is not able to separate this sharply from an asymmetrical mitosis. I too place them on a level with the displaced chromosomes, in that if

On the anaplasia of tumour cells and asymmetric mitosis

a larger number of chromosomes becomes errant, it happens in the form of an asymmetrical cell division, whereas single chromosomes within the cell can just perish. That Ribbert sees "nothing special" here

does not change the facts and would hardly be sufficient to refute my data. I have so far only discovered displaced degenerating chromosomes in carcinomata and a few sarcomata.

With reference to asymmetric mitosis, it is Ströbe who has presented most opposition to my view (Cellular processes and mitosis in tumours. Ziegler's Beiträge, vol. XI). Ströbe denies any particular biological importance of asymmetric mitoses and maintains that he has seen them also in sarcomas, in benign tumours and in various inflammatory and regenerative conditions. He says on p. 3 "In general, we recognise an asymmetry in both daughter nuclei if the latter, seen in flat plane, show different sizes." The following comment should be made here: if one views only the flat plane, that is to say, looks at it two-dimensionally, then one will certainly find asymmetric mitoses very frequently. It is absolutely necessary here, as in general in microscopic investigations, that one makes use of three-dimensional study; that Ströbe has not yet acquired the necessary practice in this is clear from the fact that he wishes to exclude all figures which do lie exactly in one visual plane. Just how seldom one encounters figures which correspond to Ströbe's postulate becomes very clear if one photographs the figures, as I have done for some time now. Only very seldom is one successful in finding daughter stars which in photographs appear equally large. But this is not the central point at all. I have always emphasised that one should not estimate the chromatin mass but the number of chromosomes. It is obvious and as I believe, for anyone familiar with these things, almost unnecessary to remark that one cannot for example estimate whether a star contains twenty-eight or thirty chromosomes. But it is certainly possible to estimate whether a star contains, say 30 or, say 10, chromosomes. For this the stars do not have to lie "in one plane" at all, if one is sufficiently practised in seeing such things; I agree totally with Ströbe when he says (p. 5): "For my part, I have reached the conclusion that it is certainly not so easy to achieve the relevant experience, even after considerable work on this subject". That one finds a sequence of doubtful pictures, I gladly admit, and one will do well to exclude the latter from these investigations.

One must, on the other hand, be particularly aware of one danger: that is the danger of the cutting through of individual cells. In every tissue with numerous mitoses one finds that the thinner the section is, the more cut through cells are seen. In my first work, I thought it hardly necessary to point out that avoiding too-thin sections was my first care (this Archive, vol 119), because I regarded it as so obvious. *A priori*, I therefore made the sections as thick as the examination permitted (seldom under 10 μ). In my second publication, I then included the following sentence, after some oral objections had been made to me: (this Archive vol. 123, p. 357) "One is always on the right track if, in estimating the chromosomal cluster, or the number of chromosomes, one chooses only those cells whose upper and lower borders are still overlapped by neighbouring cells, so that a section was not possible." Ströbe apparently overlooked this sentence because he has gathered together all other remarks from my work bearing on this, quoted them and on that basis, criticised my figures individually; this sentence alone he has not considered; otherwise, perhaps, his criticism would have reached many different conclusions.

Incidentally, I have always emphasised myself the figures in my tables which I did not regard as quite conclusive, so that Ströbe does not need to emphasise these doubts yet again, and formulate them into an attack on me. Those are probably the only points where we are in agreement with each other (Figs 8, 12). Since then I have re-studied my Fig. 15, which Ströbe doubts quite particularly, and have been able to establish that it is certainly not cut through, because cell layers are situated both above and below it.

In consequence, I believe that the difference between Ströbe and myself has arisen because Ströbe regarded the flat-plane pictures as decisive, and tried to estimate the chromatin mass, not the chromosome number; then on p. 10, he identified without further ado chromatin-poor nuclei (clearly he speaks here of resting nuclei) with hypochromatic nuclei and incorrectly attributes this view to me. Now again in opposition to Ströbe, I must repeat that I have hitherto never found an asymmetric mitosis (in my sense) in any tissue other than carcinomas. It is almost comical when Ströbe says (p. 7) that he has noted the absence of asymmetric mitoses in tumours in which absolutely no cell proliferation was to be discovered.

If asymmetric mitoses were really found in such numerous tissues as Ströbe describes, I should be prepared to dismiss the whole matter to the lumber room of artefacts, because such a finding would contradict the idea of the significance of karyokinesis too much. I cannot see my way to doing this, however, because the reports which support me – of positive results in carcinomas and negative ones in other tissues – have so increased, and I must take leave not to mention them individually. Provisionally, however, I must believe that for the most part, Ströbe has seen artefacts; I am strengthened in this view all the more because in his investigation, Ströbe used, in part, older preparations which originated in experiments by Podwyssozki, Coën and Fischer. Even if now, it is far from my wish to doubt the quality of these preparations – on the contrary, the well known works of these researchers prove that the most excellent preparations assisted them in their aims – it must nevertheless seem dangerous to use for

the present subtle investigations, preparations which were not made by oneself but which were made for a quite different aim, and whose sources of error one is quite incapable of controlling. I myself certainly exclude from my investigations all preparations which I have not fixed myself, and have treated further, so that I am *a priori* familiar with their entire genesis[1].

Karg (Concerning carcinoma. Deutsche Zeitschrift f. Chirurgie, vol. 34, Festschrift for Thiersch, pp 143–145) agrees in general with Ströbe's views, but unfortunately does not give details as to how he reached his view, so that an appropriate response is not easily possible. In the interests of the whole matter, it is very much to be wished that Karg, as well as Ströbe, would give the most accurate reproductions of any asymmetric mitosis which they have found in non-carcinomatous tissue. In the case of Karg, this would be of particular interest, because he is a well-known microscopic expert, and certainly has not limited himself to the examination of flat plane.

With reference to the following sentence of Karg, "From the epithelial cell, however, in spite of all influences which it may encounter from outside, nothing can emerge but again an epithelial cell." – which he introduces* in refutation of my theory – I can refer to what is said above (p. 443).

As I said above, I have so far only found asymmetrical mitoses in carcinomata. However, I have always pointed to the fact that probably they might be found in embryonic development as well. Hitherto I have never stated that they could only occur in carcinomata although I tend to accept that they only occur within carcinomata in adults. Above all, however, in carcinomata asymmetrical mitoses are rare, sometimes very rare.

---

[1] I said earlier that I have never seen asymmetric mitoses in sarcomas, and I have always regretted this, because from the start, I was keen to include sarcomas in the theory of cell anaplasia. Now, already in this Archive, (vol. 123, Plate X Fig. 20) a figure with degenerate errant chromosomes is pictured, which comes from a sarcoma, and since then I have often encountered** these findings. Hitherto, moreover, I have not found asymmetric cell divisions in sarcomas. Should Ströbe have been successful in really finding them, I should be very happy. In the light of his other findings, however, I must unfortunately still doubt it. Incidentally, Ströbe is totally in error if he believes that I wish, by asymmetric mitoses, to distinguish carcinomas from sarcomas. From the purely histologic standpoint, which is particularly adhered to by Virchow, there are so many transitional forms between these two forms of tumour that I doubt overall whether one will ever be able to draw such a sharp line of demarcation. This too is not at all in the interests of practice, as it is only a matter, after all, of separating malignant from benign tumours.

* sometimes a rather warlike phrase "bring into the field"
** almost certainly a misprint of "*erheben*" for "*erleben*"

This I have always emphasised; thus, I cannot comprehend how Ströbe could possibly say "I should like to believe that we should not assign to the process of asymmetrical karyokinesis the frequency that Hansemann assigns to it." In fact it is so frequent that I could not give it diagnostic importance even if it were characteristic for carcinomata. And yet there are always exceptions to this. Neelsen made an observation (and presented it to the Dresden Society for Natural Science) which I reproduce here with his permission. "A man was discharging small particles of tumour in his urine which in general displayed the characters of villous polyps (*Zottenpolypen*) *per se*, but contained surprisingly many asymmetrical mitoses." Based on this, Neelsen proclaimed the high probability that the diagnosis was a carcinoma and this diagnosis proved to be true as the disease progressed.

In general one must search for a very long time – unless one is especially lucky – before one sees a genuine asymmetrical mitosis; meaning a mitosis in which the stars contain a different number of chromosomes. It does not depend here whether the one star is a little bigger than the other, and I do not unduly credit such figures because they have neither a diagnostic nor a biological significance: but on the other hand, the only figures which are important, as far as I am concerned, are those in which one can conclude with certainty that the number of chromosomes is different or can even be counted as different.

This exhausts the common knowledge on the mitoses in carcinomata according to my experience. All other differences are only relative to the mother tissue and should only ever be discussed as forms of carcinoma in the context of the mother tissue. I reserve the right to elaborate on this further on a future occasion.

Chapter 11

"Studies on the Specificity, the Altruism and the Anaplasia of cells with Special Reference to Tumours"

(Hansemann 1893c)

Dedicated to Medical Counsellor,
Professor Doctor Rudolph Virchow,
his honoured teacher

As a sign of gratitude.

Editors' Summary of Points

Introduction

1–3 important developments in microscopy of the cell, cell division and fertilisation; 4 Hansemann's own methods of study of mitoses in human tissues – acknowledgments – surgeons, his own father, Countess Bose Foundation; 5 points on which Hansemann is opposed to Virchow.

I Specificity

6–7 Attacks the concept that "transitional forms" in histology can be used to establish sequences of morphological development – metaplasia is based on such studies; 8 despite the large number of articles, the significance of metaplasia is still uncertain – quotation from Bard's view of specificity of cells – also Ziegler's and v. Recklinghausen's views – alternative concept of histological adaptation; 9 special problems of transitional images in relation to metaplasia – Virchow's views; 10 problems of transitional forms in deciding sequences of events in cell division – special cytological features are lost while a cell divides – in this period the cell approaches its "archetype" – similar changes in dividing Protozoa – plasma cells and mast cells not seen to divide; 11 loss of functional features makes examination of mitosis easier in cells – early literature of mitosis; 12 Flemming found more than one form of mitosis in salamander testes – more literature on cell-type – specific features of mitoses; 13–14 importance of fixatives – Hansemann's methods using sublimate and haematoxylin etc; 15 photomicroscopic methods; 16 to 17 cell types which do or do not show mitoses; 18 to 19 use of "physiological regeneration" – in some tissues, they are seen only in pathological conditions – in inflammation and regeneration, the type of mitosis remains the same as normally in the cell type; 20 circumstances in which a cell type cannot be determined by the form of its mitosis – but there are individual differences between the mitoses according to cell type; 21 some mitoses do not show any tissue-characteristic features; 22 states he has defended himself against unjust attacks – *The size of the division figure* (according to cell type); 24 *Behaviour of achromatic figures*; 25–26 *Chromosomes*; 27–28 *Division space*; 29 *Cell Division*; 30–32 *The duration of the process and the period of incubation*; 33–34 *Position of the mitoses*; 35 perceptible differences in the process of cell division

179

"Studies on the Specificity, the Altruism and the Anaplasia of cells with Special Reference to Tumours"

of individual tissue types exist; 36 no transitional forms – cell lineages are retained – disagrees with v. Recklinghausen, Baumgarten, Ribbert and Schmidt; 37 transition appearances can be influenced by external conditions – Bard's summary *omnis cellula e cellula ejusdem generis* is correct – metaplasia is not a general phenomenon but occurs only occasionally; 38 specificity in relation to post-fertilisation development in the embryo – mechanical/accommodation theories are incorrect – differentiation by division of labour (internal cellular mechanisms); 39 reviews Roux's experiments on blastomeres; 40 Virchow points out identical twins come from blastomeres – movements of cells in blastulae; 41 embryological studies which support the statement that new generation stages in embryonic tissue development take place by asymmetric mitosis; 42 reviews theories of how differentiation takes place; 43 some situations in which accommodation takes place – theory of qualitative distribution of idioplasmas; 44 Weismann has taken up Hansemann's view that main plasmas and auxiliary plasmas must exist – Hertwig's view that asymmetric mitoses cannot explain regeneration in lower animals – matter to be discussed in next chapter.

II Altruism

45 Hansemann's concept of how plasmas are changed during embryological and cell development; 46 the egg as the least differentiated cell – differentiation as the result of asymmetric distribution of hereditary properties – addendum implies that all that matters is a particular "balance" of factors determining what differentiation takes place; 47 daughter cells as antagonists – lesser plasmas to explain galls – results of transplantation experiments considered less significant than previously; 48 more studies show that irretrievable separations of idioplasmas do not take place – therefore now joins with Hertwig, de Vries and Nägeli (in embryology) but asymmetric division still explains regeneration; 49 how in the egg, a balance of chromosomes is restored to previous "undifferentiated" state after "differentiation" to a germinal ovarian epithelial cell – destruction of excess plasmata in oogenesis preferred – the number of generation stages from egg to egg is the least of any cell sequence; 50 in regeneration "THE FEWER GENERATIONAL STAGES THE EGG HAS GONE THROUGH, THE EASIER REGENERATION IS POSSIBLE"; 51 regeneration can only be explained if LESSER PLASMATA IN GENERAL GO INTO ACTION AGAIN THE MORE EASILY, THE FEWER THE GENERATIONAL STAGES HAVE GONE BY SINCE THE ORGANISM BEGAN AS THE EGG" – altruism is the loss of capacity for independent existence associated with increasing differentiation; 52 altruism considered as manifest by the dependence of the whole body on each individual type of organ; 53 functions of organs seen as both positive and negative; 54 role of the pancreas in diabetes – communicates his own results here; 55 negative functions of the kidneys – destruction of the adrenal glands and "bronze disease" 56 compensatory hypertrophy of kidney – positive functions underlie altruism; 57 gonadal tissue is not altruistic – mammary hypertrophy in pregnancy as "altruistic hypertrophy" – "altruistic atrophy"; 58 altruistic interactions between mothers and embryos – death of adults after parturition or fertilisation; 59 death by exhaustion versus death by involution; 60 all this is well known – disagrees with Weismann on death being related to a fixed cell type – and with the view that ageing can be identified by histological changes; 61 altruism seen in animals as the relationship between germinal cells – altruism is a manifestation of the gain in differentiation and loss in capacity of independent existence which follows asymmetric mitoses over several generation stages.

III Anaplasia

62 chromatin level in normal cells; 63 opinions of Roux – significance of the polar bodies; 64 laws of chromosome numbers; 65 the number of chromosomes alone does not determine the type of the cell; 66 pluri-polar mitoses – fates of hyperchromatic cells; 67 reduction divisions in gametogenesis – restoration of the *status quo ante* – not seen in other cells; 68 Virchow's classification of tumours – definition of carcinomas – Amman's view of histogenesis of carcinomas; 69 methods for determining histogenesis of carcinomas – nature and definition of "epithelium"; 70 tumours and germ

"Studies on the Specificity, the Altruism and the Anaplasia of cells with Special Reference to Tumours"

layers – archiblastomas and parablastomas – no good definition in the literature; 71 Thiersch and Waldeyer on derivation of carcinomas from epithelia; 72 origin of stroma in carcinomas – sarcomas in classification of tumours; 73 distinguishing carcinomas from sarcomas – sarcomas must produce intercellular substance; 74 stromal cells of tumours – parenchymal cells give rise to tumour cells; 75 loss of characters by the mother tissue can be marked – importance for diagnosis; 76 degrees of histological change in carcinomas; 77 worse in metastases – CARCINOMAS CAN IN THEIR CONFIGURATION BE VERY MUCH LIKE THE MOTHER TISSUE OR CAN DEVIATE FROM IT TO VARYING DEGREES; THE STRONGEST DEGREE OF DEVIATION MAY OCCUR STRAIGHT AWAY AT THE START OR IS REACHED ONLY GRADUALLY IN THE METASTASES; 78 behaviour of individual cells – (in footnote) not related to cells being "younger"; 79 persisting cellular functions in carcinoma cells – motility in cancer cells – shown by Virchow and later others; 80 growth of transplants – adult cell emboli die; 81 adult cell transplants die, only malignant tumours survive – (BOTH) THE DEPENDENCY OF TUMOUR CELLS ON THEIR SPECIFIC ENVIRONMENT (AND) THE ALTRUISM HAVE WANED MORE THAN IS TO BE FOUND OTHERWISE (IN ANY PATHOLOGICAL CONDITION) IN ANY OTHER CELL TYPE OF ANIMALS OF HIGHER ORDER; 82 the carcinoma cells' ability to exist independently has increased and their altruism has decreased; as far as we know it is that which sets them aside from all other human cells, with the exception of germ cells – therefore a de-differentiation has taken place – hence "anaplasia" – but anaplastic cells are not embryonic cells; 83 clarification of anaplastic cells – in terms of plasmata theories – they are cells in which plasmata which have been in the background are now increased in relevance again – in plants with galls, the recurrence of obsolete galls can be found – germinal epithelium of ovary gives rise to follicular cells as well; 84 the process of anaplasia in tumour cells does not go so far that these cells are identical to those of normal development – but they must contain germ plasma in quantity – cell division processes in tumours – above all hyperchromatic mitoses which lead to dual and multiple division; 85 multiple divisions only occur in clumps which include other mitoses – tumour cell mitoses proceed through the same phases as mitoses in normal cells – degree of mitotic abnormalities correlates with other deviations of the cells; 86 mitoses in tumour stroma are not abnormal; in relation to regeneration, hyperplasia and inflammation – DURING PROCESSES IN WHICH THE TISSUE TYPE IS NOT ALTERED, IT SEEMS A JUSTIFIED CONCLUSION TO ME THAT THE CHANGED FORM OF MITOSES IS THE CAUSE OF THE TISSUE CHANGES; 87 thus new tissue has developed just as new tissue develops during embryonic development – chromatin considerations in differentiation – in embryos there may be no change in visible chromatin – possible involvement of non-chromatin hereditary material – after asymmetric division, which one of the daughter cells becomes the mother cell of the new tissue? 88 asymmetric division and perishing of individual chromosomes can give rise to reduced chromosomes – tumours in which asymmetric divisions have been found; 89 literature of very hypochromatic (dwarf) forms; 90 dwarf forms are not parasites – individuality of chromosomes recognised. "Now, if this lost part was exactly the one which gave predominance to a certain property in the cell, then that had to result in a less differentiated cell or in that which I called anaplasia" – plasmas may change – "or any other variation whatsoever"; 91 degrees of imbalance of properties and degrees of anaplasia – no objections in the literature are significant; 92 summary: cells in embryonic life become specific (cannot replace each other), gain differentiation, lose capacity to exist independently and increase their altruistic relationships with each other. Anaplasia is when all these changes are reversed together in an adult cell – it comes about because main plasmas are lost and minor plasmas come to the fore – metastases form more easily in proportion to the degree of anaplasia – some exceptions; 93 quantifying anaplasia – no equivalent in benign tumours; 94 the theory is not in any way about aetiology .

"Studies on the Specificity, the Altruism and the Anaplasia of cells with Special Reference to Tumours"

Introduction

1   Pliny the Younger once said: *In minimus tota latet natura*; nowhere has this pronouncement been proved more thoroughly than in the biological sciences, although the interpretation of what one understands by smallest, has changed considerably. When in 1667[1] Robert Hooke first described the cell, he meant hollow spaces in cork, that is to say, what today one can see reasonably well with a magnifying glass. He did not describe them in order thereby to present a new discovery to the public, but to show what small things could be seen with his excellent new microscopes. The cellular spaces of the cork were thus, for him, the smallest things. When the worm of trichinosis was discovered everyone talked of these small things which had been discovered in muscle and many people doubted whether such small animals were capable of producing such great disturbances. When compared with the smallest cells, they can still be called small; but now we are talking of the trichinosis worms as large powerful organisms which by that, were a long time ago forced out of the category of the smallest things. Today, when every research worker and a large proportion of doctors and even many a lay person owns excellent microscopes with the highest magnification, it is scarcely comprehensible that Virchow, who is still living amongst us and at the height of his powers, in his youth scarcely 45 years ago, had to fight the most difficult struggles for the use of the microscope in medical science, and that it was necessary to write long articles,[2] in order to defend

[1] "Micrographia or Some Physiological Descriptions of Minute Bodies made by Magnifying Glasses". London 1667
[2] On the reform of pathological and therapeutic opinions through microscopic investigations. Virchow's Archiv. vol. 1, p. 207, 1847.

2   the proposition "It is necessary that our views advance as quickly as our ability to see things down the microscope has been extended: the entire field of medicine must get 300 times closer to natural processes".

The cell was discovered and within it the nucleus and nuclear bodies (probably nucleoli – eds); it was believed that with this we had reached the limits of biological units. Since then, however, a whole mass of much smaller things has not only been seen and described, but recognised for their significance. We know that the cell which was once upon a time supposed to be the smallest of possible things is a most highly complicated apparatus in which a host of life phenomena (*Lebenserscheinungen*) are carried out. We know that apart from a thread-like substance which is contained in the nucleus, there are fine granules which carry out very complicated functions, which when separated become diseased, and which also divide and can increase. Only in recent years have we come to know a component of the cells; – the attraction granules, which are smaller than anything which has been known hitherto, for, looked at with the most powerful magnifications, they still appear as the most minute dot-shaped forms. Yet we must attribute to them a most highly complicated structure and a capacity which no other part of the cell possesses; they are able to force the threads and granules of the cell into a definite order and, finally, (are able) to compel the cell to divide itself in – emphatically – a specific way with always the same biological result. That in this they might be the purely passive middle point of the remaining cell components appears, according to observations made, to be completely out of the question. This allows us to recognise that in this respect we are still a long way from the limits of (things which) biologically stand alone (*Selbstständigkeit*) and we recall Strassburger's sentence which seems to go without saying but all the same is not sufficiently heeded:[1] "It would certainly be a strange chance if precisely now, given the proven capacity of our instruments, the lowermost frontier of life had been reached".

Now, unfortunately, with the power of our instruments, we have come close to the theoretically possible frontier. Helmholtz[2]* has shown us that the ultimate ramparts which have been thrown up, are not through the weaknesses of our technology, but by the nature of light and the limitations of our eyes, as (it is) an insurmountable hindrance. It is granted to our imagination to wander over, above and beyond this wall into a world which is so magnificent and powerful, as the real world

[1] "The Protoplasm and Irritability". Jena, 1891.
[2] Poggendorff's Annals. Jubelband (Jubilee volume). 1874. p. 557.
* a student of Johannes Müller – chapter 3 – (eds).

and whose traces we encounter at this frontier at every step. Many concepts which began as imaginative speculations have later been unexpectedly confirmed by important discoveries. We need only recall Nägeli's theories on the idioplasma[1] and their confirmation through the wonderful discoveries relating to the process of fertilisation by Hertwig, Boveri, van Beneden and others. Science cannot celebrate finer triumphs than this in the area of the smallest things.

Such results are attractive and one follows these successes with enthusiasm, and tries to evaluate their consequences for other questions too. In this, one must certainly be aware that one is always walking on the edge of a precipice of theories, to which one indubitably falls victim, if one leaves the sure ground of fact too far behind. But just as danger steels our courage, so too will we try to advance a bit further along the edge of this precipice without losing the solid foundation of fact.

These facts, however, are found in the wide and fertile territory of cell- and nuclear division, which of all microscopic studies, is the one most securely based, as the facts were gained by means of the living cell, and the sequence of pictures was placed in order by comparison with the developing change. Nowhere, however, is there such certainty in the transition pictures as in the karyomitotic cell figures; indeed I would like to say that it is the only area in which transition pictures are more than theories. Until a few years ago these cell division

"Studies on the Specificity, the Altruism and the Anaplasia of cells with Special Reference to Tumours"

processes were studied almost exclusively in lower animals with large cells or by experiments on warm-blooded animals; in the case of human material, one knew virtually only tumours, epidermis and lymph glands. Flemming said once[2] "For although there are specialist colleagues who are not inclined to approach a matter more closely until it is presented to them as a case in *Homo sapiens*, one should not make any concessions at all in this direction."

In this pronouncement lies the correct and very important meaning that no one is in a position to understand these subtle and complicated cell division processes in the small cells of humans and warm-blooded animals, if he has not beforehand completely orientated himself with the large cells of the lower animals. I, however, saw from the beginning, in spite of this pronouncement by Flemming, that one might initiate necessarily extended investigations of *Homo sapiens* if one really wanted

[1] "Mechanical-Physiological Theory of Heredity", Munich, 1884.
[2] Arch. f. mikr. Anat. vol. 20, p. 56. New contributions to the knowledge of the cell and its life phenomena.

4   to draw far reaching conclusions as to the pathology of the human being, indeed I am inclined to grant large concessions in this direction.

Only after I had acquired sufficient background by the detailed study of lower animals and by numerous experiments was I at pains to assemble an extremely rich and diverse collection of human pathological material. Naturally, you cannot do that in the post-mortem room, although it was proved by one of my students[1] that in human beings, the mitoses do not as a rule run their time after death but (literally) go to ruination, gradually by chromatolysis, in which process the achromatic spindle lasts longest. Therefore, for a long period I was a regular visitor at various surgical clinics and polyclinics, where, by the kindness of my surgical colleagues, rich and diverse specimens, normal and pathological, became available to me (flowed to me). In this respect it is my first duty to thank Professor Küster (now in Marburg) who, on the occasion of my daily presence in his operating theatre, unfailingly made available to me ample quantities of fresh tissue. No less am I grateful to Messrs von Bergmann, von Bardeleben, James Israel, Veit and many others for rich and varied material. To all these gentlemen I express my heartfelt thanks, all the more because I certainly know what it means when someone is present at an operation who wants something and, moreover, wants it immediately, as soon as a fragment has been separated from the body, not later on, whenever there might be time for it (handing over the specimen – eds).

In addition, I must particularly thank my father who put part of his physics laboratory at my disposal in order to set up the large microphotographic apparatus, the use of which would otherwise have scarcely been possible for me. For this apparatus I must acknowledge a scholarship from Countess Bose by which alone I was given the possibility of completing the expensive production of faultless photographs. I express with heartfelt feeling my gratitude as much to

I Specificity

the memory of the noble founding lady as also to the committee which regarded me as worthy of this scholarship. I am most respectfully and gratefull and in their debt.

The investigations which I was thus in the happy position of being able to carry through have led to a sequence of results which in part constitutes a confirmation of current leading theories and extend and modify the latter; in part, however, I believe, justifies new opinions. For me personally these were stimulating in the highest degree and they have given me rich intellectual enjoyment. There was only one sadness in all of this, namely, that at some points they brought me into opposition with

[1] Hammer, On the behaviour of nuclear division figures in the human corpse. I.-D. Berlin, 1891.

the view of my much honoured chief and teacher, Professor Virchow. I mean particularly on some points concerning the specificity of cells and the histogenesis of carcinomas. I should not have dared to hand over these pages respectfully and with a grateful heart to him, the founder and old master of cell theory, if he himself had not found an excuse for this in the sentence, "I willingly recognise that in many directions, in the knowledge of karyokinetic processes, such great progress has been made that thereby wholly new points of view were gained"[1]. May he judge the following remarks benevolently and mildly.

Berlin. 1892

[1] His Archiv. vol. 126. p. 8. The State of Cellular Pathology.

I Specificity

As long as one studied cells under the microscope one made use of the so-called transitional images in order to draw conclusions concerning the life of cells from the morphological presentations. The history of histology has taught us that innumerable errors were caused by the use of these methods, the extirpation of which cost much trouble and took a great deal of time, thus, once upon a time, the theory concerning the genesis of cells from amorphous blastema and of connective tissue as the matrix of all new formations, and of the origin of connective tissue out of leukocytes and so on. One can scarcely find a histological work in which conclusions were not drawn that things that lie alongside each other come from one another. In more recent and most recent times innumerable works of this kind appeared, for example, concerning the origin of tubular cells from liver parenchymal cells,[1] of lymphocytes from reticulum cells,[2] from cells out of threads and intercellular holes[3] and many others. We are not going to discuss here to what extent the conclusions of these authors are correct or not, but whether the same are at all justifiable. No histologist will give up conclusions from transition images because it is these which give life to his science, but there is in this something which surprises or even alienates one, i.e. in the expressions which are always repeated in such works. "One sees how this or that becomes". To take a few examples Herman Schmidt says in Virchow's Archive vol. 128, p. 75, "In some cells one can observe the transition in threads

[1] Baumgarten, Experimental and pathological anatomical understanding of tuberculosis. Zeitschrift f. klin. Med. 1886.
[2] Ribbert, On regeneration and inflammation of the lymph nodes. Ziegler's Beiträge vol. VI. 1889
[3] Grawitz and his pupils in Virchow's Archive vols. 125, 127, 128, 129 and in other places.

7 that is to say, the thickening of the protoplasms, the lengthening of the cell body and at the same time shrinkage of the nucleus and so on." Grawitz says in Virchow's Archive vol. 127, p. 103, "At such borders between the softening tissue and liquid pus, transition of mass numbers of tissue cells, often scarcely mixed with leukocytes, into the pus can be observed; the collapsing tissue cells in this process become mainly multinuclear and so on." Those are but two examples of many which I just happened to turn up. All that (in the papers above) is perhaps only a matter of expression, which one will perhaps judge more mildly when one understands from the presentation that the matter is not one of observations but of thoughts put into (the discussion) and of conclusions which were drawn only from those observations (considered error for "thoughts" – eds). This is essentially making the facts fit the theory rather than the theory fit the facts or making facts fit the preconceptions of the author, rather than the facts being looked at clearly for themselves. Such conclusions, however, *per se* have absolutely nothing provable. They can be made more or less probable so that in the most favourable case they achieve a certain recognition and this recognition can maintain itself until these conclusions are relieved by other more credible conclusions. Thus, only actual observations have anything binding for science, all deductions and above all transition images must arouse reservations and they have, indeed, in the highest degree been discredited through the history of histology.

Now the theory of the metaplasia of cells is based on the study of such transition images – that theory which for long dominated certain sections of pathological histology. If now one looks through works of metaplasia, the discussion is of two quite different things, on the one hand that one type of cell or one kind of cell can change into another and on the other hand that a type of cell conforms to changed circumstances and is thereby itself changed. In an essay in the Journal of Pathology and Bacteriology, May 1892, p. 673, on Transformation and descent as actual metaplasia and histological accommodation (Recklinghausen's "metatype"), Virchow distinguished these one from the other. Whilst in older works the word metaplasia was always used in the former sense, in more recent works we find it used in the sense of histological accommodation.[1]

The textbooks give relatively little information about this. In Cohnheim we find nothing fundamental about metaplasia, Birch-Hirchfeld (*sic*) just touches

I Specificity

on it in passing[2] and Klebs[3] mentions it only incidentally. Ziegler alone dedicates to it a short

[1] Compare with Posner, Virchow's Archiv vol. 118 p. 391. Schuchardt, On the essence on Ocaena, Volkmann's Hefte no. 340; Moran "Concerning transformation of epithelia", Thesis of (University of) Paris 1889 and many others.
[2] vol. 1. p. 110.
[3] "General Pathology and Morphology", pp 451, 538, 771, 773.

but yet a personal section[1]. I can certainly take for granted the standpoint of cellular pathology which at many points is concerned with metaplasia, and that Virchow now on the whole remains true to his earlier opinions is obvious from the work just quoted on the previous page (p. 7).

The little space which is allotted to metaplasia in the textbooks, compared to the extraordinarily numerous works on the same topic, is certainly no chance circumstance, but rather, is based on the research results which have made the process of metaplasia appear ever more uncertain. Most recently this question was publicly discussed at the International Congress in Berlin in 1890[2] following on a lecture by Bard entitled, "Cellular specificity and the anatomical pathological facts on which it is based". The record gives the following information on this (pages 98, 99): "Mr Ziegler: the majority of pathological anatomists may well be of the opinion that the single tissue formations in their outgrowth are not able to form tissues of another kind, that epithelium can never form connective tissue and connective tissue can never form epithelium and even connective tissue substances can only form tissues of a certain kind – Herr von Recklinghausen reminds the meeting that organisations do occur which do not accord with the theory of clearly delimited specificity, corresponding to the points of view developed by Kölliker, especially connective tissue formations from epithelial cells 1. in the alveoli of the lungs in chronic pneumonia, 2. in the connective tissue rings which emerge between Bowman's capsule and the glomeruli. The question is where the frontier of the specificity of cells and tissue is to be drawn".

It seems to me that two things emerge from this, namely, one, that such a unity as that accepted by Ziegler does not exist yet at all as long such an authority as v. Recklinghausen affirms an extensive cell metaplasia; secondly, however, that now the question is as follows: is there in the fully developed body a genuine metaplasia at all, or is everything "histological adaptation"? For the facts are not to be doubted that mucus and connective tissue can change into fatty tissue, connective tissue and cartilage into bone, ciliated epithelium into flat epithelium, which is exactly similar to the outer epidermis; none of this can be doubted. Questionable only is whether the connective tissue can change itself into epithelium as Virchow says, or epithelium into connective tissue as v. Recklinghausen presumes. Moreover, Ziegler's observation is doubly weighty, as this researcher

[1] "General Pathology". p. 232, 7th edn.
[2] Verhandlungen. vol. II, 3rd treatise, pp 92 and 98.

9 has until recently zealously defended the transformation of leukocytes into connective tissue and, thus, (supported the idea of) a genuine metaplasia. It was only through his further studies that he reached the point of denying a metaplasia at all.

The views which hitherto one had of metaplasia were acquired, as we have said, through the study of so-called transition images. There were two kinds of mishaps. Firstly, one could not be sure whether the cell forms found along side each other even if they were very similar, really transformed one into the other, that is to say, really present forms which belong together in one group; secondly, however, I see no possibility of determining by transition images whether a cell which has changed its form has also changed its kind or type, that is to say, whether it is a matter of a genuine metaplasia or only of a histological accommodation. If, for example, a tracheal cell loses its ciliated hairs, but literally develops the ability to form keratin and is now so similar as to be indistinguishable from an epidermis cell, then in the comparison of these cells there is no possibility of establishing whether the same has really become an epidermis cell or whether it has only changed its form. If Flemming in 1888[1] was able to say with a certain pride "thanks to more recent works, and particularly those of Heidenhain and his pupils, every expert pathologist can today decide in almost every case from every well fixed glandular epithelial cell to which gland it has belonged" then one cannot say this of most other cells, particularly when one takes into account the changes in cells by pathological processes in and around the same. For we judge the type of cell for preference according to the form of its nucleus and protoplasm. In his "Cellular Pathology"[2] Virchow pointed to the fact that nuclei often demonstrate great similarity amongst themselves, while the distinguishing characteristics mostly lie in the protoplasm, that is to say, in the form of the protoplasm. And it is precisely the form of cell body which is most easily changed in pathological conditions – that is precisely where a metaplasia is, if at all, mostly likely to eventuate. Therefore, we had to seek other means than those of simply contemplation of transitional forms. I proceeded from this standpoint when some years ago I approached the study of cell division. This simply had to have various advantages over the mere contemplation of non-dividing cells (passive cells, vegetative cells). One of these advantages is based on the fact that in karyokinesis, the cells attempt to assume a spherical form. This is a process which Flemming[3] indicated a long time ago.

[1] Arch. f. Anat. u. Phys. Anat. Abt. p. 287.
[2] 4th edn. p. 10.
[3] "Nuclear- and Cell Substance". Leipzig, 1882.

I Specificity

This process was found with particular clarity in his investigation of the division of pigment cells[1] and this has also been confirmed by other authors. Here we are dealing with an absolutely general law. Similarly to the way protozoa encyst themselves before division, the tissue cells retract their cell processes, so that in turn, the individual organelles of the cell move inwards towards the centre of the cell and thereby achieve a sharper distinction from their surroundings (create a sharper demarcation line). These circumstances can be clearly observed in all human organs. Thus the squamous cells of the epidermis more or less lose their serrations on cell division. One never finds a completely formed ciliated cell or goblet cell in division, no brush border can be observed in kidney epithelia, the connective tissue and mucous cells partially withdraw their peripheral processes, and so on. On the other hand, absolute spherical form is attained only very rarely in fixed tissue cells (most extremely seldom), the latter remain dependent, to a certain extent, on their environment, just as the pigment cells of the salamander do not do this. But a substantial part of histological accommodation is excluded during division and the cell approaches the ideal form of its archetype; during division it represents more its type and less its individuality. The main reason for this is that during division the cell probably gives up every other function. It neither assimilates nor does it secrete. This is apparent from a comparison with monocellular organisms[2] which not only cease to absorb nourishment, but which also before division even expel all absorption balls and partial absorption balls (*Nahrungsballen*) as well as excreting vacuoles (*Nahrungsreste*). A very interesting observation by Martinotti[3] supports this, namely, that those kidney cells which were in the act of division did not turn blue on injection with sodium acid indigo sulphate, while those which were in the so-called dormant phase (interphase – eds) demonstrated the familiar Heidenhain's reaction. Pointing additionally to this is that the combined size of the daughter cells corresponds approximately to the size of the mother cell and finally, that in cells with morphologically visible secretion, the latter reduce almost to nothing during division. Lastly, we should indicate the behaviour of the Ehrlich-Altmann granules (mitochondria – eds) during division. As I have seen in numerous preparations, these become sparser and become concentrated in the periphery of the cell bodies. In carcinoma cells and cells which were dividing, they were virtually not there at all and I never saw a plasma or mast cell in division.

[1] Arch. f. mikr. Anat. vol. 35, p. 275, 1890.
[2] Compare concerning this, Bütschli, The Protozoa, vol. 3, p. 1648 and at other places.
[3] On hyperplasia and regeneration etc. Centralbl. f. path. Anat vol. 1, p. 633.

Müller[1] too arrived at similar results, just as Luigi and Rafaello Zoja[2]. The only exceptions are, perhaps, the lymphocytes which immediately on completion of division almost have the size of the mother cells.[3]

Whilst, however, the various cells in a state of rest concern themselves with the most various types of work which are characteristic of their form, that is to say, secreting milk, mucus, water and so on, all reabsorbing it away or executing the movements of their cilia; during division, all cells complete only these processes and a great number of sources of error which could disturb a comparison are excluded.

An additional advantage lies in the movement of the cell which takes a defined exactly familiar course in karyokinesis. Thereby, all characteristics demonstrated by the dormant cell are literally pulled apart: at every phase they assume certain forms and thereby characteristic properties become visible which we were not able to observe in the dormant cell, just as a similar number of pigeons demonstrate their individualities only in their different modes of flight. In this, one has, during the process of cell division, the additional advantage that by the methods of fixation, one can capture every individual phase of division, snap shots so-to-speak of a creature in movement, similar to the photographs of a man running, a horse jumping or a bird flying*.

When the karyokinetic process right down to its details was discovered first by Schneider[4] and then by numerous researchers, amongst whom van Beneden, Eberth, Flemming, R. and O. Hertwig, Mayzel, Strassburger, Fol, Arnold and others, are most prominent, then it was in the interests of the subject to establish that all cells in the animal and plant kingdom can divide according to the same scheme, in the normal as well as in the pathological condition, and these facts can today be regarded as having been confirmed in brilliant fashion. Differences which were revealed within this scheme were often observed and described. It is known that those parts which particularly attract dyes were originally denoted as loops (*Schleifen*).

[1] Arch f. exper. Path. u. Pharmak. vol. 29.
[2] Intorno Memoire del R. Instituto Lombardo dei Scienze e Lettre. vol. XVI. VII. Dellar Serie III. Mailand 1891.
[3] Compare Flemming, Cell increase in the lymph nodes and related organs etc. Arch. f. mikr. Anat. vol. 24.
[4] Examinations of platyhelminths. Jahrb d. oberhessischen Gesellsch. f. Natur- u. Heilkunde. 1873.
* This may be a reference to the type of photography which was invented in 1878 by Eadweard Muybridge (1830–1904) – eds.

12 When it was then found that many kinds of cell exhibit no *Schleifen* then in line with Waldeyer's process the term "chromosomes" was chosen[1]. Particular forms of karyokinesis were discovered by Flemming[2] in the testicles of *Salamandra maculata* and he extensively described heterotypical and homotypical forms. The same author drew attention in 1885[3] to the smallness of the mitotic figures of leukocytes. Grawitz mentioned the same circumstance in 1890[4] and in 1891[5] I demonstrated the difference between endothelial cells, lymphoblasts and the dermis cells. Still in the same year[6] H. F. Müller, who had arrived independently at this result, used the different form of mitoses for the distinction between different cell types in the bone marrow. My further observations on this are to

I Specificity

be found in two essays "Karyokinesis and Cellular Pathology"[7] and "Concerning the anaplasia of tumour cells and asymmetric mitosis".[8] The remaining data – which are numerous in the literature – concerning mitoses which deviate from the scheme, refer to pathological forms.

In the works cited above I have asserted that one is in a position, within the familiar scheme of mitosis, to recognise differences which recur again and again in individual types of cell and which can be exactly specialised. In order to study these differences, consistently treated materials are absolutely necessary. The material must be fixed, embedded and stained in the same way, thereby a series of difficulties and sources of error arise which lie in part with the techniques and in part with the objects themselves.

In order initially to protect oneself from the bias which comes from using only one method, a long study of numerous objects, of various types and which have been treated in various ways is necessary; by that one gradually learns to distinguish what can be related to the fixation and what to the staining and one learns how to separate the artefacts from the genuine phenomena. Anyone who has concerned himself in more detail with these things will know that even within the same method there are very great variations.

[1] On Karyokinesis and its relationships to fertilisation. Arch. f. mikr. Anat. vol. 32. 1888.
[2] New contributions to the knowledge of the cell. Arch. f. mikr. Anat. vol. 29. 1887
[3] Arch. f. mikr. Anat. vol. 24.
[4] Verh. d. intern. Med. Congr. vol. II, 3, Abt p. 9.
[5] Verh. der Anat. Ges. München 1891. p. 255.
[6] Deutsch. Arch. f. klin. Med. vol. 48, p. 51.
[7] Berl. klin. Wochenschr. 1891, no. 42.
[8] Virchow's Archiv. vol. 129, p. 436.

If, however, one knows one's method precisely, then one finds that certain changes are caused in quite definite cell figures and there with a certain regularity, so that with due care one can evaluate the same to a certain extent to allow them to be distinguished. Thus, for example, at the conclusion of the diaster phase of endothelium of vessels a clumping process in the chromatin substance almost always takes place, which does not occur in other cells to that extent. In lymphocytes, achromatic spindles appear only rarely, a fact which is partly related to the fixation and so on. Whichever method one chooses – whether Flemming's, Hermann's or Fol's solutions or sublimate – is relatively unimportant; one must remember this if one wishes to compare cell figures with each other. Then one may only produce for the comparisons, such figures as have been treated by the same method.

The following data concerning forms of mitoses relate entirely to human material; they were, unless indicated, fixed directly during the operation in concentrated aqueous sublimate solution. I have found this solution to be best for human material (although it is not suitable for much animal material) as it penetrates quickly, does not deform, fixes not only the nuclei but also the cell substance and is effective for the adhesion of the stain. Therefore, I do not regard it as necessary to remove the sublimate afterwards either by washing out or with iodine. The aqueous solution is to be preferred to the alcoholic as also to the salt solution. The two latter are considerably stronger than the pure aqueous solution and, therefore, have a destructive effect on the tissue, and also the salt crystalises out in alcohol treatment and, therefore, a very careful washing with water is necessary which is not advantageous for the material and is also time consuming. I prepare the solution in such a fashion that excess sublimate is dissolved in hot, not distilled, water. On cooling, the excess is crystallised out and if the liquid is kept in a dark flask over these crystals, it will be preserved unchanged for at least 14 days. By then the amount made ready is fully used up. The pieces are to be chosen of such a size that they are completely saturated within an hour. If penetration of the sublimate to the interior takes longer than an hour, by then the mitoses have already changed so much and many organ parts, particularly smooth muscle, become extraordinarily hard with a longer period of fixation in the sublimate. After an hour I always take the pieces out and each of them is put then for 24 hours in spirits, alcohol, origanum oil, xylol, xylol-paraffin and paraffin.

Paraffin has been much reproached because it shrinks the tissue and one too easily cuts through mitotic figures. The former which often occurs in soft animal tissues

14 I have observed in human material and with the cautious embedding method used above have not seen a disturbing degree of this reached. I do not believe that any significant sources of error arise. As far as the cutting through is concerned, one can protect oneself to some extent against it by making the sections not too thin. Ten to 11 microns are absolutely thin enough, even thicker ones, for less cellular tissues are still useable. Even then, however, one still cuts through many a figure. When observing, however, one will always proceed quite safely if one only considers such cells which have other cells in layers above and beneath them. Such cells are not cut through.

As a staining method dilute Böhmer's haematoxylin was used, in which they were stained for 24 hours. The sections were stuck to the slide with egg white glycerin and these were placed upright in a bath with dye solution, in order to avoid precipitates. For the appearance of the chromosomes it is not a matter of indifference whether one takes a dilute or a strong solution just as little as the choice of dye is a matter of indifference. The stronger the dye stuff and the more one over stains the thicker the chromosomes appear to be. Where the really clear pictures are often achieved is in under-stained preparations. Comparisons should be made once more only with preparations made with the same or the most similar degree of staining possible. The counter staining was with eosin, and also here the slow method proved to be the most practical. Dilute solutions

I Specificity

applied over a long period and decolourised over a long period give the best results for the making visible of the spindle and the centrosomes. Here too strong a colouring is harmful and, therefore, for those things which are on the border of what is visible at all, orange and acid fuchsin have not proved themselves for me in human material, as these stain the cell bodies too intensively and differentiate the details to a lesser extent.

Embedding always followed in Canada balsam in which, however, my experience was in some few preparations among several thousand, that one no longer saw with the same clarity, previously quite fine details; for example, radiations to attraction spheres in normal cells after the hardening effect of the balsam. For the rest the preparations remained perfectly preserved even after several years.

Let me be permitted to say something about the photomicrographs. These, in so far as they concern individual cells (Figs 1–76), were prepared under similar conditions at about 600-fold magnification and they, therefore, permit direct comparison between them. The attached yardstick is a Zeiss objective micrometer (1 mm divided into 100 parts) taken under the same conditions. An apochromatic 2.0 immersion of Zeiss, with the aperture 1.30, tube length 160, projection ocular 2.

Bellows 50 cm was used. The photographs were carried out with the large Zeiss apparatus which was set up, shock proof, on isolation pillars. As a source of light, Auer's gas glowing light was used and was exposed for about 10 minutes with a narrow aperture (*Blende* "loophole"). This mode of lighting, over and above its easy manipulation and cheap manufacture, has the advantage over electric Circon glow light and sunlight in that with the longer time of exposure, one can better match the nuances than with short exposures. Certainly, though, shock-proof conditions are absolutely necessary as otherwise the slightest movement, particularly in the room itself causes considerable disturbances. Only Schleussner's plates were used which had been made autochromatic at the longest 24 hours by an erythrosin-ammonia bath. Zettnow's powerful light filter allows through only green and yellow light and should be tested beforehand; for this the spectroscope was used, in order to sharpen the contrasts between blue (dark) and red (light) which become weaker during photographing.

One must not expect from a photogram that it reproduces objects with the same clarity as a drawing. The shallow depth of the pictures, as a result of which only part of each cell can be clearly visualised, is disturbing. But almost more disturbing are the indistinct figures, which shine through from other levels. The scattered circles which, appearing as spots and shadows, very much affect the clarity of the pictures. Of course, we also see this phenomenon in the microscope but we are accustomed to compensate for this by use of the micrometer screw. Against these disadvantages the photogram has the advantage of greater objectivity, but only the expert will be able to see from these pictures. Anyone unpractised in these things will be able to derive very little from these pictures.

The best mode of visualising is with the magnifying glass in which, however, the unavoidable grain in the print must be disregarded. When looking through the magnifying glass this grain obscures numerous details which are visible in the originals, and while looking with the naked eye, the graininess essentially does not interfere.

In the comparison of cell divisions between each other there were in my opinion two major difficulties, the elimination of which demanded the acquisition of a specially chosen material. This was possible only in the course of several years. The one difficulty is in the circumstance that in the normal fully developed body not all types of cell contain mitoses. Where in the normal way mitoses are present, there can naturally be no difficulty in establishing the forms of these mitoses once the way (the methods) had been established. There are, however, relatively few cell types of this kind: but I include

the epithelia of all outer surfaces communicating with the exterior world, thus, primarily the outer epidermis and the cornea, the mucous membranes of the respiratory, digestive, urinary and sex organs. Further, the hair and sebaceous follicles, the crypts of Lieberkühn and the epithelial cavity of the uterus, usually called glands, finally the gland ducts and in most cases the lymphoid follicles. However, mitoses are lacking in all other tissues: connective tissue series, muscles, nerves, glia and above all in all genuine glands. The testicles and mammary glands occupy a special position of which the latter allow us to recognise a periodic appearance of mitoses[1].

As far as the cells of the connective tissue substances are concerned – particularly genuine connective tissue, fatty tissue, epithelia of the lymph and blood vessels, cartilage and so on – many people here presume incorrectly that there is here the same metabolism as in the epidermis; cells are continually disappearing and being newly formed. This is clear, eg, from Schimmelbusch's remark[2] "... how the cells of ordinary connective tissue are continually dying off in order to make place for young ones, without the cell corpses leaving any evidence and so on". However, mitoses are completely missing in these tissues in the normally developed body. Thus no morphological finding indicates a process of dying off completely and a substitution of the cell elements already present by newly formed ones. Such views – and any conclusions resulting from them – must, therefore, be regarded as quite inadmissible and I do not believe that they still have many supporters.

It is different with the glands. In these cases there is still a large group of authors who hold the view that – particularly in comparison with the lower animals – cells with secretions completely go to ruin and must be newly built up. This standpoint has also been put forward again in the tissue theory of Schiefferdecker and Kossel (p. 40, vol. 2). The findings wholly originate in the pre-karyokinetic era and are based mainly on the semi-lunar cells in the salivary glands; a fact which also converted Heidenhain[3] to this view. That this postulate, where it still

I Specificity

appears, is not based on the finding of mitoses, is clear from Frenzel's[4] work, who expressly mentions that he has looked for mitoses in vain but has frequently observed double nuclei.

[1] I have not carried out any investigations concerning possible regeneration of bones in human beings.
[2] Deutsche med. Wochenschr. no. 6, 5th Febr. 1891.
[3] Compare in Hermann's "Physiology". vol. 5. Part 1.
[4] On nuclear halving. Biol. Centralbl, no. 22. vol. 11, p. 701

In general one looks in vain in genuine glands for mitoses in those cells which are only involved in secretion; as long as the latter are normal and no longer in the process of development. Absolutely characteristic in this respect are the glands of the fundus, pylorus and duodenum. Whilst in the ducts one always finds numerous cell division figures, they are completely lacking in the secretory part. A very significant example is the much-investigated mammary gland. During the development associated with pregnancy, mitoses abound in the mammary gland. Towards the end (of pregnancy) these become ever more infrequent and during lactation they as good as cease completely. Podwyssozki[1] has already documented this and summarised his views particularly in Progress in Medicine 1886[2]. Then, in a series of essays, Coën[3] and Bizzozero and Vasale confirmed the same.[4] Steinhaus[5] too finds the same in the case of mammary glands even if, according to his data, the process is rather more complicated. Quite particularly confirming the maintenance of cells during secretion, however, is the positive data of Altmann[6] who proved that the bodies found in the secretions which one had always regarded as ejected cells, are only parts of the secretory cells without nuclei. Contrary to these results – which more or less agree with each other – are the data of Gaules[7] who found in the pancreas of a dog a few mitoses. These are to be given less credence since Nicolaides[8] could not confirm this finding. In all of this, it is naturally not asserted that during secretion a cell never dies off now and again and is then replaced by mitosis; but that such a process is not the rule and (if it does occur – eds) should be regarded as absolutely pathological.

Apparent exceptions are the crypts of Lieberkühn, the mucous membrane cavities of the uterus and the sebaceous gland of the skin. However, because of their coarsely anatomical structure, both the former are not to be regarded as genuine glands. They do not display either ducts or secretory parts – as are shown by all genuine glands – but on the contrary reveal themselves as simple mucous membrane pockets.

[1] Ziegler's Beiträge, vol. 1.
[2] Laws of regeneration in gland epithelia under physiological and pathological conditions. (no further reference – eds).
[3] Studies of the normal and pathological histology of the mammary gland, Ziegler's Beiträge, vol. 2, 1887.
[4] Virchow's Archiv. vol. 110, 1887 p. 155; Archivo per le Scienze mediche 1887, p. 195; anat. Anzeiger. III Jarhgang. 1888 no. 26. p. 781; Atti della R. Accademica delle scienze di Torino vol. XXIV. 1888.

[5] Arch. f. anat. u. Phys. Anat. Abt. 1892. p. 54.
[6] "The elementary organisms", Leipzig 1890.
[7] Arch. f. Anat. u. Phys. Anat Abt. 1882.
[8] Compare with Ogata. Arch. f. Anat. u. Phys. Phys. Abt. 1883.

18 Incidentally, that something is also secreted by the cells of this cavity does not yet prove its glandular nature because surface epithelia secrete without us denoting them – because of this – as glands. In the crypts of Lieberkühn, mitoses are primarily found in the fundus where goblet cells are almost wholly lacking. Because no mitoses appear in the epithelial cells between the crypts it is not improbable that the fundus should be regarded as the centre from which the cells arise and are gradually pushed to the surface. Originally the concept of secretion, like most anatomical concepts, was a macroscopic one: the gland secreted. Only in recent times was the concept carried over to the individual cell and thus modified. Secretion is a cell activity: dying off is not a cell activity and thus cannot be included in the concept of secreting. Therefore, one cannot include sebaceous follicles among the glands, as in them a mass of cells which are dead by regressive metamorphosis is produced. One could with equal justice say that hair is secreted by the hair follicle because in principal nothing different happens here from (what happens – eds) in the sebaceous follicles.

In those tissues in which one always finds mitoses, one usually speaks of physiological regeneration. In an essay on "Cell division in the human epidermis"[1] I have tried to prove that in the epidermis, the mitoses are to be attributed to a pathological process which is continued permanently as long as life exists. And I believe quite generally that in what we usually call physiological regeneration, a struggle of the organisms against the external world is to be seen. Thereby, above all, the localisation of the tissue is in accord with this regeneration. They all stand in direct relationship to the external world. Either they delimit surfaces or they serve to conduct secretions from the interior to the exterior. The lymph follicles constitute the only exception. Now lymph cells wander continuously through the mucous membranes as they do also through the external skin to the outside, and there they perish[2]. It is also not to be excluded that thereby a gap (in the tissues) forms, which acts as a stimulus for the exuberant growth of lymph follicles.[3]*

[1] Festschrift for R. Virchow. Berlin. G. Reimer 1891.
[2] Compare Colles. Concerning the behaviour of migratory cells in layered squamous epithelium. Virchow's Arch. vol. 86. p. 462, and Stöhr Concerning tonsils and bellows-glands. Virchow's Arch. vol. 97. p. 211.
[3] As this work went to press, I encountered the excellent investigation by Löwit ("Studies on the Physiology and Pathology of the Blood and the Lymph". Jena 1892). In it I find confirmation of this view.
* There is a suggestion here of Ribbert's "tissue tension" hypothesis (see chapter 6 – eds).

I Specificity

From this we can see that the formulation of the question was hitherto actually not quite right, although the result came to the same thing. One does not have to ask which tissues show physiological regeneration, but rather on which tissues does the external world exert a destructive influence, so that a permanent regeneration becomes necessary? All the various pathological conditions show that almost all tissues are capable of regeneration but to different degrees. In some tissues regeneration occurs so little in extent that the result is a very imperfect one – for instance, the central nervous system – but in others so strongly that they immediately react to intervention with explosive development of new cells.

If, therefore, one wishes to study the forms of cell divisions in tissues in which there is no permanent regeneration, one must resort to pathological specimens. Thereby, however, the suspicion arises that through these pathological circumstances, deceptive appearances may be created which do not correspond to any physiological process of cell division. Therefore, various processes of inflammation, hyperplasia and regeneration have to be studied in tissues which normally contain mitoses, and (also to be studied is) to what extent these are thereby changed. I have discussed what is revealed by such studies of division in pathological cells, in Virchow's Archive, vol. 123, p. 356, and I shall return to this later. Here it is sufficient to note that these investigations reveal that – as Schwarz has already emphasised for the epidermis[1] – on the whole the forms of the mitoses are not changed. Even if in the individual case some pathological deviation occurs, this can be recognised for what it is and excluded from the study.

Thus, the important result for our investigation is: IN REGENERATION, IN HYPERPLASIA AND IN THE EXPLOSIVE GROWTH IN INFLAMMATION, THE TYPE OF FORM OF DIVISION REMAINS INTACT. Like in "normal" tissue, so also in the course of these (regenerative, hyperplastic etc – eds) alterations, the mitoses are extraordinarily similar to each other with respect to size, form and organisation of their component elements; with the exception of occasional figures which are to be regarded as pathological. Simple hyperplasia and regeneration are the most similar to the physiological condition. In inflammatory explosive growths, the mitoses become somewhat larger, fuller and clearer. The individual parts – particularly the achromatic figures and the centrosomes – emerge more clearly. One finds in these preparations relatively more perfectly fixed mitoses than (one does) in normal tissue, but no essential change in the character of the mitoses takes place on account of it.

[1] On the theory of nuclear division. Virchow's Arch. vol. 124, p. 488.

From this I believe I am justified in assuming the same for those tissues in which, normally, no mitoses are present; i.e. the pathological circumstances give rise to nothing which could be understood as deviating from the usual type for the cell (type), with the exception of those relatively uncommon forms which are recognisable as pathological.

The second difficulty which was revealed by the examination of this topic was that it was frequently impossible to determine to which type of cell the observed cell division figures belonged. In all situations where the tissues are distinctly separated from each other, i.e. in all epithelia and in all more highly differentiated connective tissues – this naturally causes no difficulty. Quite different, however, are the tissues in which – especially under pathological conditions – cells of different types are present mixed together. In practical terms these are primarily the epithelia and connective tissue cells and the epithelium of the lymph sinuses and of the vessels with which these lymphoid cells then associate. However, one can disentangle these forms if one seeks suitable pathological processes in which the relevant cell-type is provided, to an extent, as a pure population[1]. Such processes occur mainly in the lymph nodes. In the normally active lymph node or in simple hyperplasia, one finds in Flemming's germinal centres, almost exclusively lymphoblasts or lymphocytes respectively. In the so-called large cell hyperplasia, which appears particularly in tuberculosis (but which can also appear without this disease), there arises an almost exclusive exuberant growth of the lymphatic endothelium. In fibrous degeneration – i.e. the induration-conditions of the lymph nodes – it is almost always only the actual connective tissues of the lymph nodes which proliferate. Thus, IN THESE VARIOUS CONDITIONS, ONE CAN STUDY THE BEHAVIOUR OF THESE THREE TYPES OF CELLS IN ISOLATION AND CAN LEARN THE FORMS OF THE MITOSES, IF ONE SEEKS OUT THE APPROPRIATE MATERIAL.

The comparative study of numerous mitoses under the most varying conditions and carried out in the manner indicated, reveals that typical differences are found which recur with great regularity in the individual tissues. This is to the extent that the relevant parts are clearly visible at all. THAT IS TO SAY, IN THE INDIVIDUAL TYPES OF TISSUE, THERE ARE INDIVIDUAL DIFFERENCES IN KARYOKINESIS, WHICH WITH SUFFICIENT PRACTICE ALLOW US TO DISTINGUISH THE INDIVIDUAL TISSUE TYPES BY THE FORM OF THEIR MITOSIS. The mitoses of individual types of cells, e.g, those of vessel epithelia, the epidermis cells and lymphocytes, are so different from each other that one can distinguish them almost at first sight.

[1] Compare with: A contribution to the origin and increase of the leukocytes. Verhandl. der anat. Gesellsch. 1891. p. 255.

However, the mitoses of other tissues, which in their (embryonic) developmental history are closely related to each other – e.g, the epidermal, sebaceous gland and hair sheath cells – are so similar to each other, that one can only distinguish them after long study.

Moreover, not every mitosis gives decisive information on the type character, as small individual physiological deviations may persist. Also, given the smallness of the objects, the position of the cell and other chance elements, all manner of artefacts may blur the type of the mitosis. One must, therefore, always examine the largest possible number of mitoses before one can be quite clear about the

I Specificity

type character. In addition, our knowledge of the cells (in general) is still really crude in comparison with the extraordinarily complicated processes which are carried out within them. If, for example, one considers centrosomes and recalls the fact that they are the middle point for typical and ordered movements of larger cell parts – and the fact that in spite of this one can only in exceptional cases perceive the details of their shapes or forms, and they, moreover, lie on the border of what is visible at all – then one realises that we only know the most coarse components of the cells while the actual details are completely concealed from us. This shows us that the variations which we still have to establish can only be concerned with relatively crude parts and, perhaps, only outer parts (of cells). These variations also often characterise only trivial processes, while at the same time the actual heart of the matter can elude us. However, that should not hinder us in registering the clearly perceptible differences which we see; and we should never refer to the individual cell but always to the results of large series of observations. Thus, let no one reproach me if for once a tissue is found which deviates from the type set down by me. If, for example, data are collected concerning form and size of chromosomes, then I know very well that both of these features can change to an extraordinary extent in the various phases (of mitosis), and also that the length and thickness of chromosomes can be very variable. However, from the observation of very numerous figures, we can establish average cases, and single individuals can be used more or less frequently as representatives, and serve as a basis of the following individual data. Such average representative individual cases (*Durchschnittsindividuen*) have also served as the basis for the photograms. In this process (of selection), I have avoided any partiality as far as possible. One also sees from this that the photograms too do not reveal more objective evidence for the correctness of these considerations than drawings would. Thus, I have not made drawings of them (the figures) only in order to make them more

credible because photograms give rise to fewer sources of errors in reproductions. 22

Now, as I believe that I have protected myself to a certain extent against unjust attacks, I proceed to the differences in individual types. These differences extend to individual, several or all formed components of the division of the mitotic figure; moreover, to the length of the single phase; and also to the whole division and to a sequence of different properties of the nuclear and cell substance.

The size of the division figure

I deliberately avoid giving numerical data concerning the size of the figures; as also later with chromosomes and centrosomes. Experience teaches that data concerning large sequences of measurements have a wearying effect and still lead to no correct result. In the shapes or forms, which are already small enough, small differences, in fact, comprise a large percentage of the total size. The variations in volume cannot be determined from any dimensions of the surfaces – which are all that can be determined with some certainty. All the same, it should be noted that in the one type of tissue, cells which have proceeded to division, differ from each other much less in size than cells not undergoing division appear to. That can be attributed to the striving of the cells (detailed above) to assume the spherical shape, whereby mistakes are made less easily in the reduction of volumes of the cells than in the often multiform non-dividing cells. Now, young cells with the exception of lymphocytes (see above) are always smaller than old cells. However, once the cells have entered the passive phase, we are no longer able to distinguish whether a cell is young or has only remained small, unless the cells possess age-related changes, e.g, prickles and fibres in epidermal cells.

Much more constant than the size of the cell bodies is the size of the nuclear division figures in the same tissues and in the same phases. Thus, in the monaster phase, one should still pay particular attention to the systole and the diastole of the chromosomes. Under this name Flemming has described a fluctuation of the chromosomes in the anaphase shortly before metakinesis.[1] Even if Flemming himself has abandoned this nomenclature for the process – in order to avoid any misunderstanding – the nomenclature still seems to me to be absolutely appropriate for the morphological condition. In the systole the star figure flattens itself down and thereby, when seen in profile,

[1] "Cell substance, Nuclear- and Cell division". Leipzig 1882, pp 212 and 213.

seems to be smaller; but when seen from above, seems bigger. In the diastole, the star figure is spread out again, and it now appears contrariwise, larger in profile, but smaller when seen from above. This circumstance is to be heeded in comparisons of two types of cell in the monaster phase.

The smallest figures are those of the lymphoblasts and lymphocytes. Let us compare the Figs 5, 14, 23, 32, 44, 53 and 62 with the corresponding figures from other tissues. The difference in size will be immediately obvious. The concern is, above all, the chromatic substance. The cell contours in the lymphoblasts are so delicate and transparent, that they are not visible in most photogrammes. These figures – which are taken exclusively from the germinal centres of lymph nodes – agree in all their properties with the mitoses of the lymphocytes in the blood or in the tissues; as have been described quite recently and ever more frequently. It scarcely needs to be mentioned that the opinion which in earlier times was very widespread – i.e. that the cells originating from the lymph nodes could not multiply in the blood – was wrong. Flemming had gone on for a long time emphasising this possibility[1]. Before that, however, it was possible to make all sorts of objections; particularly that the relevant mitoses belonged not to lymphocytes, but to other wandering cells or to endothelial cells. These objections disappear completely, now that it can be most clearly proved by the proximity of the lymphoblasts in association with both forms of mitoses[2]. The smallness of the lymphoblast mitoses is not based on a denser structure of the figures but on the smallness of its elements – which are extraordinarily soft and very exposed to artefact. Thus in no other type of cell do we see so much danger of coagulation appearing, due to fixation, e.g, even in the monaster stage (Fig. 23).

Of the types of tissue pictured, the next biggest (mitoses) are those in the crypts of Lieberkühn (Figs 7, 16, 25, 34, 46, 55, 64), then those in the hair follicles (Figs 4, 13, 22, 31, 43, 52, 61), then those in the sebaceous glands (Figs 2, 11, 20, 29, 41, 50, 59), then in the vascular epithelial cells (endothelium) (Figs 6, 15, 24, 33, 45, 54, 63), and finally, as the very biggest, in the cells of the epidermis (Figs 1, 10, 19, 28, 40, 49, 58). The remaining tissues lie between these extremes. The mitoses of the kidney and liver parenchymal cells are close in size to those of the crypts of Lieberkühn while those of the multi-layered mucous membranes are of approximately the same size as those of the epidermal cells. The mitoses of the real connective tissue cells are somewhat larger; as are those of the lymph sinus cells and vascular

[1] Arch. f. mikr. Anat. vol. 37.
[2] Compare with Verhandl. der Anat. Ges. 1891, p. 255.

epithelium – which for their part are so similar amongst each other that one is inclined to regard them as identical.

We must return later to the size of the mitoses under pathological conditions, especially in tumours.

Behaviour of achromatic figures

I have reported in the anat. Anzeiger[1] on the occurrence of centrosomes in so-called resting cells of the human being. It is very striking that one invariably finds these formations only in certain cell types; specifically in polynuclear leukocytes – which, as far as we know in humans, do not enter into mitosis – and also in the connective tissue cells. In the latter cells, later on when the mitotic figure is fully developed, centrosomes are so small that one is scarcely in a position to see them at all. In all remaining cells I was able to observe centrosomes only when the spindle is clearly developed; however, for human cells that is not before the monaster stage and is clearest in metakinesis. No formation in the cell is as much dependent on any pathological process (which might be) present as are the centrosomes. The differences in sizes of the centrosomes are, therefore, very considerable in one and the same tissue. On the other hand, they really achieve sufficient dimensions for one to perceive their details only in the epidermal cells and their derivatives. I have never seen them exceed dot size in endothelial cells. Even with the highest magnification they always remained a dot, and details cannot be perceived in them. This supports their extraordinary smallness. In lymphoblasts – probably on account of their smallness – I was not able to see centrosomes at all. In all lymph nodes and granular cells they are covered over by granules in the cytoplasm, so that they could only be seen in very thin sections, when the cell is cut through. Centrosomes become very large and shaped like a grooved bread roll. They lie obliquely to the axis of the spindle.

The spindles themselves are among the most constant formations. Once they have appeared, they appear in the same tissues always in the same form, and do not deviate from this even in tumours. In contrast, there are very significant differences – particularly in the steepness of the spindles in the monaster phase (Figs 28–39) – amongst the various tissues. In the epidermal cells (Fig. 28) they are always

[1] 1893. p. 57.

25 steepest; the internal angle being the sharpest. Here they resemble the steep spindles seen during the expulsion of polar bodies in eggs. The (spindles of the) cells of the sebaceous follicles are most similar to this (Fig. 29), while (spindles in) hair follicle cells (Fig. 31) show an essentially flatter spindle. The flattest spindles are seen in vascular epithelium and lymph cells. Whilst in the former – in spite of the fineness of their threads – they are almost always visible (Fig. 33), one mostly misses them in the lymphoblasts (Fig. 32). One reason for this is the smallness of the lymph cells, but (another reason is) because the spindle is so flat that in the diastole it is almost completely covered by the chromosomes, whilst in the systole it sticks out. The spindle was still visible in the specimen used for Fig. 32. In the photogramme – with only an amount of goodwill – one can recognise the flat triangles which close off the figure on both sides and appear as black as the chromosomes. Sometimes one finds bent spindles as in Fig. 37. Up to now, I have seen them (bent spindles) in three cases: once in normal epidermis, once in molluscum contagiosum and several times in lip cancers (from which Fig. 37 originates). In this one, I do not know whether it is a matter of artefact, (because the) figures are otherwise perfectly fixed. All the same, given the striking constancy of the spindles in other respects – including in normal and pathological tissues – I do not feel it necessary to attribute to them (bent spindles) a particular significance. Just like the centrosomes, the spindle in cells is partly (Fig. 29) or wholly (Fig. 34) covered over with granules when there is no clear division space (see later).

The achromatic connecting threads are in human cells mostly very fine and do not always appear definite. One sees them best when a clear division space is present, thus particularly in the epidermal cells. Photography is only rarely able to reproduce them clearly. What was originally present in the originals is almost always lost because of the green in printing. They, the connecting threads, are rather definite in the epidermal cells, which is particularly striking because they appear very fine in the closely-related cells of the hair and sebaceous follicles.

I Specificity

Like almost all achromatic components the latter, in the vascular epithelium, are very soft but definite; in the lymph cells, however, they are almost never visible. On the whole, however, we cannot use them much when distinguishing individual types of cell. This probably corresponds to their small biological significance.

Chromosomes

The chromosomes are most difficult to assess but yet, along with the spindle, are most important for the characteristics of the cells.

The difficulty lies in the continuous change of their lengths and breadths during division. In spite of this, however, the differences between individual cell types are extremely characteristic if one always compares cells which are in the same phases. This difference appears most definitely in the monaster phase (Figs 10–25). One finds the longest chromosomes in the vascular epithelial cells if the monaster is well developed (Fig. 24), whilst shortly beforehand (Fig. 15) the chromosomes are still rather short. Usually they form very sharply demarcated stars and in this phase they show no tendency to coagulation. The chromosomes gradually increase in size right up to the monaster stage; and the figures appear extraordinarily distinct up to the dispirem. Then, however, a striking contraction of the chromatic figure takes place (Fig. 63) through which it becomes small and indistinct. Shortly before the resting phase, however, they again become looser so that one is often able to see clearly basket structures in the field at the pole.

The epidermal cells, on the other hand, behave quite differently. Already at an early stage (Fig. 1) the chromosomes have the same length as later, and the length remains the same throughout the whole period of cell division. At all stages they (the chromosomes) are bigger than those of the endothelial cells, except in the monaster phase. Also absent are the clear diminution and contraction of the dispirem (Fig. 58) and during the final dissolution[1]. Very close to the epidermal forms are those of the sebaceous and hair follicles; except that in the former mostly, in the latter invariably, they are somewhat smaller. All these division figures are similarly very clear and transparent, like those of the vascular epithelial cells. Because of their mostly thicker and fatter chromosomes, they look stronger and more condensed. In the crypts of Lieberkühn the chromosomes are extremely thin – even thinner than in the lymphoblasts – being longer and more slender (Fig. 25). Mostly they have a tendency to coagulate, which appears at almost all phases except for the monaster, so that in the anaphase one is only seldom able to see clear figures. The chromosomes of the lymphoblasts are the shortest. I observe in them a property that I have not otherwise noticed at all. They have a tendency to form club-like swellings at their ends. It is not to be doubted that this is an artefact which, however, appears only in this one type of cell; but (in that cell type, it appears) during the most various methods of treatment.

[1] By mistake in the Festschrift for Virchow (October 1891: Concerning cell division in human epidermis, p. 5) cells of the vascular epithelial cells were mistakenly recorded where it should have been epidermal cells. It will not have escaped the attentive reader that the description did not accord with the figures. It is, therefore, important to correct this error here.

27   This phenomenon is not seen in all figures but only in occasional ones. The chromosomes remain more or less the same size and strength up to the monaster phase and do not essentially change in length up to that point. In metakinesis, they become very short and then, in the anaphase, they increase in size to such an extent that each of the daughter stars has the size of the mother star. That is based on the circumstance (already mentioned above) that the lymphocytes are, perhaps, also able to digest nourishment during their divisions. Both daughter stars move so considerably apart from each other that sometimes one can scarcely recognise them as belonging to one unit. However, nowhere is the danger of cutting off a star by sectioning of tissue – without one being able to prove it – greater than in the lymphoblasts (Fig. 53).

Nothing can be said with certainty concerning the number of chromosomes in the human being. It is, therefore, also not possible to say whether the different tissues have a different number of chromosomes. As important as this point is, I have hitherto not been able to find a method which would lead to a certain result. This anyone will find understandable if they try to count the 24 chromosomes in the larger cells of *Salamandra maculata*. What is already very difficult there – and only successful under favourable conditions – is quite impossible in the smaller and more chromosome-rich cells of the human being. This is even less possible with methods known to us. Certainly the number is higher than 24. However, I have the impression – but only only suggest it with the greatest reserve – that the number might be greater in the epidermal cells rather than in the vascular epithelial cells.

Division space

As is well known, the significance of the phenomenon of the division space is still disputed. Pfitzner[1] is of the opinion that this space represents the achromatin of the nucleus and that therefore, during division, the nucleus always remains a body closed off (from the rest of the cell). He came to this conclusion by treating the specimens with Na_2SO_4, which in his opinion colours the achromatin. Haematoxylin (when applied later) was supposed to remove this colouring, leaving only the chromatic substance tinged. Tangl[2] proved that the chromatin mass swells because of the Na_2SO_4, and

[1] On the morphological significance of the cell nucleus. Morphol. Jahrb. X.

I Specificity

[2] On the relationship between cell body and nucleus during mitotic division. Arch. f. mikr. Anat. vol. 30.

forms a peculiar figure which then is brought back to its normal appearance by the shrinking effect of the haematoxylin. Schwarz[1] does not share any of these views. He believes, with Pfitzner, that during division the cell nucleus does not give up its isolated independence, and that the division space is an artefact, which is brought about by the shrinkage of the nucleus. The cell nucleus never undertakes any connection with the cytoplasm and the entire process of division is carried out within the original limits of the nucleus. That this view – of the absolute independence of the nucleus *viz-à-vis* the cytoplasm – is incorrect is evident from all new discoveries concerning the behaviour of the centrosomes. For whether the latter primarily originate in the nucleus or whether they are part of the cell body – they are nonetheless situated at a certain point in time outside the nucleus and enter into closest relationship with the chromatic division figure via the achromatic spindle[2]. By this, a spatial mixing of nuclear and cell substance is surely proven. Specimens which Schwarz used – human epidermis – must also seem unsuitable to determine such a question. Over and above this, however, H. F. Müller[3] has proved the penetration of cell granules between the chromosomes. I therefore regard it as thoroughly improbable that the DIVISION SPACE – as I should like to call it – is identical with the nuclear margin. The question is: is the division space solely an artefact or is it based on morphological conditions of the cell, and (if so) what are they? That the division space does not exist in the life of the cell in the same way that it does in the fixed cells is beyond doubt. That it appears, however, in one type of cell with great regularity and has a different form in others – and even in certain types of cells it can be missing altogether – speaks for it having a morphological foundation. I see the same (the morphological basis) in the behaviour of the granules of cell – mentioned above – which become less numerous during cell division (see p. 10) and which (the granules) in many cells are concentrated at the periphery of the cell bodies, whilst in others they fill out the entire cell space and also penetrate between the chromosomes (Müller).

Thereby an extraordinarily clear distinction becomes apparent. In the epidermal cells and cells nearby, e.g., the hair and sebaceous follicles, we observe the divisional space sharply demarcated

[1] Virchow's Arch. vol. 124. p. 512.
[2] The literature was recently given extensively in O. Hertwig's work, "The Cell and the Tissues," pp 143-201 and I can here certainly point to it.
[3] Study of knowledge of division in leukocytes. Arch. f. exper. Pathol. und Pharm. vol. 29.

as if it possessed its own membrane (Figs 10, 12, 22, 28, 31, 40, 41, 43, 49, 50, 51, 52, 61, 69, 70, 75). Within the divisional space there is always the same chromatic figure, spindle and centrosomes, but under individually favourable circumstances,

"Studies on the Specificity, the Altruism and the Anaplasia of cells with Special Reference to Tumours"

one sees the polar radiations extending right over the divisional space. The divisional space, moreover, is never quite empty here, but it always contains a substance – which colours weakly with eosin and similar substances – but which appears more homogenous than the other cytoplasm. In a large sequence of cell-types – e.g., the vascular epithelial cells and the cells of the crypts of Lieberkühn – the divisional space is almost always present but it is irregular in form and not sharply demarcated. One sees either (i) the more intensely coloured and finely granulated border zone of the cell pushed to the fore against the divisional zone in little points, angles and edges, or (ii) the border zone becomes gradually lighter and more homogenous in the environs of the nuclear division figure. Again in other cells, the divisional space is totally lacking. To this category above all belong the lymphocytes and lymphoblasts. This is consistent with, on the one hand, Müller's data (see above) – namely, that in cells which are related to the latter the granules can penetrate between the chromosomes – and on the other hand (with the fact that) they often have such transparent protoplasm; and that, because of this, the emergence of a particular divisional space is impossible.

Cell division

The cleaving of the cell (cytokinesis) after the completion of nuclear division has no characteristic features for distinguishing between the cell-types. It happens either simultaneously from all sides or from one side more strongly than from the other. In this, there is nothing of note that would not already be known from observations of the lower animals. Only in the lymphocytes is a peculiarity (of cytokinesis) apparent, as has been already noted by Flemming (as cited above). These cells divide as a rule very early on, often when the nucleus is in the diaster phase. Thereby the daughter elements achieve early independence which, perhaps, explains the great degree of separation of the dissolution figures which has been so often observed here. I believe too, that by this the duration of division in lymphocytes is considerably shortened.

In pathological circumstances a delay in cell division occurs but this only arises when the nuclei are already in the resting phase. Sometimes cell division can simply not occur at all. That happens with particular frequency in triple and more divisions (of nuclei without cytokinesis). When more than four nuclear divisions occur, I have not observed cell division at all, whilst three divisions without division of cytoplasm are not infrequent. Thereby a series of cells with two and more nuclei is

explained. It then happens that such nuclei get ready for division afterwards, separately. Such processes I have observed several times with absolute certainty. I saw one cell where five separate nuclei were situated in the monospirem-stage. In most cases, however, the appearances indicate that multinucleate cells do not

I Specificity

originate through separate division figures from several nuclei, but by pluri-polar mitosis out of one big nucleus.

The achromatic connecting threads are tied together through cell division and form a spindle which is mostly longer and sharper than the genuine spindle in which, however, a centrosome at its apex can never be observed.

The duration of the process and the period of incubation

From the very beginning one has been aware that certain phases of cell division occur more frequently than others, and one has concluded from this that these phases must proceed particularly slowly. Thus it is known that the metakinesis of all types of cell is found much less frequently than the other phases, and so the turn around (*Umschlagen*) of the chromosomes probably occurs within a very short period of time. If, however, one now examines the tissues of various individuals and under the most varying conditions (normal and pathological), then one finds strikingly little constancy in these phenomena. Extensive counts have shown me that now the prophase is dominant, now the anaphase – in the same types of tissue but only from different individuals. I cannot decide with certainty whether here it is only individual differences or – as I am personally inclined to believe – it is the type and strength of the pathological process which is influential. Only in the crypts of Lieberkühn did I find anything of great constancy. Here the prophases and the dispirem were present in large numbers; on the contrary, metakinesis and the other figures of the anaphase were decidedly infrequent. Only isolated examples of these were found in numerous preparations from many individuals. This indicates that differences between the individual types of cell will exist; and that these differences can be blurred by pathological processes etc to the point of being unrecognisable.

On the other hand, we find considerable variations in the period of time taken by the whole cell for division between the different types of cell. Thus I believe that the mitoses of the endothelial cells and of connective tissues are carried through more rapidly than those of the epidermis. I

observed several cases of poor granulation tissue formation after longstanding inflammation, with atypical epidermal proliferation, as described by Friedländer[1]. Large masses of endothelial cells and relatively slender tongues of epidermis had formed. As the whole is formed in a short period of time, one has the definite impression that much greater masses of endothelial cells are delivered than are epidermal cells – even if one assumes if a large part of the epidermis becomes keratinised and is shed, and especially that the epidermis always takes longer for its keratinisation. Nevertheless, although the mitoses in the epidermis vary considerably, they are more numerous than those of the endothelial cells. It is also striking too that in connective tissue and endothelial proliferations – which have proceeded under the eyes of the observer, eg, tuberculosis of the oral mucous membrane – always fewer mitoses are present than might be supposed from the rapid growth and from the masses of such cells which are present. The same is true of rapidly growing fibromas, eg, the nasal polyps.

However, the number of mitoses observed does not depend only on the time for it to proceed, but it is a function of the period of rest. The relationship between these two periods determines the number of mitoses present at every moment. This is best illustrated graphically. Let us assume in a tissue space, whose size is represented by the abscissa, within a certain period a

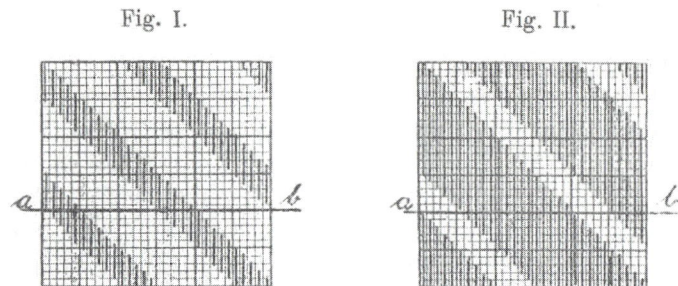

Fig. I.   Fig. II.

number of mitoses (in this example 68) occur. The time which the latter need is represented on the graph by the stripes, the period of rest by the free space in the direction of the ordinates. Now if at some point in time – which is determined by the position line ab – the further progress of the mitoses is interrupted, then in case 1 (Fig. 1) where the period of the division compared to that of the resting phase is in the ratio of 1:2; eight mitoses can be observed. On the other hand in case 2, where the ratio is 3:1, the mitoses number 18, i.e. more than doubled. In the whole period of time under consideration,

[1] "On Epithelial Proliferation and Cancer". Strassburg, 1877.

in the first case, precisely the same number of cells has arisen as in the second. From this we conclude that from the number of mitoses observed we cannot without further ado determine the number of new cells which form in the period of time. This is because, for assessing the duration of mitosis, an uncontrollable factor has to be taken into account, namely, the period of the rest pause. This factor, however, is not constant either for the individual tissues or in general. Furthermore, this factor is changed by all possible influences, although the division time itself seems to be more constant for the individual cell types, within certain limits. In order to clarify this, I isolated an infusorium belonging to the class of ciliates in a moist chamber sealed with Vaseline[1]. Here the nutrients and probably the oxygen decreased gradually. The period between successive divisions of the cells became longer, whilst the duration of the division itself did not demonstrably change. When I then placed one of these young infusoria in a new

I Specificity

moist chamber and laid on its base some oxygen producing algae, the resting pause became shorter again, indicating the possibility that the rest pause was influenced by the nutrients which were given. This is also apparent in various pathological processes, eg, the epidermis. If in a sclerosis of the skin – as is found in scleroderma and also in certain forms of leprosy – the nourishment of the epidermis is markedly reduced, the number of mitoses in it is reduced, without the latter being wholly absent. This also can be understood as nutrients affecting the rest pause. However, it may be other influences which affect the rest pause. Another phenomenon is probably relevant here, to which I referred earlier[2]. It is known that when any proliferation stimulus acts on the cells, the latter do not proceed straight away to mitosis, but that a certain time elapses which I called the period of incubation (see above). It now appears that in various tissue types (and also in various animals) this period is not the same. It fluctuates between three hours[3] and three days[4]. Suitable specimens, which are naturally very hard to come by, were not available for me to carry out comparative studies in human beings, but I was able to initiate one comparison. If one makes a small skin incision, one finds after 24 hours (probably earlier too) a perceptible increase of mitoses in the epidermis,

[1] Colpidium, Bütschli, "The Protozoa". vol. III. p. 1704.
[2] Karyokinesis and cellular pathology, Berl. klin. W. 1891. no. 42
[3] Garré: Chirurgische Beiträge von Bruns. IV. 1889
[4] v. Bügner: Regeneration of nerves. Ziegler's Beiträge. vol. 10, p. 321.

whilst during the same period of time, only an increase of the wandering cells can be demonstrated in the connective tissue. Only on the following day – or even later – do mitoses appear in the connective tissue. Thus the incubation time for connective tissue is longer than that of the epidermis. That accords with all observations which have been made in the regeneration of keratinising skin, epidermis, etc.

Position of the mitoses

A few particular things which did not find a place under the preceding headings still have to be mentioned. First of all is the peculiar process of nuclear migration in the cell prior to cell division. In all clearly bipolar cells – i.e. in the cylindrical cells of the gut, and many tumours there; in the basal cells of multi-layered mucous membranes and also in the epidermis – the nucleus shifts from the base towards the apex of the cell while it is still apparently in a state of complete rest. This phenomenon is very clear in the gut epithelia, because here all the nuclei lie at the base excepting only those cells in the process of division. They move out of the (basal) row in a step-wise fashion towards the lumen of the crypts of Lieberkühn (see Figs 7, 16, 25, 34). Only after cell division has been completed does the nucleus move in a step-wise fashion back to the base of the cell again. This process was described at the same time by Reinke[1] and by myself[2] – by Reinke for the cells of the crypts of Lieberkühn and by me for all clearly bipolar cells. In the epidermis and in the multi-layered mucous membranes this process plays a part – but only insofar as one never perceives the mitotic figure in the basal part of the cells as described by Drasch[3], but always in the top part of the cell. The process, moreover, had already been seen earlier in the central nervous system of embryos but it was not recognised that it was a case of nuclear wandering[4].

Another peculiar feature of many cells is that they only achieve division when at definite locations, so that one speaks of germinal centres or germinal layers. These very appropriate expressions were introduced first by Flemming* and have been generally accepted. For example in the epidermis and in the multi-layered mucous membranes, mitoses are found almost exclusively in the most basal cell layer,

[1] Investigations on the relationship of the nuclear forms described by Arnold to mitosis and amitosis, Dissertation Kiel, 1891.
[2] Cell Division in the Epidermis. Virchow's Festschrift, 1891.
[3] Sitzungsber. der k. Academie in Wien, 1866, vol. 93, May issue.
[4] Compare: Rauber, Nucleus division figures in medullary tube of vertebrates. Arch. f. mikr. Anat. vol. 26, 1886.
* but possibly earlier by Goodsir – see Chapter 3 (eds).

34   i.e. closest to the papillary bodies (dermal papillae). It can only be described as an error when Schütz[1] asserts that mitoses are more common in the third highest layer of the epidermis than in the basal layer. That is exactly the opposite of the real situation. An epidermis which shows more mitoses in the higher layers than in the basal layers is to be understood as pathological, and it is beyond comprehension how Schütz can add to this completely inaccurate assertion a statement that this (the erroneous assertion) is a well known fact. In addition to this, Schütz has the mitoses in carcinoma cells in the lowest cell layers, which again is absolutely incorrect, because precisely the opposite takes place. As has recently been correctly emphasised by Ströbe[2], the mitoses in carcinoma cells are distributed randomly. Nevertheless, we should not generally agree with that either, because in carcinomata which have their origin in layered epithelia, the germinal layer is just as preserved as it is in benign warts and pachydermia of the same organs. Only this germinal layer is somewhat broadened. A random distribution of the mitoses occurs, as described by Ströbe, in other carcinomata.

The same is true of the sebaceous follicles, in which similarly, the mitoses are normally situated in the basal layer and do not move upwards to any significant degree in inflammation or benign tumour, eg, molluscum contagiosum (see Figs 3, 12, 30, 42, 51, 60). On the other hand in the hair follicles, the germinal layer is quite broad from the start and does not restrict itself to the basal layer.

I Specificity

In lymph nodes, the germinal centres are exactly described in pre-karyokinetic times by His and then by Flemming (cited above). Germinal centres – which, even under physiological conditions and in each case according to the activity of the lymph nodes, show large degrees of variability in their extent – increase considerably in their size and pathological conditions and especially their mitoses. Mitoses, which are found occasionally outside the germinal centres of physiological lymph nodes, increase very significantly (in pathological conditions).

Newly-defined germinal centres are not otherwise found in the connective tissues. However, it has been confirmed by many researchers that in wounds the regeneration is striking and does not occur in the cells immediately adjacent but in the cells which are several cell places distant. Newly-delivered cells are then gradually pressed forward into the defect. In granulation tissue, on the other hand, the mitoses occur apparently quite randomly. If, however,

[1] "Microscopic Findings in Carcinoma". Frankfurt a. M, 1890, p. 14.
[2] Ziegler's Beiträge vol. XI.

one observes carefully, they almost always occur near the vessels, whose epithelia first increase in number and then become multi-layered, so that cells which derive from the capillary wall cells no longer go to the lumen of the vessels (e.g., Figs 6, 24 and 45). These cells (in the interstitium), because of the similarity of their mitoses (to those of vascular cells) are thus documented as deriving from the epithelium of the vessel or lymph sinuses. According to this, therefore, I totally agree with Billroth who says[1], "I want to assert *a priori* that the granulation tissue proceeds according to its main elements from the cells of the vessel wall". Also, Flemming[2] emphasises in salamander larvae how, in new formations of vessels, the mitotic figures are not at the apex of the vessel sprout but always one or two cells behind.

I have described the differences between the mitoses of the different cell types in relatively few types. One reason is because comprehensiveness cannot be achieved yet and another is because presentation of a larger amount of material would have a tiring and confusing effect. As one has to restrict oneself to relatively coarse parts of the cells, and the more refined structures particularly in human cells, elude us almost entirely; so the description – in the very nature of things – always revolves around the few points presented. If further material were included, one would wholly lose perspective; I will only add that apart from the tissue types mentioned, I have also studied the cells of the kidney and liver as well as the parenchymata of the salivary, mucous, sweat, labial, pylorus and mammary glands of the usual connective tissues, of the corpus luteum, of the mucous tissues, of smooth muscle and of cartilage in children. Always the special peculiarities were proved in the mitoses of these cells; even if the mitoses do not appear everywhere with the same clarity. The preceding description, together with the photograms, will be sufficient I believe to show what I would like to prove – namely that perceptible differences occur in the process of cell division of individual tissue types.

Now these differences are also expressed sharply in mixed tissues so that one can recognise them from these differences – the forms of individual tissue mitoses – e.g. in endothelium, connective tissue, leucocytes (i.e. granulation tissue), the epidermal rete; everywhere these forms are strikingly constant.

[1] "On the Influences of Living Cells of Plants and Animals on Each Other". Vienna 1890. p. 25.
[2] Arch. f. mikr. Anat. vol. 35, p. 275, 1890.

36 Nowhere are transitions from one site to another encountered – which is all the more notable because such transitions were often assumed in resting cells. Also, nowhere was such latitude for activity present than specifically in mixed tissues. Thus these findings are particularly suited to give new and weighty support to the theory of the specificity of the cell. Because it is precisely here that these transitions are completely lacking: where the cell is liberated from chance external influences, and where histological accommodation (an extremely variable entity) is reduced to a minimum. Certainly, many tissues still remain to be examined so that one is not at the moment in a position to assert that no genuine metaplasia ever occurs. The existence of the latter has become very improbable and one is forced more and more to the view that genuine metaplasia is absent – not only from epithelia in which formerly one almost assumed this specificity* – but also from connective tissues. Quite unacceptable accordingly – it seems to me – is the view of von Recklinghausen (cited above) that in the lungs and kidneys, connective tissue could arise from the epithelium of alveoli and from that of Bowman's capsule respectively; or that as Baumgarten says[1], the lymph nodal and epithelial cells participate in the formation of tubercle cells; or as Ribbert[2] and Schmidt[3] describe, lymph bodies arise from endothelial cells. The assumption may be just as improbable as that epidermis, node cells or mucous membrane epithelia derive from connective tissue cells. The simple evidence of mitoses is not sufficient to show which tissue contributes to a unified new cell formation. For it is a generally valid law that proliferation stimuli are never limited to a specific tissue but extend over a particular area irrespective of the various types of tissue. Thus in the interstitial syphilitic processes in the liver – just as was described for tuberculosis by Baumgarten (cited above) – mitoses are found in the connective tissues and the vascular epithelium, just as in the liver cells. In lupus of the skin, a significant intensification of mitoses was shown in the epidermis without it having to be assumed that the epidermal cells were involved in the formation of subepidermal tubercles. The forms of mitosis must be kept precisely separate from each other and one will never find transitions in this.

I Specificity

[1] Experimental and pathological-anatomical understanding of tuberculosis. Zeitschrift f. kl. Med. 1885, vol. 9, pp 93, 245, and 1886 vol. 19, p. 24.
[2] On regeneration and inflammation of the lymph glands. Ziegler's Beiträge VI. 1889.
[3] Arch. f. mikr. Anat. vol. 38, 1892, p. 524 ff
* probably what is meant by "specificity" here is "specific metaplastic process" (eds).

THE TRANSITION PICTURES OF THE RESTING CELLS, HOWEVER – WHICH CAN BE INFLUENCED BY EXTERNAL LOCAL CIRCUMSTANCES, BY MOMENTARY CHANGES IN NUTRITION, BY STIMULI OF ANY KIND – HAVE, ACCORDING TO THE FINDINGS OF SPECIFICITY OF MITOSIS, NOTHING TO CONTRIBUTE IN THE WAY OF PROOF OF, AND MAY NOT BE APPLIED TO, THE PROCESS OF A GENUINE METAPLASIA. 37

Thus by way of direct observation, we come to the statement which was put forward by Bard[1] on the basis of more theoretical considerations: "*omnis cellula e cellula ejusdem generis*".

If I am now inclined – on the basis of the previously mentioned investigations – to deny a genuine metaplasia, and on the other hand to assume extensive degrees of histological accommodation; one could easily gain the impression that the concept of histological accommodation had replaced metaplasia, but that the matter itself remained unchanged. Now that is naturally not the case, as can be immediately recognised if one examines it more closely. I exclude all transitions from epithelial cells to connective tissue and vice versa as impossible and find myself in agreement with the majority of histologists on this. That ciliated epithelium can translate itself into squamous epithelium; or the epithelium of the ducts of the pancreas in the case of ranula into ciliated epithelium; or that cysts with multi-layered epithelium and the like can develop from testicular tubules; is well known and has been interpreted as histological accommodation. However, it would be incorrect if on the basis of these findings one were to assert that the flat epithelium in the trachea or on nasal polyps is really epidermis, or that the ciliated epithelium of the ranula is identical with that of the trachea. It is certainly doubtlessly correct that bones or fatty tissue and so on can be formed from connective tissue. However, with Ziegler (cited above), I believe that not every connective tissue can transform itself into either bone or fatty tissue, but that only specific types of connective tissues can do this. If, for example, mucous tissue of the foetus transforms itself into fatty tissue while the mucous tissue of the vitreous humour does not, then that alone is a sign that we are dealing with two different types of mucous tissue. That connective tissues are not everywhere the same is clearly already evident from ordinary examinations: for example, compare the connective tissues of the skin with those of the ovary; here also the mitoses show considerable differences. Indeed, I am inclined to assume that the connective tissue in every organ is a specific one and particularly on the basis of the forms of mitoses.

[1] Arch. de Physiologie. 1886. Tm 7. Series III. p. 406.

38 However, my material is not yet sufficient for me to embark upon a classification of the forms of connective tissue and that is also the reason why I have refrained from setting down any single mitotic sequence characteristic of connective tissues. The idea of the unity of connective tissue does not stem from morphological agreement but mainly from the idea of a unified connective tissue germinal cell. However, because the paraplast theory has lost more and more supporters and it has been shown that connective tissue can be formed in the most various places of the embryo, so then one will be the more easily converted to the view that connective tissues are not identical everywhere. Moreover, the idea of the specificity of the different connective tissue types contradicts the theory of a unified connective tissue germinal cell as little as the specificity of epithelia contradicts the idea of a unified derivation of the latter.

If one now assumes such a specificity of cells, one must also formulate an idea as to how this specificity comes about because all cells once upon a time derived from the same cell – the mature fertilised egg cell. There are two theories on this: (i) that the cells are brought into position by mechanical means and that their character is determined thereby, whilst (ii) assumes a differentiation proceeding from intracellular mechanisms. The first view, however, also actually assumes a histological accommodation, which then leads to a lasting inheritable property of the cells. Other researchers furthermore, amongst whom O. Hertwig publicly declares himself in his text book "History of Development",[1] take up an intermediate position, in that they assume differentiation via histological accommodation in consequence of mechanical change in situation; and also propose a differentiation by division of labour.

The foundation of the idea of the independent development of the individual tissues is to be traced back to Remak[2]. Then the purely mechanical theory (of this) found its main proponent in His, who in his well known work on body form explained the mechanical influences on the shape of the embryo in an elegant and most vivid way. But just as little as the beautiful and interesting attempts of Quincke[3] and Bütschli[4] convince us of a purely mechanical concept of

[1] 3rd Edition 1890. pp 66-72
[2] "On the development of Vertebrates".
[3] Sitzungsber. der Acad. der Wissenschaften zu Berlin 1888. vol. 34.
[4] Investigations of microscopic foams and the protoplasm. 1892.

39 movements of protoplasm – at least in the present state of the sciences[1] – so too, a purely mechanical concept of cell differentiation cannot satisfy us.

The second view of physiological division of labour and the differentiation arising thereby was really the next step, and to my knowledge was first precisely expressed by Bard[2]. Bard's essay, however, remained completely unheeded and was very little known. It was also unknown to me when I developed similar views in a lecture on polymastia[3] and in Virchow's Archive[4]. These ideas are so important for what follows that I must go into the matter somewhat more precisely.

When the egg cell is fertilised and begins to divide, two things can happen: either the division is a like one or an unlike one. If the division is a like one, then both of the first cleavage spheres are like each other, but not like the mother cell. This is clear from a sequence of embryological observations. Roux[5] proved in frogs that after the destruction of the one cleavage sphere, a hemi-embryo arises. This hemi-embryo later in development makes some contribution towards regeneration of the other half. Van Beneden and Ch. Julin[6] showed how in *Ascidia* – and Kowalewsky[7] in bony fish – the first cleavage of the egg divides the embryo into right and left body halves. Driesch[8] saw that in echinoderms after destruction of the one cleavage sphere, a complete but dwarf-like embryo arises; Hertwig[9] observed that from the cleaving spheres of *Triton taeniatus* and *cristatus*, the front and back halves – most frequently the belly and the breast – of the embryo developed. From all these, and still more observations – which amongst themselves have fanned the flames of the dispute concerning isotropia and anisotropia of the egg – it is collectively clear that every cleavage sphere forms either a part or a dwarf form, and only both of them together yield the normal embryo.

[1] See also on this, Verworn, "The Movements of Living Substance". Jena 1892.
[2] Cellular specificity and histogenesis in the embryo, Arch. de Physiol. 1886. vol. 7, Section III. p. 406.
[3] Verhandlungen der Berl. anthropol. Gesellschaft. Issue of 18 May 1889, p. 439.
[4] vol. 119, p. 315.
[5] Virchow's Arch. vol. 114.
[6] Arch. de Biol. 5. 1884.
[7] Zeitschrift f. wiss. Zool. 1886.
[8] Ditto vol. 53 1891.
[9] "Old and New Theories of Development". Berlin 1892.

Thus a genuine division of labour has taken place, because if differentiation depends only on both cleavage spheres remaining together and, therefore, each takes on only part of the work, i.e. IF IT WERE A MATTER OF THE FIRST STEP IN A HISTOLOGICAL ACCOMMODATION, then each of the cleaving spheres would have to provide alone a complete and normal embryo. This can happen in exceptional cases; that not only the egg but the mother cell too can divide into similar cells. In this way twins can arise, as has been expressly recognised by Virchow in his essay on Origin and Pathology[1].

If a primary differentiation of the first cleavage spheres can be shown in the so-called "equal egg cleavage", this is still more apparent in "unequal egg cleavage".

It is well known that this (unequal egg cleavage) is found in very many animals, for example, the platyhelminths, the orthonectides and dicyemides, the nematodes, the rotatoria, the annelides and so on[2]. A really splendid example is the development of *Rhodites rosae*[3] which was precisely investigated by Weismann. One part of the cleaving nucleus moves to the front pole of the egg. The hind part divides first and forms the blastoderm. Only then does the front part divide and the so-called inner germinal cells arise; these form the wall of the middle gut and add themselves to the mesoblast. This process is absolutely classic in the dicyemides and orthonectides. The first cleavage spheres are distinguishable by their size. The smaller one alone for the moment, continues to go on dividing, so that the larger cell becomes surrounded by the descendants of the smaller one. In the dicyemides now, the larger cell remains undivided until after completion of the ectoderm: it then disintegrates into individual developmental cells. In the orthonectides, two other cells separate themselves from the large cell, and these become muscle fibres; whilst it (the large cell itself) divides into a heap of cells which mature either into ovarian or testicular cells. How the chromosomes behave in such an unequal division has been, as far as I know, studied only in one case; by Häcker[4] as has been illustrated there on Plate 24, Fig. 5. He describes the process thus: the germinal cell divides into the proto-genital cell (A) and the proto-mesodermal cell (B). Chromosomes in both are in equal numbers (8), but different in form and behaviour when stained. The A cell has long, large and faintly-staining chromosomes; the B cell

[1] His Archive vol. 103.
[2] See also "Textbook of Comparative Developmental History" by Korschlet and Heider.
[3] Contributions to Anatomy and Embryology. Festgabe for Henle. Bonn 1882, p. 80.
[4] The nuclear division in the mesoderm- and entoderm formation of Cyclops. Arch. f. mikr. Anat. vol. 38 p. 556.

has short small and intensely-staining chromosomes. These cells pass on these properties to their successors. In the cases in which an asymmetric division takes place at the outset, there can be no question of histological accommodation. It must be a process based in the nature of the cells that leads to this differentiation – in which the daughter cells are neither the same amongst themselves nor the same as the mother cells.

But also in primarily equal divisions, a clear unequal division of all cells constituting the cleaving sphere often takes place early. Thus in the blastula phase, the cells of the vegetative pole are clearly distinguishable from those of the animal pole by their size and their content in yolk components. This is important not merely in cases of primarily unequal cleaving – where mostly an epibolic gastrula is achieved; i.e. where the vegetative cells become surrounded by the animal cells – but also in cases of primarily equal division. In these divisions, an invagination gastrula is formed, so that the vegetative cells are differentiated from the animal cells before the infolding process. Thus differentiation precedes the infolding process; hence differentiation is not the consequence of the change of location because it is not brought about by the infolding. One sees this very clearly, although quite schematically, in the *Amphioxus* blastula, as was described

I Specificity

by Hatschek; and still more clearly in the so-called amphiblastula phase of *Syncandra raphanus*[1]. Numerous other examples are available to prove the same fact. There is no reason to look for a different explanation for the meroblastic eggs, in which these circumstances are not as transparent as in the holoblastic ones.

Here, right in the initial stages of egg cleaving, a principle is apparent which can be followed through the entire embryological development. Every unequal division is followed by a sequence of equal divisions. These latter have the purpose of enlarging the group of cells formed by the previous unequal division. Thereby, in the development of an organ or of a group of cells of equal value, certain phases can be established to which I have given the name, generation stages[2]. THUS, GENERATION STAGES IN THE FAMILY TREE OF A CELL-TYPE ARE ALWAYS THOSE TIMES WHERE UNEQUAL DIVISIONS TAKE PLACE. THESE LEAD IN TURN TO A NEW CELL GROUP – AND THENCE TO THE FORMATION OF A NEW ORGAN.

Every new generation stage is accompanied, or soon followed, by a change in the growth direction. We see this again most

[1] v. Belfours, "Handbook of Comparative Embryology", translated by Vetter. vol. 1, p. 135
[2] Virchow's Archiv. vol. 119, p. 315.

clearly in the lowest animal forms, but we can also observe the same in the development of vertebrates. The infolding of the vegetative cells of the blastula and the gastrula arising from that is the first example. We see the same in the formation of the spinal marrow canal out of the medullary plate; the eyeball and lens pit; and particularly in the development of glands – e.g., the liver, lung, skin glands and so on. In this, the effect is wholly the same: whether in the formation of the new type of tissue the new type sinks into what is already present, or the new type grows around it; just as whether a gastrula is achieved by invagination or by epiboly.

There is a series of theories about how this differentiation of cells comes about, which (the series of theories) are built up wholly on the assumption that the hereditary properties of the cells – the idioplasmas – are tied to definite anatomical components of the cells; i.e. the idioblasts. O Hertwig[1] puts forward the view that each cell of an organism receives the basic hereditary material from the egg cell, and that the particular nature of each cell is only determined by the fact that the idioblasts – each individual part of the hereditary material – become effective for each cell according to the conditions deriving from the whole complex of hereditary material, whilst the other idioblasts remain latent. Particularly Nägeli[2] and Hugo de Vries[3] have declared themselves in favour of this view. In order now, however, to gain an idea of how it is that the cells – although possessing all hereditary loci – can still bring individual loci into action: Nägeli has thought out a rather complicated dynamic theory in which the individual idioblasts or micelle groups, as he calls them, get into particular tension-and-movement states, whereby the plastic and chemical processes of the cells are regulated. De Vries on the other hand assumes that only specific idioblasts – which he calls pangenes – become active, increase in number and move from the nucleus into the cell substance, whereby they determine the form and function of the cell and lead to a hereditary capability outside of the cell nuclei. All these theories, however, presuppose that the cells first achieve this changed situation and only then change their properties. Thus one would have to seek first a further reason for the change of the situation and – even if with His, one wished to recognise purely mechanical reasons for many cases – then such mechanical reasons would still be lacking in by far the majority of cases.

[1] "The problem of Fertilisation and Isotropy of the Egg". Jena 1884, Comparison of egg and sperm formation in nematodes. Arch. f. wiss. Zool. vol. 36, 1890. "Cell and Tissue". Jena 1892.
[2] "Mechanical-Physiological Theory of Heredity". Munich 1884.
[3] "Intracellular pangenesis". Jena 1889.

To this should be added those cases in which morphological changes in the cells become apparent prior to the change of location. Even if one did not wish to acknowledge this, then the unequal cleavage of the egg would be left over; which cannot possibly be explained as a result of the location, because it represents a primary state. In addition, however, these theories contradict the specificity of cells, which is based on positive findings and consistent with histological accommodation. Even then, one would need yet another theory to explain why the cells hold on so firmly to a property which has been achieved by accommodation, and pass it on to posterity, as they do in fact.

It should be asked now whether there are no examples at all to be found of a histological accommodation through change of location in the developmental history. In favour of this, however, there are now two quite unambiguous examples. The first of these, and the clearest for me, has always been the development of the epithelium of Bowman's capsules in the kidneys. If the kidney anlage has advanced so far that the convoluted tubules are closing up awkwardly (*krümmen*) at their ends, then they move into relationship with the tangles of the vessels, which are developing at this point. The cells from the convoluted tubules grow around the latter to a certain extent, in that the cells from the small canal come to lie firmly alongside the tangle, and the tangle grows in front of and against the small canal. In this process, for the moment, no kind of differentiation of these cells, in contrast to the remaining tubular epithelium, takes place. The differentiation of the cells only begins when the glomerulus is completely formed. Here the change in direction of growth is a passive one, brought about by the vessel tuft and the change in the cells which appears later is a consequence of the changed location. Thus we also see that in inflammation and proliferative phenomena, the epithelium of Bowman's capsules and (the epithelium) of the vessel tangle return to the character of the tubular cells and these tubular cells also proceed through the same sort of changes. For the same reason, however,

I think that it is very improbable that these cells, as is often maintained, are supposed to serve only as filters. On the contrary, I believe that they produce an independent secretion, even if, perhaps, to a more limited extent than the tubular epithelium. Whether further alongside of this, filtration takes place is another question.

Another theory maintains that a qualitative distribution of idioplasmas amongst the cells takes place from the start; that a continuous fragmentation of the egg anlagen proceeds and only the generative cells reconstitute the entire anlage complex. However, whilst Bard (cited above) reaches the conclusion that only those plasmas necessary for the characteristics of the cells get into the corresponding cells, I have stated the

view[1], with which Weismann[2] has recently associated himself THAT ALONG WITH THE MAIN PLASMAS, FURTHER AUXILIARY PLASMAS REMAIN BEHIND IN THE CELLS, AND THAT THE SPECIFICITY OF THE CELL IS BASED ON WHICH MAJORITY OF MAIN PLASMAS HAS BEEN CREATED BY QUALITATIVELY UNEQUAL DIVISION. Just as such an assumption does not contradict the facts from plant biology given by Hugo de Vries (cited above), neither does it at all call into question a hereditariness of the body cells outside the cell nuclei. But it does explain further the reservations set out above against the view on accommodation of cells (Hertwig, Nägeli, de Vries). Hertwig[3] says that the assumption of qualitatively unequal divisions contradicts the fact that in plants and lower animals almost every group of cells can reproduce the whole organism. It is also in contradiction to the fact that cells can change their function as taught by the study of regeneration. I will try to demonstrate in the following chapter that these reservations are only sustainable if, with Bard, one denies the auxiliary plasmas; but can be easily dispersed if one accepts auxiliary plasmas.

[1] Virchow's Archiv. vol. 119.
[2] "The Germ Plasm: A Theory of Heredity". Jena, 1892.
[3] "Cell and Tissue" p. 286.

II Altruism

In the previous chapter, the specificity of cells was explained as the result of either unequal or halving divisions of cells during development. The assumption was that after unequal divisions, each cell must possess main plasmata which determine the character of a cell, as well as lesser plasmata, which are pushed into the background by the main plasmata.

This concept of mine will have to be defended against two lines of criticism; the one by Hertwig and the other by Bard. The former states that all kinds of plasmata are evenly present in all cells but only some become active. The latter says that each cell contains only those plasmata, which characterise its nature. Weismann[1], who by and large shares my view, has built his theory on the examination of large amounts of zoological material. It is now my brief to explain how pathological anatomy underpins this concept.

This is how I envisage the development of the specificity* of cells. The ovum contains all kinds of plasmata of the future organism in an even way, so that all plasmata are in balance and none outweighs the other.[2] This could be expressed in a simplified scheme where we assume there were only three different kinds of plasmata: – – – – – · · · · · | | | | |, or 6a + 6b + 6c, where "a", "b" and "c" denote the type of plasmata.

[1] "The Germ Plasma, A Theory of Inheritance". Jena, 1892.
[2] I may remark that this does not mean to comment on the isotropy or anisotropy of the ovum, because no assumptions are made as to how the plasmata are distributed within the egg cell, other than that they are all there, regardless of shape or form or localisation.
* i.e. of embryological lineage commitment (eds)

This means the (fertilised – eds) egg is the least differentiated cell and is able to fulfil all necessary functions all by itself. Then at first unequal division – the first generational phase – this cell divides in such way that two new cells are generated of the composition (4a + 3b + 3c) and (2a + 3b + 3c). When these cells are completely grown they will comprise (8a + 6b + 6c) and (4a + 6b + 6c)*. The sum of these cells equals the sum of two (fertilised – eds) egg cells. However, the idioplasmata are arranged in such a manner that in one cell, plasma type "a" is predominant, whereas in the other one, it is "(b + c)". To be able to generate the sum of functionality, these two cells must belong together. Should they be required to exist without the other the first cell would suffer "(b + c)" deficiency, whereas the second one would suffer a lack of "a" plasmata. If the first of these hypothetical cells then divides unequally, the offspring may look like this: "(6a + 3b + 3c)" and "(2a + 3b + 3c)" and in the adult stage: (12a + 6b + 6c) and (4a + 6b + 6c)*. This demonstrates two things: firstly, in one cell the "(b + c)" plasmata are increasingly outweighed by "a" plasmata. Thus, with each generation there is a stronger differentiation. The second cell, which sprang from the first division has to double as well, otherwise the sum would not make up to a multiple of the (fertilised – eds) egg (number). Thus, we will end up with 4 cells: (12a + 6b + 6c), (4a + 6b + 6c), (4a + 6b + 6c), (4a + 6b + 6c). The sum of these four will be (24a + 24b + 24c) – equivalent to four times the original (fertilised) egg cell. This sum must be an exact multiple of the egg number, otherwise not all functions of the body will be preserved. If one division was missing, the second generation of cell would look like: (12a + 6b + 6c), (4a + 6 + 6c), (4a + 6b + 6c). The sum would be (22a + 18b + 18c), thus plasmata "a" would outnumber "(b + c)", potentially resulting in an incomplete organism. There are many variations of this scheme but all would have similar results. If the second generation were (4a+4b+4c) and

II Altruism

(4a+2b+2c), or fully grown (8a+8b+8c) and (8a+4b+4c) it would be required of the second cell (4a+6b+6c) to double to be able to achieve a total of (24a+24b+24c). In this latter variation, the four-cell organism would be: (8a+8b+8c)+(8a+4b+4c) + 2(4a+6b+6c). Instead of simply doubling, the second cell may divide unequally; as long as it divides and does not remain in its first generational phase.[1]

[1] The scheme outlined above is, of course, nothing but a theoretical construct and I am not saying cells would really occur like that. The fact that in real life there are not three but many, many types of plasmata already implies a near infinite number of variations, of which I arbitrarily picked just one. Likewise, the choice of a number of 6 is entirely arbitrary, any other even number would have done. It simply serves the purpose of illustrating whether the types of plasma, "a", "b" or "c", are balanced or not. However, it has to be an even number, because each ovum capable of differentiating consists of two equipotent halves, of male and of female origin.
*Hansemann seems to believe (incorrectly) that the chromosomes replicate after nuclear division, not before.

From this it can be concluded that the resulting relationships between cells are close ones. The term describing this relationship will be named "altruism" and we could view the sister cells – which sprang from the qualitatively unequal cell division – as complementary opposites. These ideas came from two observations, both of which were not easily explicable by Hertwig's theory. FIRSTLY, THE FAILURE OR LOSS OF ONE CELL TYPE CAN BE SUFFICIENT TO CAUSE THE DEATH OF AN INDIVIDUAL. SECONDLY, PROLIFERATION OF A CELL TYPE IS ACCOMPANIED BY PROLIFERATION OF ITS COMPLEMENTARY OPPOSITES.

Prior to analysing this a little further we must first oppose Bard's view of absolute differentiation. I do agree with Hertwig[1], that the assumption that cells contain only main plasmata fails to explain many phenomena in lower animals and plants in regard to propagation and regenerative processes. This dilemma led me to postulate the existence of lesser plasmata years ago.[2] It was mainly findings from plant biology that sparked this idea. For example M.W. Beyerink[3] showed, that *Poa nemoralis*, under the influence of galls, could sprout roots where they normally never would sprout. Furthermore, galls of *Salix purpurea* could turn into roots, which are identical to young roots of the same type of willow.[4] The results of the transplantation experiments (mentioned earlier) appeared more important to me in the past then they probably are. That is because in these, a true recurrence of lesser plasmata – as found in metaplasia – is not actually happening after closer scrutiny. Frog skin and rabbit cornea, when transplanted into humans, are able to stimulate existing tissues to proliferate and close over a defect but get resorbed in the process. This also happens to mucosa transplanted into epidermis and the wall of atheroma. Likewise I have discarded Friedländer's[5]

[1] "Cell and Tissue". p. 286.
[2] Virchow's Arch. vol. 119, p. 318.
[3] The gall of *Cecidomya Poae*. Botan. Zeitg., 1885, vol. 2.
[4] On the Caecidium of *Nematus caprae*, Botan. Zeitg. 1888, vol. 1.
[5] Physiological and anatomical examinations of the uterus, Arch. f. Gyn. vol. IX, p. 22.

48 example of the regeneration of uterine mucosa from glands as proof of the existence of lesser plasma, since I realise now that these so-called "glands" are not real glands, but very much like Lieberkühn's crypts – simply recesses of the mucosa. Thus these cells are expected to possess the same idioplasmata as the mucosa cells themselves. Apart from seminal findings in plants and several lower animals – which are carefully collated by Weismann (as mentioned above) in an excellent fashion – it is what happens in tumours, which makes me confident about postulating lesser plasmata. The same is true of regenerative processes and the altruism of cells.

Of the findings in lower animals, the most important one seems to be budding, as it has been described recently by Albert Lang[1]. Lang found in investigations initiated by Weismann that the budding in these animals is not – as was previously thought – (a process of) extending from the ectoderm and endoderm of the original animal, but from ectoderm only. Because of this, the latter endoderm of the bud is the offspring of the ectoderm of the original animal. Since the bud is an exact copy of the original animal and because the endoderm is no different from that of the mother animal, the only explanation for this must be that in the ectodermal cells – or at least the one cell from which the bud springs – the idioplasmata of the endoderm must have persisted as latent lesser plasmata. I am of the opinion that this example should suffice to form an insuperable contradiction to Bard's view of the absolute separation of idioplasmata.

Thus I am joining with Hertwig, de Vries and Nägeli in this matter. Let us look at a few facts relating to regeneration, where we will find much more to support Weismann's and my theory of the qualitatively unequal cell division than will support the view of those researchers who believe in *post facto* regulation through main and lesser plasmata.

From the scheme mentioned above (pp 45 and 46) it follows that a cell is the more differentiated, i.e. (particular) main plasmata out-number the lesser plasmata, in proportion to the greater number of generation stages through which the cell has passed since the egg. Therefore the lesser plasmata will find it harder to regain active status the more generation stages have elapsed since the very first division of the egg. If such a law-like relationship could be practically proven, then that fact should underpin

[1] On budding in *Hydra* and some *Hydropolyps*. Zeitsch. f. wiss. Zool. vol. 54, p. 365, 1892.

49 my and Hertwig's views which would not be explicable by a progressive differentiation alone.

As far as maturity goes, if the egg cell is a somatic epithelial cell, it should contain as main plasmata the idioplasmata of an epithelial cell. In addition, it is considered to contain all lesser plasmata of all other possible idioplasmata, because it can develop into the complete organism. During maturation, the excess of one plasma must somehow be counter-balanced, to the effect that the resulting

II Altruism

cell is a completely non-differentiated egg cell. How this state could possibly be reached has not been explained. Weismann[1] was originally of the opinion that once the first polar body was expelled, the excess plasmata had disappeared. Possibly influenced by the arguments of Boveri[2], he abandoned these ideas later on[3]. For a cell to assume one state after another, a balance of plasmata has to be reached; this can only be achieved either by all plasmata except one increasing so that any particular one does not become predominant, or by losing some of one type of plasmata. The first possibility is so complicated that we cannot even try to imagine how such a process could function. Therefore, only the second possibility remains; which is that expulsion or other form of destruction of the excess plasmata occurs. I do not wish to speak against the better insight of Boveri and Weismann, but I must admit that Weismann's first idea sounds more plausible to me, although he has now revoked it: it did seem to cover the observed facts better than does this other theory which is now the only idea still standing.

However, for the process of generation of eggs – meaning de-differentiation of the somatic cell to form the undifferentiated egg cell – to happen, one has to maintain that during this process, plasmata – which were once pushed into the background due to the predominance of another type of plasma – come into action again. Where ever we can follow germinal cell lines at all, we find that IN NO SINGLE SOMATIC CELL IS THE NUMBER OF GENERATIONAL STAGES SMALLER THAN IN THE DIRECT SEQUENCE FROM EGG TO EGG. For example in diptera, many worms and other animals, there is a single generation stage between egg and primordial gonadal cell, and in daphnides – according to Weismann – about five generation stages; in other animals a few more. However, just the fact that one is able to count generational stages at all is already

[1] "On the Number of Polar Bodies and their Significance for Heredity". Jena, 1887.
[2] "Cell Studies". Jena, 1890.
[3] "Amphimixis". Jena, 1891.

proof of a relatively low known number of them. THUS, IN THE EGG THE REAPPEARANCE OF AUXILIARY PLASMATA IS COMPATIBLE WITH A LOW NUMBER OF GENERATIONAL STAGES.

What is happening with regeneration? Where a tissue regenerates itself from left over foci of the same type, no one mentions the occurrence of auxiliary plasmata but they do where, after loss of complete parts of the body or whole organs, the remainder of the body regenerates the lost parts. We find the largest regeneration potential in the simplest, so-called lower order animals. A polyp can form a new individual animal out of almost any piece of it, and as Loeb[1] has shown, all that is required is a simple cut into the stem of the animal, to start a complete regeneration. Some worms, for example, lumbriculus and nais can regenerate the head from the tail end, and the tail from the head end. Several lower order vertebrates are capable of complete regeneration of extremities, for example, of a lost tail; we even see occasionally in the lizard the growth of two new tails in place of the original single tail. Furthermore, the embryo has a greater capacity for replacement (of lost parts) than the fully formed animal[2]. In higher vertebrates, regeneration only happens to a very limited degree. Thus, we still find traces of this phenomenon. For example in birds, regeneration of the feathers; in stags regeneration of antlers. In respect of this replacement in higher vertebrates, the extent is significantly less than what a polyp or a triton can achieve. Thus, the dogma formulated by Spallanzani[3] holds: the more complicated organs are, the less easily they can be regenerated. All I have to add is that the word "complicated" is a rather non-specific term. We would have to say now: THE FEWER GENERATIONAL STAGES THE EGG HAS GONE THROUGH, THE EASIER REGENERATION IS POSSIBLE. Thus, it is clear that the polyp needs a fewer number of generation stages to be completed than the worm; the worm needs fewer stages than the triton and the triton needs fewer stages to become a triton than the vertebrates need to become vertebrates. One might counter that argument saying that this observation may well be right in its entirety but the details do not always fit, because animals which are phylogenetically closer to lizards – for example, turtles, crocodiles and snakes – have virtually no ability to regenerate lost organs.

[1] "Organ Formation and Growth". Würzburg, 1892; "On heteromorphosis". Würzburg, 1891.
[2] Fraisse*: "The Regeneration of Tissues and Organs in Vertebrates, especially Amphibia and Reptiles". Cassel and Berlin, 1885. * author's name (eds)
[3] "Experience to serve the History of the Generation of Animals and Plants". Genf, 1786.

51   This counter argument, however, would not hold water (*stichhaltig*): first, "phylogenetic relationships" is a rather loose speculation and, in addition, says nothing about the number of generational stages (needed for each species to progress from an egg to a complete adult animal). More importantly though, one needs to remark that, as the scheme presented on p. 45 demonstrates, great diversity can arise from the qualitatively uneven division. On account of this, even with a small number of generational stages, potentially the circumstance could occur where some plasmata greatly outweigh the others, and auxiliary plasmata would not have a chance to come into action. For example, that would be the case if the (fertilised) egg cell ($6a + 6b + 6c$) did not form ($4a + 3b + 3c$ and $2a + 3b + 3c$), but instead $5a + 3b + 3c$ and $1a + 3b + 3c$. Only if divisions in all animals were to happen according to an identical template – an assumption which is not known to be true at all – could we say that the potential for regeneration would be strictly proportional to the number of generational stages. Thus it would be sufficient to show that with increasing numbers of generational stages, the ability to regenerate decreases, without the necessity for every single case to fit this principle perfectly. This would be because, with an increasing number of generational stages, the degree of differentiation increases but not the reverse, so that one can deduce the degree of differentiation from the number of generational stages. The only way in which we can explain how one kind of tissue regenerates out of another kind of tissue is – as Weismann (has discussed) exhaustively (above) – if one

II Altruism

postulates the existence of auxiliary plasmata in cells that must have been latent and then suddenly become active again. We must put forward the statement: AUXILIARY PLASMATA IN GENERAL COME INTO ACTION AGAIN MORE EASILY, (WHEN) FEWER GENERATIONAL STAGES HAVE GONE BY SINCE THE ORGANISM BEGAN AS AN EGG.

As I said above, I was prompted to construct these cell division schemes with qualitatively uneven divisions by the intriguing balance of relationships which the different kinds of cells maintain in the body – a circumstance which I named *altruism*. If we now assume that with increasing differentiation of the cells, some of the plasmata become more and more dominant, we would have to say that the functionality of certain cells has to become increasingly more one-sided and restricted and thus, more and more complementarity is required to serve all the rest of the functions of the body. This, by definition, makes every cell type dependent on its complementary opposites; and equally, each cell type individually dependent on every cell type in turn to remain in existence. A single type of cell loses its ability to exist independently with increasing differentiation. If it was true, however, as Hertwig, de Vries and Nägeli wish to believe, that each cell contains all potential anlagen and only some of them are active at one time, such altruism could not be explained at all. It would be hard to understand, why the plasmas which are still present in sufficient numbers but are inactive, would not fill the gap.

Altruism as I have defined it, is a state which is present in a fully-grown body everywhere – although it might have begun at the first cleaving (of the egg) – and has not been sufficiently studied.

When the kidneys are out of action either due to disease or surgical removal, the individual perishes. The same occurs if a person suffers bilateral pneumonia; or the lungs are destroyed by tuberculosis; or are compressed out of action due to large pleural effusions; or, for example, when the liver is destroyed due to either connective tissue proliferation, or atrophy or neoplasms. No one finds that surprising because the functions of these organs in regard to preserving life are sufficiently understood. No one, therefore, has (bothered to) come up with theories why the body perishes if these organs no longer function. The empirical knowledge of the fact has satisfied the scientific thirst. In contrast, we find it odd that death (and I mean death independent of secondary processes like sepsis) occurs after an extensive scalding of the skin. People have speculated that it could be shock or circulatory problems – for example thrombi – that cause such death. What is entirely inexplicable, however, is when people die after loss of an organ whose function is unknown to us, – for example the thyroid gland or the adrenal gland – and that death happens in an odd but very constant kind of way. Although all these questions have not been clarified as yet, one cannot doubt that the thyroid gland and the adrenal glands must be equally essential for life as the lung, liver and kidney. The thyroid gland seems to have a very constant relationship[1] with myxoedema, idiocy and hyperthyroid cachexia[2]. Somewhat less certain are circumstances pertaining to the adrenal glands. In my mind a very clear relationship has been described by Tizzoni[3] whose experiments prove that Addison's disease has to do with the adrenal glands. In practice, caseating disease of the adrenal glands and bronze disease occur strikingly commonly, although exceptionally one can occur without the other. There is another striking relationship of the adrenal glands to the central nervous system; this is the atrophy of this organ in anencephaly. Weigert[4] was the first to draw our attention to this fact, and I have

[1] See the recently compiled literature by Horsley in the essays in scientific medicine. Festschr. f. Virchow. 1. p. 376.
[2] Kocher, Surgical Congress. Berlin, 1883.
[3] Ziegler's Beiträge. vol. VI, p. 1, 1889.
[4] Virchow's Arch. vol. 100. p. 176 and vol. 103, p. 204.

been able to confirm his observations in four documented cases. The adrenal glands in many cases weighed less than 100 mg; only once approximately 150 mg, whereas normal adrenal glands in the new-born should weigh two to three grams. For such a relationship between organs of unknown functions in the rest of the body we have no explanation whatsoever so far, but yet this is not different at all from the deaths which occur when there is loss of function of the lungs, the kidneys or the liver. This demonstrates only the loss of one cell-type which cannot be survived by the complementary opposites. This is a manifestation of altruism in the fully-developed body.

Now there is another matter arising whose concept has so far has not been discussed at all. It is the dual functions of organs. These can be divided into negative and positive. Without prejudice to the manner in which these functions are performed, I call those ones "negative" where certain substances are eliminated from the body. Here it should be stated that such substances which are excreted through negative functions, e.g, bile and saliva, can later on find another use in the body. In some organs we know both type of functions. The most precisely researched are probably those of the lungs; the negative function of this organ is to excrete carbon dioxide and the positive function is to add oxygen to the body. We know that the epithelium of the gut secretes mucus and makes chyle. We know – since the investigations of Claude Bernard – that liver cells make glycogen for the body in addition to secreting bile. For some time we have known the intermediate cycle of lipids in the liver[1] and Schröder[2] believes that urea is synthesised in the liver. Very interesting experiments have been conducted by von Meister[3] in rabbits which had a large part of their liver excised. The total excretion of nitrogen through the urine was initially decreased with the effect that the ratio of these to the total nitrogen was also decreased. At the same time, however, the amount of excreted substances increased so that the ratio of those to the total nitrogen increased. The decrease in the amount of urea was proportional to the amount of liver excised. With increasing regeneration of the liver the amount of urea rose again. A. Fränkel has reported a case[4] of atrophy of the liver where the excretion of ammonia in the urine

[1] Virchow's Arch. vol. 123, p. 187 and vol. 11 (sic – eds), p. 574.
[2] Schmiedeberg's Arch. vols 15 and 19.
[3] On regeneration of liver cells and on the participation of the liver in the formation of urea. Centralbl. f. Path. II. No 23.
[4] Berl. med. Ges. Am 15. XI. 92.

increased five-fold. Such investigations are invaluable in such a field of darkness.   54
 Considering all this, who would not think of the pancreas which very recently has come to the forefront of interest through works of Mehring and Minkowski[1] and the large body of literature[2] stimulated by them. Results of animal experiments all seem to point to the fact that diabetes is not caused by a lack of excretion of abdominal saliva (pancreatic secretion) – i.e. the negative function of the pancreas – but, in fact, by the lack of internal secretion of the body of the pancreas as was described by Lanceraux and Thiroloix[3]. If one transplants the gland into another place within the body but still completely separates it from the gut, diabetes is prevented. Only when the transplanted piece is removed (from the body) does diabetes follow. While this might be very clear experimentally, unfortunately it is not quite as clear from human studies. For a long time, I have been observing the relationship between the pancreas and diabetes and have come to the following preliminary results, which I am happy to communicate here because it is important for the questions which we are dealing with. Nevertheless, I would like to come back to the topic in a more detailed publication later. In diabetes it is quite common to find a macroscopically recognisable atrophy of the pancreas both in the diabetes in advanced age, and in that which afflicts young individuals with coma. The atrophy – which is sometimes linked to cirrhosis or polysarcie and occasionally to cyst formation – is only occasionally advanced enough to say there is a near complete loss of pancreatic parenchyma. Furthermore, once looked at under the microscope, the cells appear little changed. In other cases, where there is a total destruction of the pancreas secondary to necrosis, diabetes had not occurred. All cases of either extensive atrophy or of total necrosis of the pancreas will lead to death. If one were to draw conclusions from that, it seems that the relationship of the pancreas to diabetes is a little weaker than between the adrenal glands and bronze disease – especially if one views diabetes not as a disease but as a symptom of diseased organs. A lot of questions remain in this field.
 The negative functions of the kidneys

[1] Arch. f. exper. Path. vol. XXVI. p. 371.
[2] See Minkowski, Berl. klin. Wochenschr. 1892. No 5. p. 90.
[3] Académie des Sciences 1. August, 1892.

55 have, perhaps, been the best-studied of all the organs to date. The question is now whether or not they display any positive functions. In this respect I would like to point out the relationship between kidney disease and cardiac hypertrophy, and the one between hydrops, anasarca and uraemia. The myocardial hypertrophy (in these cases) has mostly been explained by dynamic factors. However, the rapidly-occurring oedema of the skin – especially of the eyelids – and all other symptoms of uraemia are by no means well understood at the present time. These phenomena are not sufficiently explained by simply stating that the body is overloaded with substances which would normally be excreted in the urine, because also by injecting such substances it has never been possible to create these clinical features experimentally. There is some unknown factor missing to explain all this. Of course, it is not self-evident that this unknown factor will be a positive function of the kidneys. However, there is something else that lets me speculate that that might be so.

It has been known for some time, that with caseous destruction of the adrenal glands, bronze disease occurs and this rarely happens when the adrenal glands harbour cancer. The same can be said of the pancreas, where even total malignant transformation (obviously I am talking only of primary cancer of the pancreas) still does not lead to diabetes. In my view, the explanation is as follows: the cancer cells are offspring of the organ cells and still possess sufficient function for the body to satisfy the needs of the body. So such patients then do not perish because they lose the organ but because of other injurious effects of the cancers. Lewin in his compilation[1] had only one such case (number 25). Cases 36 and 150 are very dubious: the first was most likely primary bowel cancer; in the second, it was very doubtful that bronze disease was actually present. The author stated: "One can tell with certainty that tumours of the adrenal glands are extremely rare in bronze disease". This does not preclude the possibility that there may be cancer cells whose function is not sufficient to meet the requirements of the body. However, the rule is as stated above: in caseous disease of the adrenal glands, bronze disease is common; in carcinoma it is the opposite. There is something similar about the kidneys which to my knowledge has not been brought to anyone's attention. What is known is that compensatory hypertrophy of the one kidney occurs after the other one is lost. In recent years I have had three cases of unilateral, total, primary renal carcinoma without any hypertrophy of the other kidney –

[1] Charité Annals 1892. p. 537.

56 the last of these cases I only dissected very recently in the Augusta Hospital. The weight of the kidney was normal and it had a slightly dull appearance. The measurements of the kidney (male of 54 years) were 11 cm in length, 6 cm in width and 3 cm in greatest thickness. Vierordt[1] gives the following values for the dimensions of a normal adult kidney: "Length 10.8–11.4, width 5.4–6.3 and at the top part of the kidney often 7.2, and thickness 3.4–4.5." One could object

that – like the way in which hypertrophy of the right ventricle does not occur in weak consumptive invalids, whilst hypertrophy of the heart is often significant in strong individuals – then a cachectic patient suffering from cancer would not be able to develop a renal hypertrophy. In the first two cases, above, no information concerning their nutritional status is available, but in the last case there was significant weight loss – but not a significant cachexia – and it is known that even in feeble individuals significant hypertrophy of kidneys can occur in other diseases. I remember a special example where secondary ovarian carcinoma was present in the left kidney, causing a massive hydronephrosis – and on the right side a significant hypertrophy of the kidney. This was although this female of approximately 60 years was severely cachectic. Thus I think it is possible that the loss of negative function of one kidney is not sufficient for the compensatory hypertrophy of the other kidney. However, perhaps in addition, other – presumed positive – functions must be destroyed (for hypertrophy to occur). Possibly cancer cells deriving from the renal parenchyma can produce those (factors responsible for positive function) sufficiently (to prevent compensatory hypertrophy).

When reflecting on the dual function of the organs, we have so far only talked about organs with secretory functions, to illustrate their positive functions. Organs without secretory functions have naturally only a positive function, e.g, the muscles, the lymph follicles, the central nervous system, the spleen, the adrenal glands and so on. In any case it is not the negative functions of the organs that proves their altruism, but their positive functions. What matters is what positive function one cell group provides for the others – if they provide anything at all – and therefore my aim was to characterise all the positive functions in those organs where we habitually only think of their negative functions.

Now we have to talk about a special type of cell which highlights especially the concept of altruism in relation to the rest of the body, namely the gametes. These differ principally from all other somatic cells in the sense,

[1] "Dates and Tables". Jena 1888. p. 63.

that they are removed from the body without any pathological events and independently of the will of the individual. If our theory about altruism of cells is correct, somatic cells should perish after losing these germ cells.

The influence of the development of gonadal cells on the body is widely known. When they develop at puberty, new organs form – for example hairs – and the whole body changes its function, whereas until then, there had only been a simple increase in the mass of existing organs. There is also something new in principle happening. What also falls into this category is the enlargement of the mammary glands during pregnancy. We could label these phenomena altruistic hypertrophy, in so far as with the growth of one cell type, the complementary opposites also grow. This would maintain the above-mentioned scheme (p. 45) which demands such altruistic hypertrophy, should the body lack certain func-

"Studies on the Specificity, the Altruism and the Anaplasia of cells with Special Reference to Tumours"

tions which it needs for perfect existence, and such qualities as the egg guarantees, as are necessary. Which cells are actually the complementary opposites of the germ cells in each case will be difficult to establish *a priori*, because we do not know most of the germ lines in animals. In those animals, for example, the diptera – where even the first cleavage of the egg leads to the primordial stem cell – the whole rest of the body can be regarded as in complementary opposition to the germinal cells. The altruistic hypertrophy, thus, certainly forms in opposition to the compensatory hypertrophy. In the latter, the loss of one cell group is followed by the hypertrophy of another similar cell group; in the other example the enlargement of one cell group leads to an enlargement of the complementary opposites.

The reverse of this is altruistic atrophy[1] which transpires from investigations of the function of adrenal glands, the pancreas, the thyroid and so on. The same is also evident in gonadal cells. Here we know of changes which follow the loss of gonadal cells as in castration or the insufficient development of the gonads. The clearest examples are found in lower animals. I would like to join Götte[2] and Weismann[3] and to agree with the observations of Julins[4].

[1] The terms hypertrophy and atrophy are not meant to imply that the process itself is always a true hypertrophy or atrophy, but only that the net result on the one hand is more, and on the other hand, less, than normal.
[2] "The Origin of Death". Hamburg and Leipzig, 1883.
[3] "On Life and Death". Jena 1884. p. 30 ff.
[4] Contributions to the history of Metazoans. Researches on the organisation and the embryological development of Orthonectides. Arch. de Biol. vol. 3, 1882.

58 The latter describes how the ectodermal cells of orthonectides undergo atrophy before the embryo is born and Weismann draws the conclusion that the atrophy is a condition *"sine qua non"*. He (Weismann) overlooks, however, that they exist as independent beings long before they are born (when they are – eds) within the mother animal and thus, there cannot be any talk of altruistic interaction between the cells of the mother and those of the embryos. The ensuing atrophy and subsequent death cannot be following on reproduction; a view that Götte holds and Weismann rightly disputes, but it has to involve the loss of the germinal cells, which is obviously not the same thing.

In plants also we see death of the individual after the emission of the gametes. One has to focus naturally on simple individual plants, and not groups of plants, which are called corms. This is well known in annual plants and also Winter plants like our Winter crop and Winter canola. Biannual plants, for example, *Oenothera biennis* (the wine flower), or *Cynoglossum officinale* (the dog tongue) germinate in Spring and bring to full development their vegetative parts by Autumn. The flowering and fruiting stages happen the year after, and after this, the plant dies. A very characteristic example is the so-called hundred-year aloë (*Agave americana*), which in its native land, takes five to 10 years to achieve

II Altruism

flowering and fruit stage, after which it dies. In our gardens, however, it takes 50 to 100 years to reach this flowering stage. What we see here is that the duration of life is significantly longer when the time to blossoming is artificially delayed.

To return to animals; matters here are not quite as clear, which is probably related to the different mechanisms of fertilisation and giving birth which have evolved in different species. One could interpret, for example, in the orthonectides – and perhaps also in the dicyemides – that the death of the ectodermal shell – which is all that is left after the embryos are delivered – is an adaptation of parasitism. This is because both of these types of organisms, according to some researchers[1], could be seen as regressed, developmentally crippled, flat worms. Likewise, among insects, death has often been interpreted as exhaustion following the act of fertilisation or the laying of eggs. This is not really surprising when one takes into account that there are insects whose eggs can only be delivered by a process of bursting of the body; and that *Termes lucifugus* – a kind of termite in southern France – is capable of laying 80,000 eggs in one day[2]. However

[1] Whitman. Communications of the Zoological Station, Naples, 1883, vol. 4.
[2] Lubbock, "Origin and Metamorphosis of Insects". Jena 1876.

regularly the death of insects follows the loss of gametes – not only in females but also in males, who survive the act of copulation rarely longer than a few days – there are some species where there is no reason to believe that exhaustion plays a role. Furthermore, in insects there are such situations as among the Agave. Insects can remain in the pupal stage for extremely long periods of time. For example, I once kept a cocooned satin moth for four years because of its beautiful cocoon and presumed it long dead, when all of a sudden it emerged in front of me as an *Imago*. I personally cannot see any principal difference between death by exhaustion and death by a preceding process of involution – as Weismann[1] would like to believe – but rather (I see it) simply as a matter of degree. The word "exhaustion" has been used only for animals such as insects anyway, in whom the gametes take up such a large portion of the body mass; and in which the body appears to be simply a shell surrounding the former. The higher we ascend the animal kingdom, the more gametes decrease in terms of relative volume, in relation to body weight, and in humans they form only a tiny percentage (0.08 per cent) of the body weight – as testicles, and 0.9 per cent of the body weight – as ovaries. Thus, the loss of those could not be so directly destructive on the complementary opposites as in animals in which the volume of gametes make up one-quarter or one-half of the body mass – and sometimes even exceed the volume of the rest of the body. Experience also teaches that postmenopausal women as well as castrated persons can survive the complete loss of their gonadal cells for a long time, and to my knowledge, castrati do not have a shorter average life span than normal individuals, either in man or in animals. One could also object that older people of more than 70 years are still able to procreate – meaning that they are still in possession of their germinal cells. These contradictions can only be resolved if we improve the precision of our definitions. What we have observed is that humans and animals grow older and lose their germinal cells. What I claim now is that ageing and physiological death – meaning the necessity of dying – is following on from this loss. It is obvious that we understand two things about ageing; one being constant damage secondary to illnesses which have been survived, but leave quasi scars; and the second being changes that come with time, in the absence of any diseases whatsoever. Among the latter we could count changes of the skin; loss of elastic fibres; changes in bones and muscles; atrophic states of the kidneys (smooth atrophy); and also in the spleen, the liver, the heart; and some changes in the central nervous system and so on.

[1] "On the Duration of Life". Jena 1882, p. 27.

60   I do not need to describe all of this in greater detail, because it is so well known. These states are never encountered in isolation, but always occur together to a greater or lesser degree. Together they form the real symptoms of ageing and are so similar to the features of cachexia after losing both adrenal glands, or the thyroid gland and so on, that one would naturally like to search for an organ, the loss of which could be responsible for this generalised atrophy. If one now went about starting a compilation on the relationship between the ability to procreate and the symptoms of ageing, one should only focus on such beings who display relatively little scarring from the struggle with the environment. Given the difficulty – perhaps the impossibility – of compiling such statistics, the assumption that physiological death follows on the process of loss of gametes, is probably going to remain just a theory for ever, at least in higher animals and especially in humans. However, theories – like all ideas in natural philosophy – will have their believers and their opponents. If one looks, the anatomy of lower animals and plants seem clearly to support this view, and I would like to disagree with Weismann[1] who says: "Death happens because the duration of life has been predetermined to a fixed time". This obviously explains absolutely nothing. And then he continues: "And in particular, until such time as procreation is completed". Considering the time-relationship which this researcher seems to acknowledge, it is completely amazing that he still argues directly against the causal relationship between the loss of germinal cells and physiological death. This view of his, I think, can be explained two-fold: he has not developed his concept of altruism properly – as is evident from what is said above. Secondly, because his assumption is "that processes of life of larger animals are intrinsically linked to changes in morphological elements of the tissues"[2]. I have previously argued against this view many times[3] and just as above, again and again, have tried to prove its untenability.

Anyone looking at everything I have said above about the altruism of cells will immediately recognise that the central point of this is not new, and only that

II Altruism

the way of looking at it has changed. The facts themselves are already to be found in the provisional hypothesis of Darwin concerning Pangenesis[4]. Darwin's small germinal structures (gemmules) – which, as he

[1] "On Life and Death". Jena 1884. p. 32.
[2] "On the Duration of Life". p. 27.
[3] Karyokinesis and Cellular Pathology. Berl. klin. Wochenschr. 1891. no. 42.
[4] "The Variation of Plants and Animals under Domestication". vol. 2, Chap. 27.

has already pointed out, probably do not exist at all – explained the phenomena in such a surprising manner that it was widely thought to amount to a hypothesis, the basis of which could be established from positive observations. The same attempt should be made in relation to observations of the altruism of cells. Any intrinsic relationship between the somatic cells amongst themselves and with the germinal cells seems to me, from all existing experience, to be a postulate, and I see this connection as the altruism of cells, as I have defined it. I further believe that what naturally follows on from this is how acquired properties can have some sort of influence on heredity, where nothing else seems to happen but an exchange of metabolism between different kinds of cells. Not in a sense that cut-off tails* or fingers are passed on by heredity – these are things which only a few would believe occur nowadays – but in the sense that different life styles, different climates, pathological constitutions, and so on, are able to modify genetic material. The possibility of this assumption Virchow also has emphasised several times on different occasions[1].

In the chapter above I would have liked to have shown that this altruism of cells can only exist if it is assumed right from the beginning that qualitatively unequal divisions of cells occur, and through that process, that cells can gain in differentiation. Further, (after this, it is to be assumed that) cells lose the ability to exist independently, the more so the more generational stages the cells are away from the egg. This all goes to prove that the scheme which I outlined (p. 45) is justified.

[1] See Origin and Pathology, Virchow's Archiv vol. 103, pp 1, 205 and 413.
* Weismann's famous experiment, see chapter 3 (eds).

III Anaplasia

(Translation of this section of "Studies ..." was provided by Mr Thomas Kruckemeyer – see Acknowledgments)

62 For some time now, mitoses under pathological conditions have justifiably received special attention and a great deal of very interesting works on regeneration and hypertrophy has come about, especially from the institutes of Arnold and Ziegler. However, it is not the occurrence of mitoses under pathological conditions which is to be discussed here, but rather their form in pathological processes. These forms as well have already been investigated by many researchers and with regard to any literature published on these matters up to 1890 I refer to the details I have provided in Virchow's Archives vol. 119, pp 300 and 301.

However, there are still a few points requiring special clarification. It is a widespread opinion that the nuclear division process is initiated by the increase of chromatin within the so-called resting cell. On this, please compare with the multiple works in Ziegler's articles on pathological anatomy and the same statement can be found in Schmaus[1] and many other places. There is no doubt that, during the so-called resting phase, the nucleus steadily becomes more rich in chromatin. However, I cannot see at all that such a process represents a process which especially initiates nuclear division. All information found in these locations gives the impression that one has to regard a nucleus particularly rich in chromatin as one which is just about on the cusp of dividing. Firstly, though, it is impossible to determine the chromatin level within a resting nucleus and, secondly, one is unable to predict what is to become of a resting nucleus rich in chromatin. It may divide into two or even more parts, but it does not have to divide at all or it may die through chromatolysis. Therefore, one is unable to predict anything at all about the significance and fate of such a nucleus.

1) "Outline of Pathological Anatomy". p. 72.

63 In order to avoid this problem, I have already several times pointed out,[1] that there is only one way to determine correctly the chromatin level of a nucleus and that is not during the so-called resting phase, but rather during division. But even here it is not the length and thickness of the chromosomes which is of importance, but only their quantity.

Since Roux[2] has claimed that it must be the purpose of nuclear division figures to distribute chromatic substances onto the daughter cells as evenly as possible, this claim has been generally accepted despite the fact that Roux himself entitled his small and very interesting brochure 'a hypothetical discussion' and this hypothesis is indeed so simple, clear and accurate that one hesitates to deny it one's endorsement. However, one gets into strange conflicts when one rightly adheres to another sentence, which is also accepted by a great number of researchers, namely that chromatin is the carrier of hereditary factors in the cells. There is a (type of) cellular division in which the daughter cells are totally different from each other and in which, at least in most cases by far, chromatin is nonetheless distributed evenly as per the standard rules of karyokinesis. That is the formation of the polar bodies (*Richtungskörperchen*) in the ovum. This process, which has been studied extensively in recent times, always provides the same result: by way of regular symmetrical nuclear division two cells of totally different appearance and behaviour are formed, a larger one which is able to be fertilised and to develop, as well as a smaller one which dies. Depending on the type of animal, fertilisation takes places before, but generally only after ejection of the polar bodies. The polar bodies contain exactly as much chromatin as is left behind in the egg and, yet, only a little cytoplasm collects around the chromatin of the polar bodies and the cell does not remain viable. Sperm cannot electively effect this since the process takes place without consideration of the act of fertilisation. However, the chromatin also cannot be responsible for this effect since it was divided into two completely equal parts for the egg and the polar bodies. But even if we were to follow the Nägeli-Hertwig opinion, then either such conditions would have to exist – which after all can be neither detected nor suspected during ejection of the polar body nor during the unequal egg cleavage – or here, too, some idioblasts would have to receive a stronger valence from

[1] Virchow's Archiv. vol. 119 p. 299 ff, vol. 123 p. 356 ff, vol. 129 p. 436 ff.
[2] "On the significance of nuclear division figures". Leipzig 1883.

the mother cell than others, i.e. once again an asymmetrical nuclear division without asymmetrical chromosome division would have to take place. Hereditary characteristics cannot lie exclusively within the chromatic substance, but rather they need still another basis. Therefore, an even distribution of chromosomes cannot at the same time be a guarantee for an even distribution of idioplasmata.

This is also supported by the strange laws of the chromosome number as it has been determined to date. It is a known fact that the same has been shown with enormous constancy for various classes of animal. For example, Flemming[1] found 24 chromosomes for salamander larvae, a number which was confirmed by Rabl[2] for epithelia and the connective tissue bodies of salamander larvae. Retzius demonstrated 16 chromosomes for the epithelia of the *Proteus*[3]. Schwarz[4] found 24 chromosomes in the cleavage spheres (*Furchungskugeln*) of trouts and Plattner found the same number in the testicular cells of pulmonates.[5] Boveri[6] provides the following information for the cleavage spheres of various animals: *Ascaris megalocephala* (Typ. van Beneden) 2, (Typ. Carnoy) 4, *Coronilla* 8, *Spiroptera strumosa* and *Ophiostomum mucron*. 12, *Filaroides mustelarum* 16, *Echinus microtuberc* and *Sagitta bipunctata* 18, *Tiara* 28, *Pterotrachea, Carinaria* and *Phyllirhoe* 32 chromomsomes. Häcker[7] found for all *Cyclops* species 8 on the somatic and 4 on the genital cells. All mammals have a far larger number of chromosomes and since these chromosomes, especially in humans cells, are extremely small, counting has so far not been successful. Hauser[8] states the number of chromosomes in stomach carcinoma to be 8–12. I have described several times that cells with such a small number of chromosomes occur in carcinoma. However, they are rare and could not be classified as a type. The overview of such numbers indicates that they alone do not allow us to come to any conclusions with regard to the species of animal nor the tissue. Two conclusions may be drawn nonetheless: that the number of chromosomes in somatic cells must always be an even one. This fact is based on the process of fertilisation as we have recently come to understand it through van Beneden, Hertwig, Fol and Boveri. Especially the last named has, through his interesting fertilisation experiments of nucleus-free egg parts,

[1] "Cell substance, nuclear- and cell division". Leipzig 1882.
[2] Morphological Yearbook. vol. X.
[3] "Biological Investigations". Stockholm and Leipzig 1881.
[4] Medical Yearbook 1888, p. 315.
[5] Arch. f. mikr. Anat. XXVI pp 343 and 599.
[6] "Cell Studies". Jena 1890, Issue 3, p. 60.
[7] Arch. f. mikr. Anat. vol. 39, p. 556, 1892.
[8] "The Cylindrical epithelial carcinomas". Jena 1890. p. 72.

provided conclusive proof that the chromosomes are carriers of hereditary characteristics and that their number is of significance for the form of the embryo. Yet, in *Echinus microtuberculatus* as well as in *Ascaris megalocephala,* Boveri[1] has also found exceptions which seem to have completely irregular chromosome numbers. Even with his attempts at explaining these numbers in a simple manner and at portraying the cells as capable of normal further development it has not as yet been proven that these are no pathological forms.

What does transpire from all this is that, even if the number of chromosomes obviously plays an important role in cell genetics, this number alone does not determine the type of cell. On the other hand, we cannot assume that the chromosomes within a cell may arbitrarily increase or reduce in number without this changing the type of cell.

It seems to me that this conflict can only be resolved in such a way that the body which we term a chromosome in accordance with Waldeyer's process and in which we see a certain organ of the cells is, in effect, not identical with chromatic substance or chromatin. Chromatin is part of the chromosomes, but chromosomes consist of more than chromatin. In fact, chromatin might not even be the essential [part] in chromosomes – a view which, after all, has already been expressed repeatedly.

If we take a survey of the field of normal developmental history, we will encounter chromosome increase only where ovum and sperm come together and thereby the number of chromosomes is doubled. No other such increase in chromosomes is known in normal cells. However, it is certainly well known that

III Anaplasia

under pathological conditions, chromosomes can increase of themselves. While previously one might have considered that here too, a kind of fertilisation process had taken place – which was in fact maintained by some authors[2] – recently a convincing explanation has sprung from Hertwig's experiments. This researcher has demonstrated[3] that under the impact of external stimuli, a cellular division which has already begun can be suppressed, in which case the nucleus returns to the resting stage. Once the

---

[1] Cited above, pp 35 and 61.
[2] Klebs, The formation of nuclear chromatin. Fortschritte der Med. VI 1888, and Schleich, "On the Aetiology of Tumours". Berlin 1889.
[3] "On the Fertilisation and Division Process of the Animal Ovum under the Impact of External Agents". Jena 1887. On Pathological Changes to the Nuclear Division Process as a Result of Experimental Interventions, Internationale Beiträge zur wissenschaftl. Med. 1, p. 195.

---

effect of the stimulus has ceased, division takes place which then, however, with increased chromosomes, is often into four parts. This discovery seems to me to be of utmost importance for our examination, since it provides sufficient explanation for the pluri-polar mitoses as they have often been described in the past and as I show them in human material in Figs 69–71 and it characterises them as products of a pathological process. They occur both in animals and humans with pathological regeneration, hyperplasias (Figs 69 and 70), inflammation and especially often with carcinomas (Fig. 70). Much more difficult to interpret than these pluri-polar giant cells are the bipolar hyperchromatic figures. I have seen such several times in tumours, both benign and malignant, and provide examples of such in Figs 75 and 76. Fig. 75 is from a normal wart from a child's neck. Fig. 76 shows the largest human cellular division figure which I have ever come across. It stems from a sarcoma of the adrenal gland and came to fixation only 30 hours after death. It is clearly visible how well the achromatic spindle has still been preserved. By the way, this is the only figure out of them all which was not fixed while at living body temperature. The question which arises now is whether one is confronted here with a new type of cell or whether these are just pathological forms which have originated from the normal cells through an inhibitory stimulus. Since these cells occur always in isolation I feel it is right to assume that the latter is the case, that these are cells which need to divide, whose division has been inhibited for so long until the chromosomes have increased to a large number without the attraction spheres having divided. What may also occur, however, is that the chromosomes are scattered throughout the whole cell, in which case the chromosomes take on an irregular shape and finally dissolve within the cell. Such cells are especially frequent in carcinomas and I have shown one such in Virchow's Archive vol. 123, Plate X, Fig. 15. Hyperchromatic cells, i.e. such with an increased number of chromosomes, have therefore mainly two fates: either the chromosome number is returned to its original state through pluri-polar division or the cell dies. In exceptional cases, hyperchromatic filial cells may also form.

So, what is happening with the reduction in chromosome numbers? From a historical development perspective, we only know this process in the so-called reduction division. This has been demonstrated for many animal species in the ovum and sperm cells by Flemming[1], Platner[2],

[1] Arch. f. mikr. Anat. vols 29 and 37.
[2] Arch. f. mikr. Anat. vol. 33.

Henking[1], Hacker[2], Jschikawa[3], Boveri[4], von Rath[5], and for plants by Guignard[6]. The name stems from Weismann[7] and the process plays a paramount role in the maturation of ovum and sperm[8]. What it means is that a cellular division, even before the nucleus returns to the resting state, is followed immediately by a second cell division whereby the number of chromosomes is reduced by half. This leads to the ovum requiring fertilisation, the sperm cell being capable of fertilisation, and through the coming together of these two cells the definitive number of chromosomes is then restored again. Boveri (cited above) has observed that the total number of chromosomes may also be reduced through the death of individual chromosomes. During this process of chromosome reduction, which is the only one we are actually aware of in normal cell life and can observe with some certainty, the cell is substantially altered in its nature. During this process – whether through the process has as yet not been proven – from a somatic cell another one emerges with independent existence and the capacity for development. The chromosome reduction has therefore a decisive influence on the character of the cells which we cannot grant to pluri-polar cell divisions even though they also represent a chromosome reduction, in a manner of speaking, because this effectively represents only a restoration of the *status quo ante* while the actual reduction division is about a change of cell type.

Now, reduction divisions as in sex cells are, even under pathological circumstances, totally unknown in other cells, i.e. no proof has ever been presented that a cellular division has been followed immediately, without resting state and without repeated halving of the chromosomes, by another cell division. What is known, however, is a reduction of chromosomes, and this occurs in malignant tumours.

Before we take a closer look at the cell division processes in tumours it will be necessary to come up with a definition for these and especially for the term of carcinoma. Some, led by Virchow, provide a definition from a purely morphological point of view. They see carcinomas as alveolar tumours,

[1] Zeitschrift f. wiss. Zool. vols 49, 51 and 54.
[2] Zool. Jahrbücher vol. V., Abt. für Anatomie.
[3] Compare Weismann, "On the Number of Polar bodies". Jena 1887.
[4] "Cell Studies". Jena, 1887, 1888 and 1890.
[5] Arch f. mikr. Anat. vol. 40.

III Anaplasia

[6] Annales des sciences nat. Botanique I. 14. 1891.
[7] "On the number of polar bodies and on their significance for heredity". Jena, 1887.
[8] Compare also Hertwig, "Cell and Tissue", p. 189 ff.

which invade other tissues heteroplastically. Carcinomas mimic organs and are therefore described as organoid. In contrast, sarcomas are histoid tumours which form an intercellular substance around each cell and are formed like a tissue, but can at the same time also advance heteroplastically. This definition, which had initially been given very clearly by Virchow, was shifted by the fact that proof was furnished that carcinoma cells originate from epithelial cells, and this was followed soon after by the second proof that sarcoma cells originate from cells of the connective substance series (*Bindesubstanzreihe*). In reality, though, proof of this was provided only for some of the tumours and from now on such heteroplastic tumours as were derived from the epithelia were described as carcinomas, those from the osteoid substances as sarcomas. However, since among the latter also many alveolar tumours of typically organoid structures could be found, the term sarcoma did not suffice any more and one had to generate new words. That is how the alveolar sarcoma came about. In view of the predominant uncertainty with regard to the histogenesis of a tumour, it could certainly not be maintained that one had come up with anything practical here and this opinion is confirmed the more one peruses the more recent literature on such matters. For example, in Amann Jr.[1] one can read: 'We must therefore only speak of a carcinoma where we have absolutely certain proof that the new formation originates from an epithelium, while for a tumour which might well be of the same general form, but whose origin has been demonstrated to stem from the endothelia we must speak of an endothelioma.' Well, if that had been demonstrated that would be very nice and we would be no longer in any trouble, but in how many cases is that really possible? If that was as easy as Amann, despite his extensive and very thorough examination, makes it out to be, this argument on the histogenesis of carcinomas and sarcomas would probably never have arisen or would have long been decided. However, each tumour always contains new difficulties, each one offers different circumstances, and in addition one only very rarely finds a tumour so complete and under such favourable conditions as Amann demands them; and yet, there is a demand on the anatomist for a diagnosis and it must be met.

The method of achieving this, as described on p. 51 of the same work, would hardly seem manageable in practice: 'Obviously, for the determination of this fact it is not sufficient

[1] "New formations of the Cervical portion of the Uterus". Munich. 1892. p. 50

to examine some smaller pieces from just any area of the tumour, but rather one will have to go to exactly those locations which show the early stages of the tumour formation, one will have to pay great attention especially at the edges of the tumours to the behaviour of the various tissue elements, i.e. connective tissue, endothelium, epithelium, both in the healthy and the altered tissue, and above all the task will be to demonstrate the transition of the organ's one or other tissue elements into the tumour elements and to illustrate the proliferation processes of the tissue type in question through the appropriate multiple mitoses findings.' In exceptional cases, it might perhaps be possible to meet some of these requirements, but I must absolutely refute that one could observe the transition of the organ's tissue elements into the tumour elements, however thorough the examination under the microscope. One might well put forward theories and voice assumptions on the matter, but one will not get a grip on the classification of tumours in doing so. Mr Amann may forgive me for using his work out of all to exemplify the issue. It just so happens that his very thorough examination, which I have no wish to doubt or to degrade, is the most recent monographic work of this kind which has come before me. It is no different in many others which cannot all be cited here.

Furthermore, another difficulty arising from these considerations is the question of what should be seen as epithelium and what as osteoid substance. The term epithelium which is known to have been coined by Ruysch and which means nothing but the skin on the mamilla[1] was equally[2] transferred to the mucous membrane of the bowel.[3] Now, as long as one used epithelium, depending solely on the situation, to describe any skin lining a cavity, and epithelial cells for the cells making up this skin, everything was clear and understandable. Only when one started to use epithelium for a certain kind of tissue, when one put the word in principal opposition to the osteoid substances, the confusion arose. Normal anatomists soon understood this flaw. Consequently, Quain as early as 1882 in the ninth edition of his book, and Gegenbaur in his textbook of 1885 both returned to the purely localistic meaning of the word and described everything lining a cavity or covering a surface as an epithelium. In Kölliker's classic "Handbook of Histology" (vol. I 1889), the word epithelium

[1] Thesaurus anat. III. Amstel. 1703. p. 26.
[2] same reference X. pp 11, 13.
[3] see Virchow on the correct spelling of the word "Epithelial". His Archiv. vol. 11, p. 465.

is no longer to be found under the classification of tissues. The pathologists, however, hung on to the epithelium as tissue type with great tenacity and since no sufficient definition could be found except by the location, they went back to the historical germ layer theory and tried to trace the tumours all the way back to the germ layers. This led to the terms archiblastoma and parablastoma.[1] From now on, carcinomas were to belong to the archiblastomas and sarcomas to the parablastomas. However, it is undeniable that thereby this new term carcinoma does match neither the old morphological one nor the later genetic one (stemming from the epithelium). Since the parablast (as used by Waldeyer) forms exquisite epithelia from which alveolar tumours can come forth, such as in the adrenals and on the brain's vascular plexus; and the archiblast forms a tissue which on completion must most definitely be counted towards the osteoid substances, this is the glia substance; but nobody would dream of counting the gliomas among the carcinomas. Klebs therefore made things easier for himself by further setting aside neuroblastomas as a third class while Ziegler[2] has the gliomas simply develop from the middle germ layer and counts them among the osteoid substance tumours. However, since the whole parablastoma theory has begun to falter again, the basis of such a tumour classification appears also highly uncertain. But neither can we accept differentiations such as epithelioma and endothelioma as long as epithelium and endothelium cannot be recognised as tissue type. As soon as a tumour develops from an epithelium layer or an endothelium layer – if one wants to keep this term which after all has been proven in practice – then these cells lose exactly those characteristics which allow us to describe them as epithelia and endothelia.

In fact there is no other way for me to find a common definition for all epithelia than that which starts from the cell situation, and I can find nowhere in the literature a reasonably adequate attempt to that end, despite the fact that epithelial and even epithelioid cells are mentioned everywhere. As Waldeyer says: "I use the term epithelia here in its broader sense whereby it is understood to mean all those cells which owe their development to the upper or lower germ layer or the so-called germ epithelium."[3] Assuming this origin can be determined everywhere with absolute certainty, how does one now distinguish these cells from those of a different origin? While the justifiability of such a classification

---

[1] Klebs, "General Pathology". Jena 1889. pp 573, 737 etc.
[2] "General Pathology". 7th edn, 1892.
[3] Sammlung klin. Vortrage. No 33, On the Cancers. p. 176

---

may be conceded, I do not understand how one can deduct from this the concept of an 'epithelial character'. 'Character', after all, is a property which is inherent in an object and which must find some expression through form or function, even when one observes this object, detached from its surroundings, all by itself. Therefore, it cannot be the situation which is decisive here, and neither can the origin. But now, even the term epithelial character is transferred to tumours. For example, Ribbert[1] states that carcinoma cells, even in the youngest metastases, maintain their original epithelial character, and Karg says: 'Despite all influences which might impact on it from the outside, the epithelium cell can never turn into anything else but another epithelial cell.'[2] But even the most ardent supporters of these theories get somewhat embarrassed when asked how they want to go about differentiating these cell types. How is one to recognise a cell as an epithelial cell if it is completely surrounded by others like it or by other cells, which is exactly what all those people demand who also describe the carcinoma cells, for example in a lymph node metastasis, as epithelial? Such questions are always answered by the same reply as Amann (cited above) gave it: one cannot distinguish the epithelial from the endothelial cells, but one must determine their histogenesis.

As far as such origin is concerned, it has made without doubt enormous progress since Thiersch[3] has proven that skin cancers developed from the epidermis and since he very carefully voiced the suspicion that similar conditions may also apply to the other carcinomas, a fact which has been demonstrated by Waldeyer[4] who simultaneously showed for a number of carcinomas that their metastases developed through direct protraction of cells from the mother cancer. The Thiersch/Waldeyer views have been confirmed by numerous works, especially more recently through the very thorough examinations undertaken by Hauser.[5] If, very generally, one understands 'parenchyma' to mean such cells of an organ which characterise the same, i.e. as liver parenchyma those cells secreting bile, as kidney parenchyma those cells secreting urine, as skin parenchyma the epidermis, as mucous membrane parenchyma the mucous membrane epithelia etc, then one could say that the

[1] Deutsche med. Wochenschr. 1891. No 42, p. 1183
[2] Deutsche Zeitschrift für Chirurgie. vol. 34, p. 144.
[3] "Epithelial Cancer", Leipzig 1865.
[4] Virchow's Archiv vol. 55.
[5] "Cylindrical Epithelial Carcinoma". Jena 1890.

works of the aforementioned scientists have demonstrated that THE PARENCHYMA OF CARCINOMAS HAS DEVELOPED FROM THE PARENCHYMA OF THE MOTHER ORGANS, THE STROMA OF CARCINOMAS FROM THE STROMA OF THE SAME. As far as I can see this sentence may be deemed to be definitive, and I want to add straight away that I would also consider another certainty, which is namely, at least as far as carcinomas and the majority of sarcomas are concerned, that metastases develop through transplantation from the primary tumour. If I exclude those few cases in which an event of transplantation can be proven directly, then it would seem to me that this view is supported especially by the cells' specificity. It (the specificity) makes it impossible to explain how the same forms of cancer cell are to develop, for example, from lymph node-, liver-, lung cells etc. as are in a primary oesophagus cancer, or how cells with mucus goblets can form in a lymph gland in the case of a primary intestinal carcinoma.

In this context, how about sarcomas? I believe that here much is thrown together which should be strictly kept apart. For example, I am of the opinion that over time one will separate those forms of lymph sarcomas which lead to a general diffuse 'sarcomatosis' from real sarcomas and will group them with the infectious tumours, similarly as is already done with cholesteatomata (*Perlsucht*) and gummas and as one also tends to do with leukaemic tumours. For all sarcomas, however, which develop from a specific osteoid substance such as cartilage, bone, lymph glands, periosteum etc. or from muscles, glia, vascular epithelia etc. one can clearly, just as with carcinomas, differentiate between two types of tissue: a stroma which serves as supporting substance and holds up the vessels, and a parenchyma according to which we describe the tumour as chondro-, osteo-,

III Anaplasia

glio-, lympho-, myxo- etc. sarcoma. The reason for the parenchyma often being less clearly distinct from the sarcoma than is the case with carcinomas lies in the fact that such tissues are far more closely related to the stroma connective tissue, both in their developmental history and, especially, in their ability to form an intercellular substance. Where this relationship is very close, such as with fibrosarcomas, myxosarcomas etc., it will often be very difficult to separate parenchyma from stroma, and in some cases where the vessel walls partake directly in the formation of the tumour, the vessels in the sarcomas have no specific walls and blood circulates simply within the cavities of the tumour itself. However, where the relationship is a very distant one, such as with vessel epithelia and connective tissue, sharply separated alveolar tumours develop which have been described as alveolar sarcomas or endotheliomas and which, in my view, with the

same justification can be counted among the carcinomas and possibly even must be. This shows that even apparently histoid tumours can, in reality, be organoid because I can in principle see no difference in whether the parenchyma of a tumour consists of issue from the epidermis, the liver parenchyma, the intestinal mucous membrane etc. or of the bone, cartilage, endothelial cells etc.

Here, we are faced with the actual problem of distinguishing between carcinomas and sarcomas. Even if one subscribes to the purely morphological classification principle one will time and again be confronted by forms for which one cannot state with any certainty whether they are to be counted among carcinomas or sarcomas. Indeed, what these reflections reveal is that there is neither a morphological nor any other dividing line in principle between carcinomas and sarcomas. This boundary will always be shifted arbitrarily and, in fact, one would hardly find 2 researchers in this field who place it in exactly the same place. Therefore, one has perhaps to ask oneself the question whether it is of any significance at all to retain these two words. For the practitioner this is of very little interest, he wants to know whether a tumour is benign or malignant; which is why, in practice, we very often find the term cancer for all malignant tumours, without any worry about the histological structure. Therefore, the only ones concerned are the anatomists and I for one have no scientific qualms about relinquishing these terms which, after all, do not reflect our current understanding of "cancer damage" (*Krebsschaden*) and "flesh tumour" (*Fleischgeschwulst*). If I nonetheless approve of retaining them then this is due to the respect for historically assured terms which enable us to bring about a mutual understanding. And even if it is impossible in some cases to come to a decision on whether one has to do with one or the other, in dealings with practitioners these terms have proved exceptionally worthwhile. However, should one retain the carcinoma and sarcoma terminology then I can see only the one differentiation principle, namely the purely morphological one, without concern for histogenesis and aetiology. A definite aetiology would without doubt lead to another and potentially better classification principle, but in that case the terms carcinoma and sarcoma

73

would most likely disappear. I shall therefore in the following take carcinoma to mean such tumours whose parenchyma cells do not form any intercellular substance and thereby do not set up an organic contact with the stroma, while I shall describe as sarcomas those whose parenchyma cells do form an intercellular substance and thereby take up direct continuity with the stroma. To this must be added in both cases the concept of

malignancy about which I will say more later. To me, this seems to be the only possible way of extracting oneself from the chaos of adenocarcinomas, carcinomas, alveolar carcinomas and sarcomas etc.

Now if we compare the stromal cells to those of the mother tissue, we will not find any difference here except that which is caused by inflammation or regressive metamorphoses and which we have to consider to be secondary and not directly related to the issue. Such mitoses as occur in the stroma of tumours show indeed no divergence from the cell division processes which occur during inflammation, regeneration and hyperplasia in the connective tissue and the vessels. I add further that the stroma formation in the metastases cannot be put down to the mother organ. In my experience, the stroma of metastases is always identical to that of the organ in which the metastases are found and must therefore be derived from that. The form of the mitoses contained therein only strengthens my view.

It is a different matter, however, in the parenchyma. Since it has been discovered that tumours are not made up of something which is foreign to the body, but rather of genuine body cells, and especially since one endeavoured to deduce the origin of the tumour parenchyma from the parenchyma of the organ, one has always emphasised the similarity between tumour and organ cells, and the idea of this correspondence seems to have won the upper hand to such a degree that the effectively existing differences were often seen to be irrelevant or accidental pathological changes. This is also indicated by the above quotes (p. 71) of Ribbert and Karg concerning the preservation of the epithelial character of carcinoma cells. As I have already stated elsewhere[1] as well as in the above (p. 70) with regards to the term epithelium, I only take it to mean (just as is done in Disse's "Outline of the Tissue Theory", Stuttgart 1892) the continuous cell layers which cover cavities or surfaces whose individual cells are cylindrical, cubical, ciliated or whatever, but otherwise have no common characteristics, and they cease to be epithelia when they encounter another situation, for example, in the case of medullary cancer, when they form dense piles of cells which fill the tissue gaps or, in the case of scirrhous tumours, when they are arranged individually or in long rows completely surrounded by tough connective tissue.

Of course, one could reply that this is just an argument about words and that "epithelial character" means the prevailing

[1] Virchow's Archiv. vol. 129, p. 442.

III Anaplasia

property of that epithelium from which the cancer has just sprung. However, I cannot support that view either, but rather have to assume that often the character of the mother parenchyma is totally lost in the cancer parenchyma, and indeed that even the character of the metastases does not always match that of the primary tumour. Of course, there are carcinomas which imitate the mother tissue with surprising accuracy. Fig. 77, for example, shows an epidermis cancer from the edge of the lip which has the complete structure of a normal epidermis. Only, the epithelial cones are longer, they stretch deeply into the cutis which displays a rich infiltration by round cells. Such a tumour's surface is covered by malpighian cells, normally tends not to be ulcerated and is at most somewhat excoriated, but tends to spread more and more with centrally progressing scar formation. Such carcinomas are not exactly common, but are well known by surgeons and really can only by diagnosed by their course. The same applies to large bowel cancers, one of which is shown in Fig. 80. The mimicry of the normal intestinal mucous membrane goes so far that the epithelium of the clear ductules of glands (*Drüsenschläuche*) even contains goblet cells. The diagnosis of carcinoma was justified only by the course which in this case ended in the patient's death through relapse – the histological picture could hardly be discerned from those of a polypoid mucous membrane hypertrophy. The same conditions can also be observed in other organs if the cells have morphologically well characterised functional properties, i.e. if one can tell a fixated individual cell's function in life, such as the keratinisation of epidermis cells or the mucous secretion in intestinal cells. Many other cells, however, do not have such properties and for these it is difficult or impossible to demonstrate to what degree the carcinomas originating from them have retained the tissue's primary characteristics. Yet in exceptional cases one succeeds nonetheless. For example, I have observed a primary liver cancer, and published in the Berlin klin. Wochenschr. 1890 no. 6, whose parenchyma cells still showed a clear secretion of a green liquid similar to bile. In one of Perls' cases[1] this secretion was found to be still existent even in metastases.

However, now we move on further to carcinomas whose parenchyma is considerably more different from that of the mother tissue, but not yet to such a degree that its origin can no longer be determined with some degree of certainty. In Figs 78 and 81, I provide two carcinomas of the epidermis and the bowel as examples. Fig. 78 shows a

---

[1] Virchow's Archiv. vol. 56, p. 436.

---

typical cancroid of the cheek. Keratinisation is near complete, but differs from that of Fig. 77 in that there are hardly any cells with keratohyalin granules. Furthermore, it shows itself to be less resistant against external damage since the surface of this carcinoma was extensively ulcerated. While Fig. 77 leaves one hardly in any doubt that this is a tumour of the epidermis, Fig. 78, in the absence of any other information, might raise doubts on whether one has to do with a cancroid of the epidermis, the oesophagus or any other organ. We find something similar in the case of bowel cancers. Fig. 81 shows a cylindrical cell cancer of the colon. Glandular lumina are still clearly visible, the epithelium – which here can still be described as such – is single-layered in some places, multi-layered in others. Goblet cells or other cell properties usually characteristic of the intestine are absent, such as the distinct double-contoured cell edge still clearly visible in the cancer of Fig. 80. One could take this carcinoma of Fig. 81 just as easily for a cylindrical cell adenoma of another organ. An even greater deviation from the mother tissue is displayed by the carcinomas of Figs 79 and 82. Fig. 79 is once again an epidermis cancer of the edge of the lip. Fig. 82 is a carcinoma of the colon. The cells only remind one very faintly of the mother tissue. In the lip cancer, one finds only in places weak signs of keratinisation, rare traces of indentation on the cell edges point to their origin from squamous cells (*Riffzellen*). In the colon cancer the cells are by now only vaguely cylindrical, mostly cubic or polymorph. Distinctive glandular lumina are only sparsely to be found. The cells line cavities in several layers and, in places, form solid cones. The pure medullary cancer has nearly been reached. What these 6 examples, 3 each from 2 organs, therefore show is that the cancer parenchyma does not always mimic the mother tissue's character in the same way, that it may resemble it very closely, but that it can also be distinctly different from it, and one can differentiate between various degrees of deviation so that one could set up a scale which would start with carcinomas of least deviation and conclude with those of the most.

Now, if one examines different metastases from one and the same cancer and to that end chooses a carcinoma which, in the primary tumour, shows only a slight deviation from the mother tissue and which develops from an organ whose cells have morphologically well characterised biological properties, then it is not all that rare to find that similar changes occur from metastasis to metastasis as we have shown them in the above series of individual carcinomas with increasing deviation from the mother tissue. Let us, as an

example, take a cancroid from the oesophagus. The primary tumour is shown in Fig. 83. In the picture we see large parenchyma cones with cell pearls and central keratinisation, similar to those in the skin cancroid of Fig. 78. Fig. 84 has been taken from a mediastinal lymph gland which was located not far from the primary tumour. Here, the keratinised pearls are far more rare, and the parenchyma is arranged in large cell accumulations whose individual cells show polymorph forms. Fig. 85 belongs to the same case and stems from a mesenteric gland. The carcinoma's configuration has been completely altered, the parenchyma forms a multi-lobular structure interspersed with rare tracts of connective tissue. Some concentrically arranged cells still point towards a tendency to form onion-shaped cell balls which are no longer fully developed, however. At this stage, the cancer has a similar appearance to the somewhat more magnified image at

III Anaplasia

Fig. 79. In Figs 86, 87 and 88 another example is provided from the stomach. In Fig. 86, we have the typical adenocarcinoma from the stomach with its cylinder-shaped cells. Fig. 87 has been taken from a tumour mass of the same case which partly blocked the portal vein. The figure shows that the cells have largely lost their characteristic cylindrical form, the glandular lumina have decreased in size and the epithelium is multi-layered in places. Furthermore the figure shows an extremely scanty stroma, the glandular tubes are in places connected only by single-walled capillaries which is definitely due to the localisation in a vessel where the tissue is not suitable for the generation of a more plentiful stroma. Fig. 88, finally, shows a liver metastasis from the same case. The glandular lumina are far more indistinct than with the primary tumour and the thrombus, the cells are mostly multi-layered and, in places, form solid cones. If we compare these three figures with Figs 81 and 82 we find similarly pronounced deviations from the mother tissue. At times one finds various degrees of deviation from the mother tissue already in the primary tumour. However, the two examples from which Figs 83–88 have been taken stem from such cancers where the primary tumours have been fairly uniformly structured.

By way of the examples provided in Figs 77–88 I wanted to prove THAT CARCINOMAS CAN IN THEIR CONFIGURATION BE VERY MUCH LIKE THE MOTHER TISSUE OR CAN DEVIATE FROM IT TO VARYING DEGREES AND THAT THE STRONGEST DEGREE OF DEVIATION MAY OCCUR STRAIGHT AWAY PRIMARILY OR IS REACHED ONLY GRADUALLY IN THE METASTASES. I would still like to make special mention of the fact, though, that it is not at all obligatory that the degree of deviation increase with each carcinoma or with each of its metastases.

It is indeed far more common that the character of the primary tumour is preserved in all metastases. However, I have never once found that the character of a tumour in metastases or the further stages of a carcinoma has approached that of the mother tissue again. That is to say, where a strong deviation from the mother tissue existed already in the primary tumour, this was never less so in the metastases, in which case the tumour here would have looked more like the mother tissue than in the primary tumour. In my experience, that does not occur.[1]

If we now have a look at how individual cells behave during these changes of the configuration of carcinomas then considerable deviations from those of the mother tissue can already be found in the resting cells. Here too we start off with cells with morphologically well characterised functional properties since these allow for a much clearer demonstration of any changes. With the epidermis carcinomas various deviations of the keratinisation type can be found. For many of these, this takes place in a type-specific manner which even includes the formation of keratohyalin granules. A small discussion in Virchow's Archiv vol. 128 pp 368 and 542 between F. Franke and J. Steinhaus has once again confirmed this already known fact. For other carcinomas, however, no formation of keratohyalin takes place and therefore the keratinisation is no longer the same as with the normal epidermis. It effectively occurs abortively through skipping of some transitional forms. Even the spinous cell formation may be pushed very much into the background or disappear altogether so that any similarity between the carcinoma cell and the epidermis cell can no longer be demonstrated. However, spine-formation and keratinisation are signs of old age

[1] After completion of the manuscript I read a report on my paper (in Virchow's Arch. vol. 129) by Hanau in Fortschritten der Med. 1893, no. 1, p. 13. The author is of the opinion that the differences which I emphasise in metastases as compared to the mother tissue can be attributed to the cells being younger. Accordingly, they would have to assume the character of the mother tumour once they are older. That, however, does not tally with the observation that even very large and old metastases display the same deviations from the mother tumour as do the younger metastases of the same organ. It is not only the age of the cells which has an effect. It might well have an influence on the form of the younger layers of a tumour, but not on the whole tumour since one always finds older portions next to younger ones there, regardless of whether it is primary or the secondary tumour. In that way, the oldest sections of a metastasis might be older than the youngest ones of the primary tumour. By the way, Hanau does not make such a consistent argument since he later fully agrees with my view which he only puts into somewhat different words: 'The biological independence of tumours from their breeding ground shows all kinds of degrees.' Which is exactly what I endeavoured to prove and to support by morphological manifestations.

in the epidermis cell and one could therefore make the point that this will not eventuate in carcinomas because the cells do not reach the necessary age for it and die off in various ways already prior to that and are replaced by young offspring. We discover further that colon carcinoma cells can still secrete mucus, liver carcinoma cells still bile-type fluid. Mostly, however, this will not occur any more. Carcinoma cells alter the specific function of their mother cells; with colon cancers they lose the double-contoured edge and often also the cylindrical shape, with cancers of ciliated epithelia the cilia-hairs etc. But here, too, one could argue that this does not represent a true change of cell type, but rather a histological accommodation since even a keratinised ciliated epithelium – for example in the case of a chronic catarrh of the trachea or a nasal polyp – functions differently, excretes no mucus and no longer has cilia. These changes therefore tell us nothing about the internal processes during the development of a carcinoma cell from the normal tissue mother cell.

Some carcinoma and sarcoma cells, however, also show a rather strange and, as I see it, not sufficiently acknowledged property, which is the active motility of tumour cells. On this, only four observations are available. The first was carried out by Virchow[1] on an enchondroma, the second by Lücke[2] on round cell sarcomas, the third by Carmalt[3] on carcinomas, and lastly the fourth by Grawitz[4] on lymphosarcomas. Waldeyer makes the comment: 'If one examines fresh cancer cells on a warm slide in the blood serum they often appear to be of round shapes, occasionally with blunt processes which display slow sluggish movements.'[5] It refers to Carmalt's observation who expressly states that – besides himself –

III Anaplasia

Waldeyer, Weigert and a few others had also seen for themselves the cells' mobility. It is therefore hardly proper simply to refute this observation, as Grawitz (cited this page) tries to do, who himself was unable to show movements in carcinoma cells. Such investigations seem not to have been carried out anymore since then, at least I have been unable to find anything else on the topic. I myself only once had the opportunity to examine the freshly extirpated carcinoma from the mamma of a bitch and here I was able clearly to observe slow movements on a few large cells, which could not be mistaken for leucocytes,

[1] His Archiv. vol. 28, p. 238.
[2] "Handbook of Surgery" by Pitha. II vol, 2nd issue, p. 181.
[3] Virchow's Arch. vol. 55, p. 486.
[4] "Two Infrequent forms of Tumour" etc. in Dissertation Berlin 1873.
[5] Volkmann's Sammlung klin. Vortr. no. 33, p. 169.

in a heated microscope cabinet. However, these consisted only of a change in form, but not of a change in locality. The number of cells moving, however, was only the odd one as compared to those where no change in shape took place. I am of the opinion – and that was the reason why I did not pursue this important question any further by experimental means – that this mobility is a quality of all young cells which has just been generated by division and is by no means anything carcinoma-specific.

Irrespective of whether cells actively wander into tissue gaps or are carried off by the blood or lymph stream, it is a fact that they can also multiply in body locations other than those where they were generated and that they are capable of forming new tissue which is like or similar to the old one. No other tissue is able to do so with the exception of that of the so-called malignant tumours. However often attempts are made[1] to let tissue heal on at a different location, any lasting and continued development of the transplanted tissue will be successful only where exactly the normal tissue conditions prevail. If one transplants periosteum into the lungs then there will be indeed a bone of similar consistency developing for a while, but then it will be absorbed again after a short time. I have repeatedly transplanted skin pieces from very small rabbit embryos into the frontal eye chamber of other rabbits. The pieces took well; they even continued to develop without any substantial loss of progress so that, after a while, one could detect hairs on them. Then, however, growth ceased suddenly, the piece shrank more and more, and after a few weeks everything had been reabsorbed without the occurrence of any pus or any other inflammation. Furthermore, it is a well-known fact that skin transplants from one animal succeed only in another of the same or a closely related species. The same applies to those earlier blood transfusions from animal to man which produced such horrendous results. More recently, cell embolisms have also repeatedly been found, e. g. liver cell embolisms by Jürgen[2], and Klebs[3], and embolisms of chorion cells in eclampsia by Schmorl[4]. In these cases one never sees anything of the proliferation processes, but rather the cells die off gradually, while in the case of tumour cells lying free in the vessels, e.g. in fresh portal vein thrombi

[1] For example by Cohnheim and Mako, who introduced periosteal fragments into the lung. Virchow's Arch. vol. 70, p. 161, especially p. 167, or by Kaufmann "Enkatarrhaphie of Epithelium", J. Dissertation, Bonn, 1884.
[2] Verhandl. Deutsch. Naturf. Berlin. 1886.
[3] "General Pathology". vol. 2, p. 120.
[4] Verhandl. der. Ges. deutscher Naturforscher 1891 in Halle.

81 in stomach cancer, one quite often finds numerous mitoses. The same rule applies everywhere: any tissue transplanted onto foreign ground must die. The only exceptions are malignant metastasising tumours. It is not a rare occurrence that carcinomas and sarcomas thrive in equal abundance in the lungs, the kidneys, the liver, the bones, the central nervous system, the subcutaneous fatty tissue etc. This points without doubt to a greater ability to exist independently by these cells than that of any other somatic cell within the human body. THE DEPENDENCY OF TUMOUR CELLS ON THEIR SPECIFIC ENVIRONMENT, THE ALTRUISM HAS BECOME LESS THAN WE FIND IN ANY OTHER CELL TYPE OF ANIMALS OF THE HIGHER ORDER. Metschnikoff[1] has shown for animals of the lower order that wandering cells can turn into fixed tissue and from that he concludes that people now, when even Ziegler has reverted from his view re the formation of connective tissue from wandering cells, have plunged into the opposing extreme and refute this process altogether (p. 156). What Metschnikoff forgets, however, is that the migratory cells of frogs, of *Bombinatogneus*, of axolotl larvae, etc do not match the leucocytes of higher order mammals in their biological value. On the contrary, it is exactly this statement from such a formidable observer which offers support for the view that the cells of lower order animals possess a lesser specificity than the cells of higher order animals, due to them being removed by fewer generational stages from the egg, and that therefore their altruism towards neighbouring cells is lower than in these and that they are therefore capable of forming tissue in other locations also. They support the view that only cells of lesser altruism than the cells of higher order mammals, and especially those of humans, can leave their original position and are able to settle in other locations and turn into fixed tissue, as we see with carcinoma cells.

One could object to that by maintaining, as has been done by Justinian von Froschauer[2] that cancer cells have a lesser viability than normal tissue since they die in such great numbers. If we put the question, however, why so many cancer cells are destroyed one has to put it down to the fact that pathological processes develop so easily in cancers. And that again has its reason in two conditions. Firstly, carcinoma cells are lacking the mother organ's characteristic protective devices of keratinisation, ciliary movements, edge membrane etc.

[1] "Leçons sur la pathol. comparée de l'inflammation". Paris, 1892.
[2] "Two proposals concerning the infectious and cancer disease". Vienna, 1872.

III Anaplasia

After all, where these things are still present in carcinomas such as of the epidermis, one does not find any substantial ulcerations.[1] Secondly, the milieu which metastases especially find does not always offer as much appeal to the cells as it might appear and they are insufficiently nourished. Therefore, the standard cancer cell is not necessarily more frail than the normal tissue cell, but rather the external conditions in which it finds itself hold greater dangers for it to fall ill.

We have therefore found that the ability of carcinoma cells to exist independently has increased and that their altruism has decreased, and as far as we know it is that which sets them aside from all other human cells, with the exception of germ cells.

Based on what I have said in the previous chapter about altruism, it logically follows that such cells of lower altruism and greater independence are less differentiated than the body cells from which they have sprung. Therefore, a de-differentiation has taken place. For that process, I[2] have suggested the term 'anaplasia'. Anaplasia therefore means a changing of the cells in the sense that they are less differentiated than their mother cells, and this decreased differentiation manifests itself through a reduction in altruism and an increase in their ability to exist independently. This state finds its most complete expression in germ cells where the altruism ceases altogether and de-differentiation is complete.

The anaplastic cell must not, however, be confused with the embryonic, and clear distinction between these terms is essential. In view of the extensive use so often being made of the word 'embryonic cell' I cannot at all agree with Billroth[3] that this is a 'fight against windmills', especially since embryonic cells have a clearly defined meaning and cannot be confused with juvenile cells either. This latter misuse of the word has already been attacked by Rabl[4] with whom I wholeheartedly agree. Embryonic cells are cells of the embryo,

---

[1] Although Hanau (Fortschritte der Med. 1893. No 1. p. 14) maintains that this does not accord with other experience, I must nevertheless affirm that the severity of ulceration of a cancer is on the whole in proportion to the development of the protective organs of its cell. That this relationship, because of external circumstances, can vacillate within certain limits, is self-evident, because even an ordinary wart can ulcerate, and yet no one will maintain that an ordinary wart is an ulcerated tumour. See note on p. 78.
[2] Virchow's Arch. vol. 119, p. 321.
[3] "Effect of Living Plant and Animal Cells". Vienna, 1890, p. 19.
[4] On the Principles of Histology. Verh. der Anat. Gesellsch. 1889, p. 62.

---

i.e. cells which are as yet not fully differentiated, or at least do not need to be. Juvenile cells are cells which have just been generated by division. Anaplastic cells, finally, are such which have lost in differentiation, i.e. which had been more highly differentiated previously. Anaplasia is therefore the opposite of the embryonic in that the latter takes off where the earlier is finished, i.e. in the egg. Therefore, there are juvenile embryonic and juvenile anaplastic as well as juvenile fully differentiated cells. Furthermore, it does not follow automatically that anaplasia must take the same road back as that taken by the development, the prosoplasia. Even if an anaplastic cell on occasion could match an embryonic cell with regard to its developmental state, this would always have to be considered a special coincidence.

In order to now examine this process of anaplasia in the light of plasma theories, we have to express it thus: in anaplasia, plasmas which up to now had been pushed into the background are now gaining in relevance again. In plants, we are able to illustrate this process especially clearly for tumours after we have been successful in growing plants from galls which would not have grown on the same unaltered part of the plant. With regard to such processes I refer to Hugo de Vries' interesting work 'The Intracellular Pangenesis'. For animal and especially human tumours the recurrence of obsolete plasmas cannot be demonstrated in the same way as in plants since, for them, we are not aware of the property of layers to the same extent. There is, however, one case where we can take a look at this quality of human tumour cells, at least to a certain degree.

It is a known fact that eggs and follicles of the ovary develop from the germinal epithelium in such a way that two cell types are formed with one of them maturing into the egg and the other one forming the follicle epithelium. Now, from the latter develop not infrequently malignant tumours, which really have only very little similarity to a carcinoma; this is why they have also been described as cystadenoma malignum or adenoma malignum and the like. They express their malignancy through their progressive nature, the ability to form metastases in lymph nodes, skin etc. and to cause death through general cachexia. Among the cylindrical or cubic epithelium of these cystic or gland-like tumours, one finds occasionally cells of particular size or position. These are sometimes encircled by a ring of epithelium cells so that they lie as if within a follicle or they are hanging, as shown in Fig. 89, and are still connected by a cell process to the connective tissue

and are only moving towards being cut off. Such cells are so very similar to primordial eggs that so far nobody had any hesitation about describing them as such. We therefore can see that here germ plasma finds expression in the offspring of cells which, as purely somatic epithelium cells, no longer revealed anything of such a plasma. Dr. Emanuel will in the near future publish two such tumours in Virchow's Arch. and collate the literature. I have gained much more certainty about the process of anaplasia especially through the study of these tumours. Obviously, nobody will make the assumption that these large cells are completely identical to primordial eggs from which mature eggs could develop in the most favourable case. As I have pointed out above, my ideas concerning anaplasia do not go so far that cells could be formed by it which would be identical to those of normal development. Nevertheless, cells are formed which are so similar to primordial eggs that one has to assume that they contain germ plasma in noticeable quantity, even though they develop from cells which separated

III Anaplasia

already at an early stage from true germ cells and thereby took a developmental path which is completely different from that of the later eggs.

The changes in the cells of malignant tumours as compared with the mother tissue consist therefore in the anaplasia, i.e. in the reduced differentiation, and in connection with an increased ability to exist independently. However, we have here once again a quality which cannot initially be detected in the individual cell, but rather finds expression only in the general behaviour of the body's cells. It is therefore important to examine whether, in mitosis, differences in principle from the mother tissue can be found. Because, since we have seen that human body cells maintain their specific forms of mitosis even with inflammable growths, regeneration and hyperplasia, any changes of this type in malignant tumours must be of utmost importance. That such a change cannot be found in the stroma has already been mentioned earlier (p. 74). However, if one wants to study these conditions in the parenchyma cells then one has to stay with the healthy tumour cell and has to leave aside all forms which in comparison with normal growth processes have shown themselves to be pathological. I am talking here above all of hyperchromatic mitoses which lead to dual and multiple division. After all, these are without doubt far more common in carcinomas and some sarcomas than with other growth processes, and this process corresponds to the stronger growth stimulus prevailing in these tumours. They have nothing, however, to do with the generation of tumour cells, with new biological

properties, are but simply the expression of pathological cell functions. Accordingly, multiple divisions are never found in isolation, i.e. in such way that they are the only cell division figure far and wide, but are instead lying in whole clumps of other mitoses. Only, as Klebs[1] expresses it quite correctly, in malignant tumours they look usually far more untidy than in other tissues. Fig. 69 for example shows a 3-way division from an epidermis growth on the edge of poor granulations after phlegmon of the finger. Fig. 70 is a four-way division from the same section as Fig. 69. The fourth star lies on a different level and is only discernable as a shadow. Fig. 71 shows a four-way division from the carcinoma at Fig. 79. One can see two large stars with a strong difference in chromosome length. A third star of the same size lies on another level and can be seen as shadow. The fourth star at the upper right is hardly half the size of the three others. It is of special importance here to exclude carefully all signs of degeneration in the mitotic figures which, after all, occur frequently. Among these are particularly the various forms of lumping together of the chromatin and the chromosomes and the well-known processes of regressive metamorphosis which cause the formation of vacuoles and inclusions and which have recently been discovered time and again and, in parts, have been interpreted in the most fantastical manner.

Now, with regard to the average tumour cell, it must first be very generally pointed out that its division proceeds exactly in accordance with the known pattern of karyokinesis; each individual stage can be exactly located and all details of the attraction spheres, achromatic figures and chromosomes can be viewed in exactly the same way as with physiological body cells. However, depending on the specificity of the cells and especially of the cell division process, as it has been described above, one is forced to view the mitotic processes of malignant tumours not in general, but rather must compare each type of tumour specifically with its mother tissue. But even by doing that one does not achieve consistent results if, for example, one treats the carcinoma types which can develop from one tissue all mixed together. Carcinomas with slight deviations from normal tissue reveal only slight deviations in the type of their mitoses, while those with strong deviations display such a considerable change to their mitoses that one is no longer reminded at all of the type of the mother tissue and, due to the circumstance that in some tumours various deviations from the normal tissue may occur in juxtaposition, the most varied forms of mitoses are also to be found here.

[1] "General Pathology" vol. II.

Therefore, no specific norms may be set for these deviations since new forms are present in each and every carcinoma so that no longer at all can one speak of certain types and can only state: forms no longer correspond to those of the normal mother tissue. In order to provide proof of the claim just made I shall give an example. To that end I have put together the mitoses series from the carcinoma in Fig. 77 with slight deviation, and that of Fig. 79 with strong deviation. Both are epidermis carcinomas from roughly symmetrical locations on the bottom lip and even from the same individual; one of the tumours sat on the right, the other on the left of the bottom lip. Figs 8, 17, 26, 35, 47, 56 and 65 stem from the carcinoma at Fig. 77 with slight deviation, Figs 9, 18, 27, 37, 38, 39, 48, 57 and 66 from the carcinoma at Fig. 79 with strong deviation. If one now compares these figures to each other as well as to the well-defined figures of the normal epidermis as shown in Figs 1, 10, 19, 28, 40, 49, 58, one will find that the group going with Fig. 77 deviates far less from the standard than the one belonging to Fig. 79. Furthermore, the first carcinoma (Fig. 77) displays a far greater evenness of forms than the second one. This disappearance of the type can be seen fairly clearly in the four mitoses of the same phase in Figs 37–39.

The same thing which was seen in this example of two epidermal cancers with slight and strong deviation can be found in all carcinomas which I have been able to examine. These were made up of a greater number of epidermis, bowel and mammae cancers as well as a few laryngeal and vascular carcinomas (endotheliomas), a chondrosarcoma and some lymphosarcomas. IN THE STROMA ONE FINDS EVERYWHERE THE EQUIVALENT MITOTIC COURSE AS IN THE STROMA OF THE MOTHER TISSUE; IN THE PARENCHYMA ON THE OTHER HAND THE CHANGES IN MITOSES AS COMPARED TO THE MOTHER TISSUE'S PARENCHYMA ARE THE STRONGER, THE MORE THE OVERALL DEVIATION HAS DEVELOPED.

III Anaplasia

From this it is obvious that a close relationship exists between the degree of deviation of the carcinoma in question from the structure of the mother organ and the form of the mitoses. However, since we indeed miss such deviations in principle during regeneration, hyperplasia and inflammation, I.E. DURING PRO-CESSES IN WHICH THE TISSUE TYPE IS NOT ALTERED, IT SEEMS A JUSTIFIED CONCLUSION TO ME THAT THE CHANGED FORM OF MITOSES IS THE CAUSE OF THE TISSUE CHANGES. In view of this connection between altered mitoses and altered tissue, the new form of mitoses can neither be related to coincidental pathological states nor the changes in tissue to a histological accommodation.

Rather, we have to assume that some new tissue has developed just as new tissue develops during the development of an embryo at the boundary of a generational stage through new cell differentiation. This similarity goes so far that for both carcinomas and organoid sarcomas as well, just as with a new generational stage, the growth direction changes, a fact which caused Thiersch[1] to assume a lower resistance of the connective tissue and which was also accepted by Boll[2] and others. Furthermore, this also demonstrates that the form of mitoses in carcinoma does not automatically entitle one to assume knowledge as to its mother tissue.

All this leads one to the conclusion – and I have no hesitation in drawing it – THAT THAT WHICH I HAVE UP TO NOW DESCRIBED AS TISSUE CHANGES IN CARCINOMAS AND ANAPLASIA ARE ONE AND THE SAME THING; THAT THE CHANGE IN THE CARCINOMAS IS AN ANAPLASTIC ONE AND THAT IS OPPOSED TO NORMAL DEVELOPMENT INSOFAR AS THIS REPRESENTS PROSOPLASTIC CHANGES TO THE CELLS.

The question now is whether one would be able to comment on the way in which this new tissue with new cells grows from the old one. As we have seen above (p. 65) in our discussion of embryonic cell differentiation, cells of various kinds can develop without differences in the chromatic substance being noticeable in the daughter nuclei, and one must therefore conclude that the cell's hereditary qualities are not linked solely to the chromatin visible to us. Vice-versa, though, we must assume that, whenever the chromatic substance is divided into two unequal parts and this asymmetric nuclear division is followed by an asymmetric cell division, cells with different biological properties emerge and one can only argue about whether the cells generated thus will be able to become the mother cells of new tissue or whether they are pathological forms which will lead to the obligatory demise of the cells. A third possibility, given the constancy of chromosome numbers in normal division and in lower order animals where one can have a clearer perspective of these conditions, I cannot perceive. Therefore, any change in chromosome numbers will necessarily cause other cells to develop so that the question remaining is: what biological significance do these have?

[1] "Epithelial Cancer". Leipzig 1865.
[2] "The Principle of Growth". Berlin 1876.

88 However, in carcinomas and sarcomas one will find two occurrences which lead to a reduction of chromosomes. One is the asymmetric cell division and the second the perishing of individual chromosomes within the cell. In addition, one will find cells with a reduced number of chromosomes.

The irregular distribution of chromosomes within the cell was first pointed out by Klebs.[1] I then described the asymmetric cell division at first in Virchow's Archive, vol. 119, p. 229, and followed that with further notices on the matter in vol. 123, p. 356 and vol. 129, p. 436. The points of argument which sprang from this discovery have been sufficiently discussed in those three articles. Since then, one further article by Vitalis Müller[2] has been published on the topic. By and large, this author comes up with the same results as myself. He finds asymmetric mitoses in carcinomas, twice doubtfully in sarcomas, once (at least a hypochromatic figure) in an angiosarcoma whose form is not specified in more detail and might belong to those which I describe as carcinomas, and finally no asymmetric forms in benign tumours. Nevertheless, he does not share my views 'since both in his benign tumours as well as in the sarcomas, mitoses are present in overall very low numbers.' At present, the matter is at a point where some of the authors[3] find asymmetric mitoses everywhere, award them no significance whatsoever and tend to view them as artificial products. Others[4] find the asymmetric mitosis only in malignant tumours and award it special biological significance. Yet others[5] again accept my findings as basically being correct, but for a variety of reasons deny them any special significance. I would like to present my own views here once again. I describe that cell division as asymmetrical in which two daughter stars of differing chromosome number are formed and where, if cell division has already occurred, cells of various size develop. In most cases, the number of chromosomes can only be estimated, for example in Figs 67 and 68, and in very rare and exceptional cases may also be counted. Such asymmetric

[1] "Pathological Morphology".
[2] Virchow's Arch. vol. 130, p. 512.
[3] Ströbe, Ziegler's Beiträge vol. XI, Schütz, "Microscopical Findings in Carcinoma". Frankfurt a. M. 1890 and Karg, Deutsche Zeitschrift f. Chirurgie vol. 34.
[4] Alberts, Deutsche Medicinalzeitung 1890 no. 93, p. 1043, Klebs, Deutsche medic. Wochenschr. 1890 No 24; Kruse, Deutsche med. Wochenschrift 1891 and I myself.
[5] Ribbert, Deutsche med. W. 1891 p. 1183, no. 42. Hauser, "Cylindrical cell carcinomas". Jena, 1890 p. 72 and Müller, Virchow's Archiv. vol. 130.

89 mitoses I have to date found only in carcinomas (as per my definition above), but they have also been observed in sarcomas by Ströbe (cited above) and by Vitalis Müller (cited above). The first has frequently mistaken artificial products for asymmetric figures, which I have tried to prove in Virchow's Archive, vol. 129, pp 346 ff. His findings in sarcomas are therefore not reliable. Müller admits himself that the two asymmetric mitoses which he observed in sarcomas were dubious. As yet, my reports that asymmetric mitoses have so far only been

III Anaplasia

noticed in carcinomas are therefore justified. By the way, I would like to repeat here once again that it is not at all my intention to find a specificity for carcinomas as opposed to benign tumours or even sarcomas. I am only interested in examining the biological properties of cells, and whether the results will later be of any practical value or not is up to the future to demonstrate. In addition to these asymmetric mitoses, one finds hypochromatic cells, i.e. cells with a remarkably low number of chromosomes, in the same tumours as the asymmetric mitoses. I have found hypochromatic cells or dwarf forms, as for example in Fig. 36 (from the carcinoma at Fig. 79), mainly in carcinomas and a few times in sarcomas. Vitalis Müller (cited above) confirms these findings as well. Finally, to these cell division images is added a further third form which is that of scattered chromosomes. I stated in Virchow's Archive, vol. 129, p. 444, that these chromosomes were initially described by Retzius[1] as 'peripherally situated ribbons'. However, that was an error which Prof. Flemming was kind enough to point out to me. That researcher had already described them in Archive of Microscopic Anatomy, vol. 16, p. 377 and vol. 18, 1879, pp 201 and 202, and shown them in the latter reference in Figs 8, 9, 35a, b, 43–44. Flemming initially took them to be normal and only Schottländer[2] declared them to be pathological. These chromosomes, which have sharp contours and are connected to the achromatic figure, are without doubt normal formations and are only later integrated into the figure. However, there are also lost chromosomes, which lie completely outside the divisional figure or even outside the divisional space, whose contours often appear faded (Figs 72–74), which are definitely condemned to die. As long as such chromosomes are still connected to the achromatic figure, as are the two bottom ones in Fig. 74, and show clear contours it is impossible to say whether they are still to be integrated into the figure at a later stage. In Fig. 74, one can quite clearly

[1] Biologische Untersuchungen, 1881 no. IX..
[2] Arch. f. mikr. Anat. vol. 31. p. 457.

make out the difference between the simply lost and between the lost atrophic chromosomes. Such figures can be found in carcinomas and sarcomas. In view of their whole appearance and colour reaction it is doubtlessly correct that these are indeed chromosomes since they can only be found in cells which are just in the process of division, and never in resting cells. I especially protest against these forms or the hypochromatic and asymmetric mitoses being seen as parasites. The serious researcher can harbour no doubts that these are certainly forms which are part of the human tissue, and it is only for curiosity reasons that Adamkiewicz[1] will be quoted here who considers all carcinoma cells as parasites (*Coccidium sarcolytus*), and states: 'We now know that this asymmetry of mitosis is exactly characteristic for the single-celled human organisms as opposed to the physiological cells.'

These three forms: the asymmetric mitosis, the hypochromatic cell and the cell with atrophic scattered chromosomes are the actual findings in carcinomas and many sarcomas. Everything else is hypothesis which I considered to be useful for the explanation of the development of new cell types which, to me, also seems assured. I imagined that both, through asymmetric cell division as well as the atrophy of individual chromosomes, individual parts of the cell get lost. Just as the individual chromosome, the smaller cell part is condemned to die. I was confirmed in this by finding cells which had very few and at times dissolving chromosomes.[2] Now, if this lost part were exactly the one which gave a certain property predominance in the cell, then that had to result in a less differentiated cell, or in that which I called anaplasia. This follows from the pattern described in the previous chapter (p. 45) whose justification I have attempted to demonstrate. If we assume a cell of form (12a + 6b + 6c), de-differentiation, i.e. a reduced predominance of individual plasma types, may occur due to the fact that individual parts, e. g. 4a, are expelled and cell (8a + 6b + 6c) is left over. Up to that point, such a cell might not have been present in the body, but it must have a lower differentiation and a greater ability to exist independently than cell (12a + 6b + 6c) in accordance with the statements made in chapter 2. However, a de-differentiation might also be caused by asymmetric division in such a way that, for example, two cells (6a + 2b) and (6a + 4b + 6c) result or any other variation whatsoever.

[1] "Investigation of Cancer". 1893.
[2] Virchow's Arch. vol. 119, Plate IX, Figs 17 and 18.

Cell (6a + 2b) would then not be able to live and would correspond to the smaller part in which I have repeatedly observed degenerative signs of the chromosomes which pointed towards a demise of the cell. The 2nd cell (6a + 4b + 6c), however, would be a cell of lesser differentiation than cell (2a + 6b + 6c) since two plasma types balance each other out while the 3rd deviates less than in cell (12a + 6b + 6c). Obviously, this is only an image which might help us to make sense of the potential process. And, indeed, I do not maintain at all that this is the way it is, or even that it has to be like that, but rather only that it could be like that, and I consider it a hypothesis worth discussing which does justice both to the findings and the results as well as the prevailing biological opinions in that is seeks an explanation for the coming about of anaplasia. So far, nobody has become closely involved with this hypothesis which I had developed in essence already in vol. 119 of Virchow's Archive, and all authors who have looked at my article have dealt mainly with an absolutely trivial comparison which I had used by chance. At that time, Weismann's theory was still under discussion, according to which the egg in the first polar body discharged its somatic properties and only through doing so became a freely mobile egg cell. To draw on this as a comparison seemed most appropriate to me. Even though Weismann himself has now in his "Amphimixis" given up his earlier view, it is nonetheless obvious that this has nothing in common

III Anaplasia

with my hypothesis on the development of carcinoma cells. Ribbert (cited above), Ströbe (cited above), Nöggerath[1], Hauscr[2], Karg (cited above) all cling to my comparison with the polar bodies without going into more detail concerning the crux of the matter, possibly for the reason that, of all the examples and arguments from zoology and botany provided by me, medical doctors are most familiar with the discharge of the polar body. Here, I have therefore left out any comparison with reductive divisions, even though I have no misgivings – even after Weismann's retraction – in considering the processes of reductive division and asymmetric mitosis from one perspective.

We can therefore summarise the previous results as follows: during their embryonic development, body cells achieve a far-reaching specificity which prevents them from replacing one another *mutatis mutandis**.

[1] "Contributions on the Structure and Development of Carcinomas". Wiesbaden 1892.
[2] Münchener med. Wochenschrift 1892, 7 June p. 411.
* performing each other's function (eds)

In physiological cell life, this specificity once achieved will have become definitive with the conclusion of the development. This specificity is acquired in such a way that the properties which are tied to certain body components of the cell, and which we describe as idioplasmata according to Nägeli or as pangenes as per Hugo de Vries, are distributed to the cells in such a manner that one type of idioplasma is prevalent in numbers, but others – minor plasmas – are still present in the cells in reduced numbers. In developing its specificity, the cell gains in differentiation and declines in its ability to exist independently. Since in each cell type a certain group of idioplasmas is dominant, but independent life requires the equilibrium of all idioplasma types present within the egg, the cells take up a kind of altruistic relationship to one another: each cell type needs all the other ones, all the other ones need each individual one for their existence. Under certain conditions which we must describe as pathological for the overall body, the cells' specificity may be altered and if so it is reduced. A number of findings would confirm that this alteration, 'the anaplasia', comes about due to the fact that main plasmas are ejected and this causes minor plasmas, which had already been pushed into the background, to gain once again in significance. Through this, the process acquires a certain similarity to the budding in lower animals, but differs from it in that the anaplastic cells distinguish themselves from other body cells through a lesser degree of altruism and from their mother cells through a greater ability to exist independently. THROUGH THE ANAPLASIA OF THE CELLS NEW ORGANS ARE FORMED WHICH, JUST LIKE THE MOTHER ORGAN, CAN HAVE EITHER A POSITIVE OR A NEGATIVE FUNCTION WITHIN THE BODY.

Now, two potential conclusions suggest themselves for the explanation of tumours: one is that the degree of anaplasia is identical to the degree of malignancy, i.e. that the tumour can form metastases the easier the more anaplastic it is. However, I would take that conclusion to be a misapprehension since that would integrate into the anaplastic process a concept of usefulness for the life of the cell. Yet, about that we know nothing whatsoever and that is not at all what the term of anaplasia is about. In addition, though, such a conclusion would in practice be of no significance at all since the degree of anaplasia may change both within the primary tumour as well as in the metastases at any moment and indeed often does so. It is not rare that one is given tumours for examination which display such a low degree of anaplasia that one could have reservations about describing them as carcinomas. If one were then to assume that these tumours had no tendency towards relapses or metastases, one would

be subject to a disastrous error since it happens often that the relapse which occurs very shortly, or a long time, after the first operation reveals a very high degree of anaplasia, or that general metastases with severe anaplasia lead to the death of the patient. And anyway, nothing is more common than carcinoma relapses displaying a more severe anaplasia than the initially extirpated tumour.

A second conclusion which one might draw from the statements made above could be that one would put all genuine tumours down to an anaplasia of the cells and would maintain that benign tumours are those with the least anaplasia; if the anaplasia gains in strength the tumours turn malignant. Especially the fact that benign tumours may turn into malignant ones – which might happen less often than is generally assumed, but should at least have been proven beyond doubt for a number of adenomas – might make such a conclusion very attractive indeed and I tried for a long time to find something that could provide a positive basis for it. In benign tumours, whether they are those which develop from epithelia or those from connective substances, no changes can be found in either resting or dividing cells which could be brought in any way into line with those explained as anaplastic in the above. Of course, even in tumours which without doubt have nothing to do with carcinomas and which to the best of our knowledge will never turn into carcinomas, strange deviations of the mitoses from those of the mother tissue can be found. As an example, I have shown in Figs 3, 12, 21, 30, 42, 51 and 60 a series of mitoses from a molluscum contagiosum which are comparable to series 2, 11, 20, 29, 41, 50 and 59 from a sebaceous follicle. Especially when one sees a great many mitoses, however, these changes are not as substantial and above all not of such a principal nature as in malignant tumours. Obviously, one could reply to this that in carcinomas with low anaplasia the deviation of the karyokinesis is not very substantial either. I myself would not have regarded this slight deviation in carcinomas with low anaplasia as proof had I not observed the gradually progressing stronger deviation in carcinomas of stronger anaplasia, and one must remember that the first beginnings of anaplasia are very minute and imperceptible just as it is a well-known fact that one is unable to recognise histologically every carcinoma without exception as just that. Nothing equivalent

III Anaplasia

to the anaplasia in malignant tumours has as yet been detected in benign tumours so that one – I may indeed say unfortunately – must issue a *non liquet* ("not proven") since there is,

as yet, no basis whatsoever for a general application of the theory of anaplasia. 94
    Please allow me one concluding comment. A number of authors who have looked into my theory of anaplasia, among them especially Alberts[1], Ströbe[2], Nöggerath[3] and Hauser[4], portray it in such a way as if it were an attempt to explain the aetiology of tumours. That this is a misunderstanding I would hardly have to emphasise since all I speak about anywhere is that cells do change and in which direction they do so. No discussion at all took place, however, on how this change was brought about, and that was intentional since my research did not provide me with any grounds whatsoever for such contemplation. My views, therefore, do not collide in any way with any aetiological theory. On the contrary, they provide plenty of space for any direction taken in this regard.

[1] Deutsche Medicinalzeitung 1891. no. 34.
[2] Ziegler's Beiträge vol. XI.
[3] "Contributions on the Structure and Development of Carcinomas". Wiesbaden 1892.
[4] Münchener med. Wochenschrift 1892, 7 June p. 411.

"Studies on the Specificity, the Altruism and the Anaplasia of cells with Special Reference to Tumours"

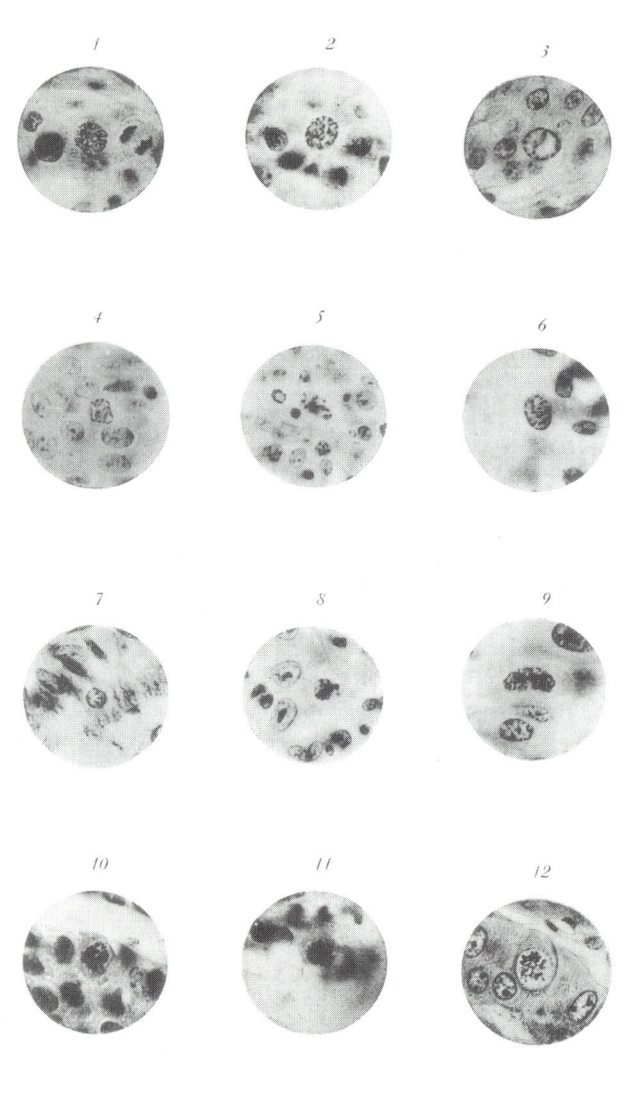

Plate I

Plates

Hansemann, Zellstudien. Taf. II.

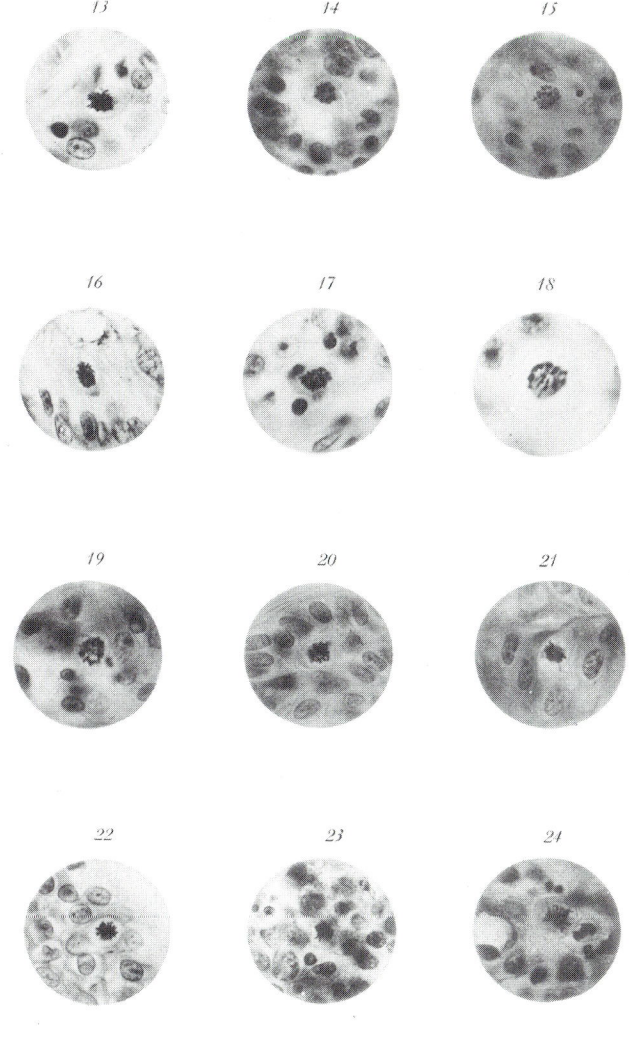

Lichtdruck von Alb. Frisch, Berlin.

Plate II

"Studies on the Specificity, the Altruism and the Anaplasia of cells with Special Reference to Tumours"

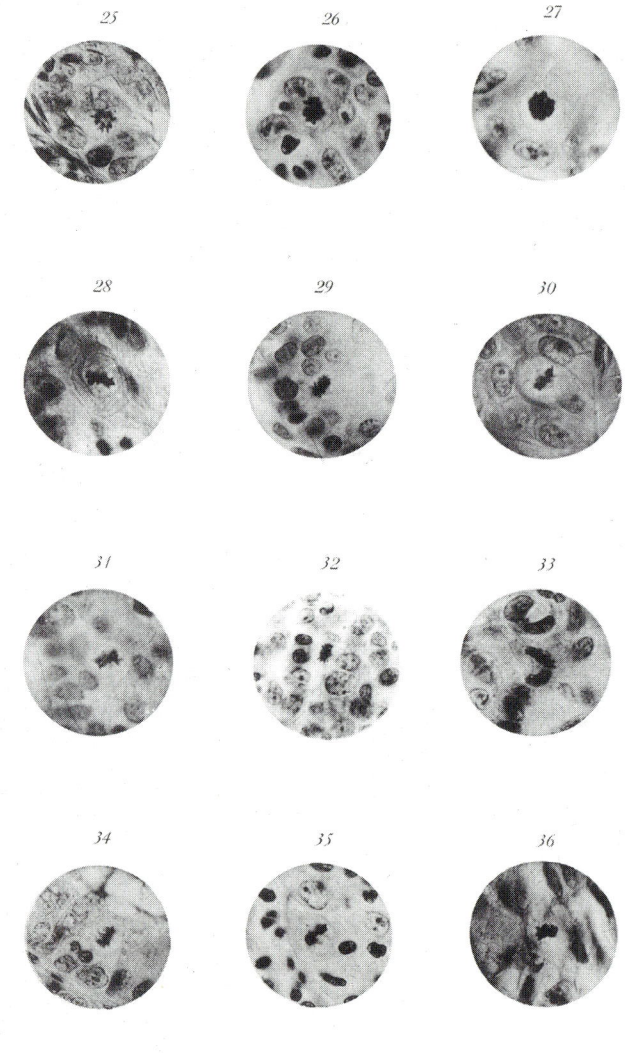

Plate III

Plates

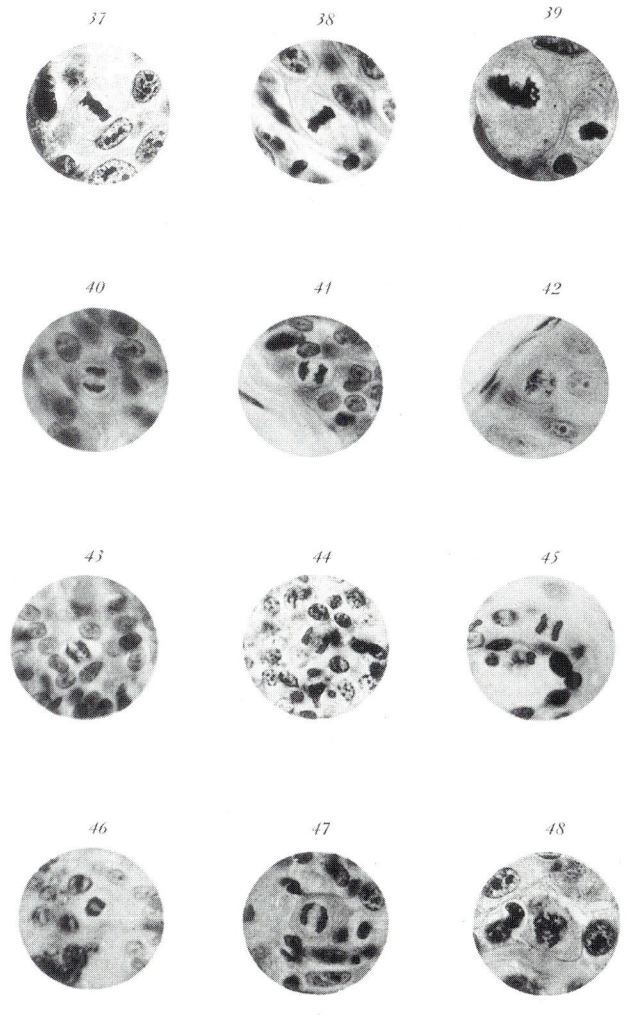

Plate IV

"Studies on the Specificity, the Altruism and the Anaplasia of cells with Special Reference to Tumours"

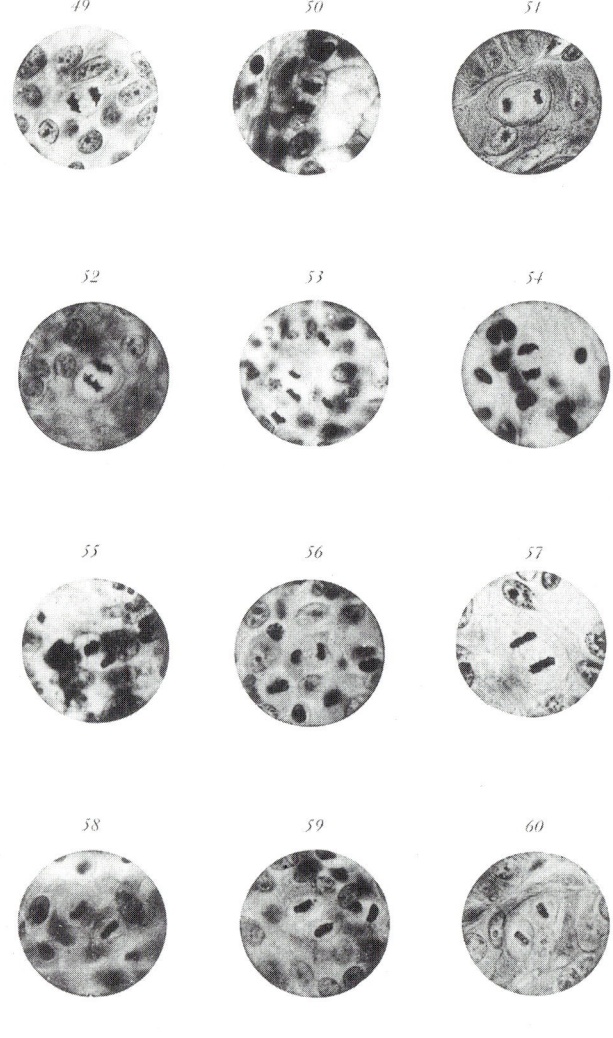

Plate V

Hansemann, Zellstudien. Taf. VI.

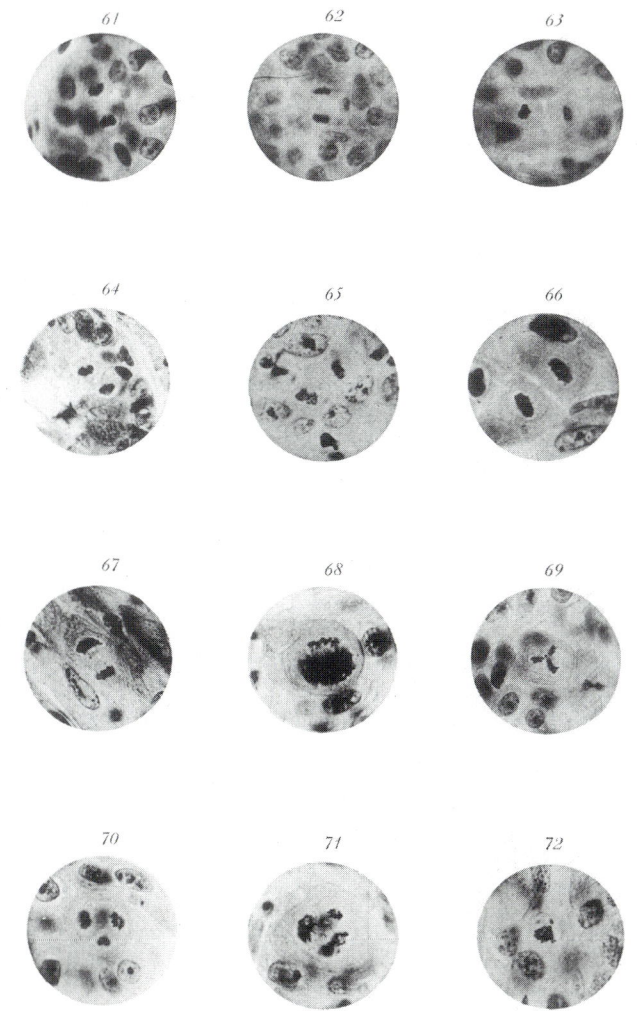

Plate VI

"Studies on the Specificity, the Altruism and the Anaplasia of cells with Special Reference to Tumours"

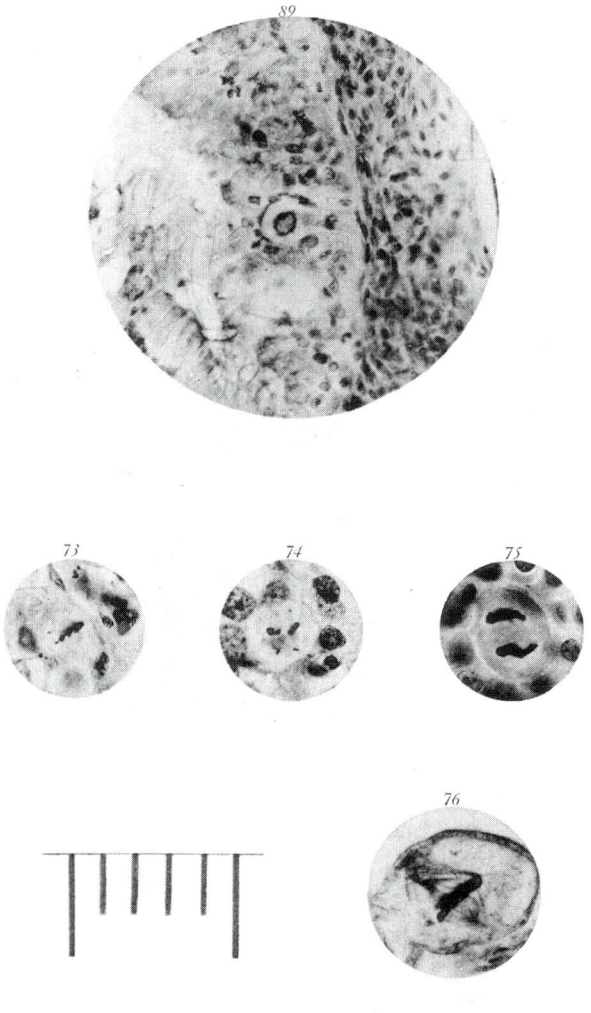

Plate VII

Plates

Hansemann, Zellstudien. *Taf. VIII.*

77

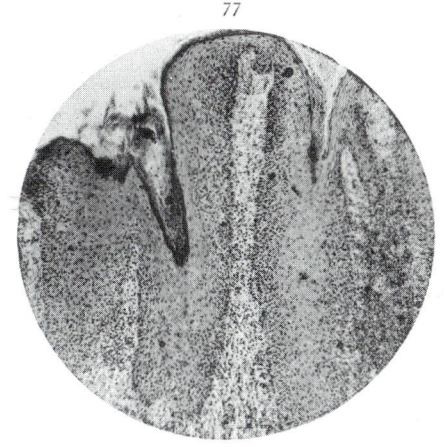

78

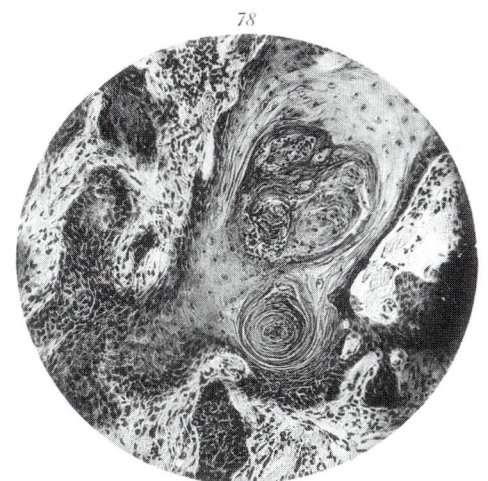

Plate VIII

"Studies on the Specificity, the Altruism and the Anaplasia of cells with Special Reference to Tumours"

Hansemann, Zellstudien. *Taf. IX.*

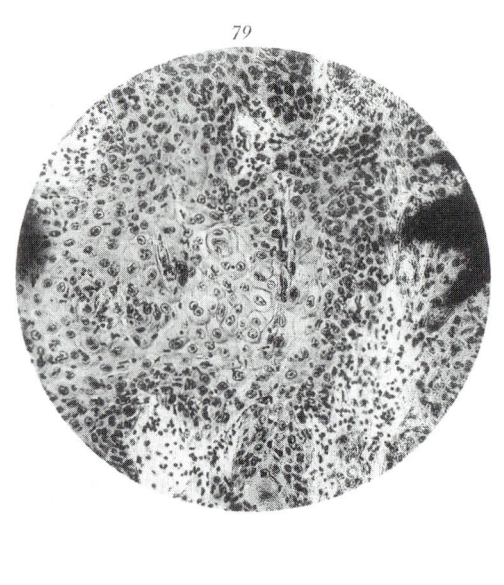

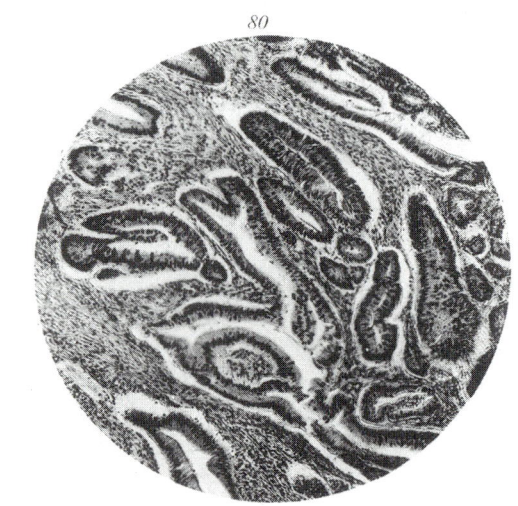

Plate IX

Plates

Hansemann, Zellstudien. *Taf. X.*

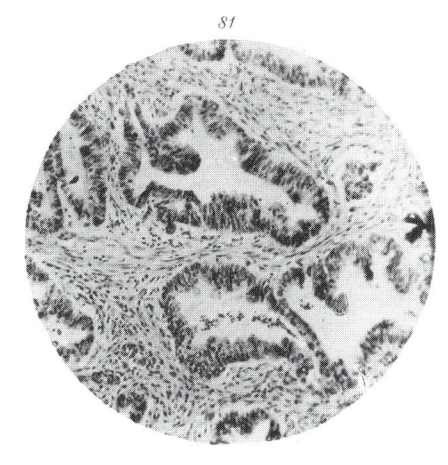

81

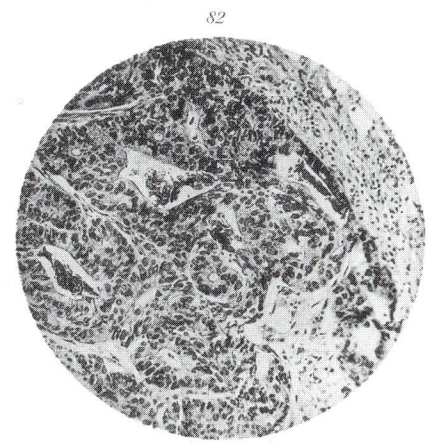

82

Plate X

"Studies on the Specificity, the Altruism and the Anaplasia of cells with Special Reference to Tumours"

Hansemann, Zellstudien. Taf. XI.

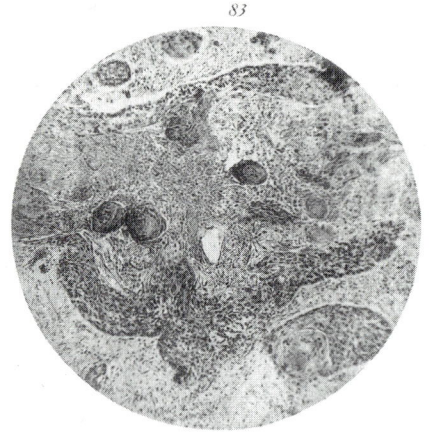

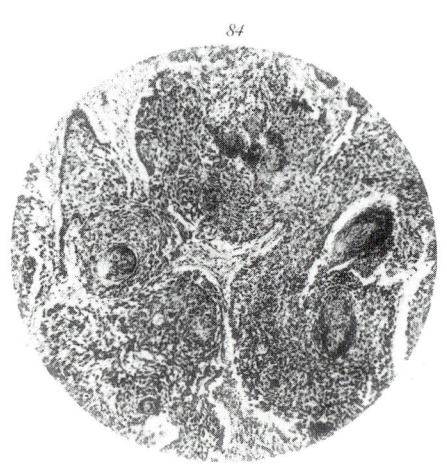

Plate XI

Plates

Hansemann, Zellstudien. *Taf. XII.*

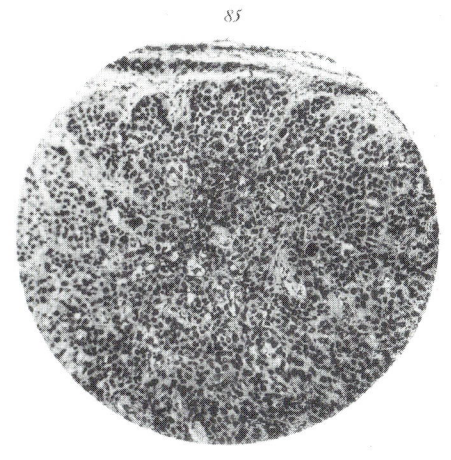

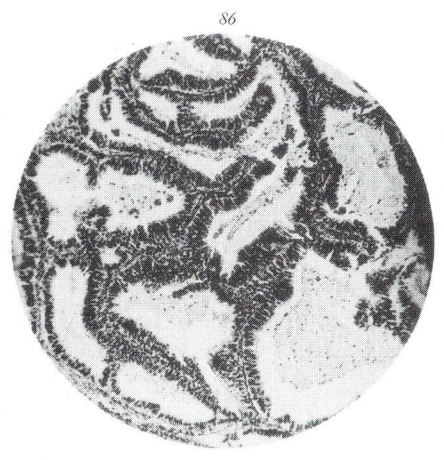

Plate XII

"Studies on the Specificity, the Altruism and the Anaplasia of cells with Special Reference to Tumours"

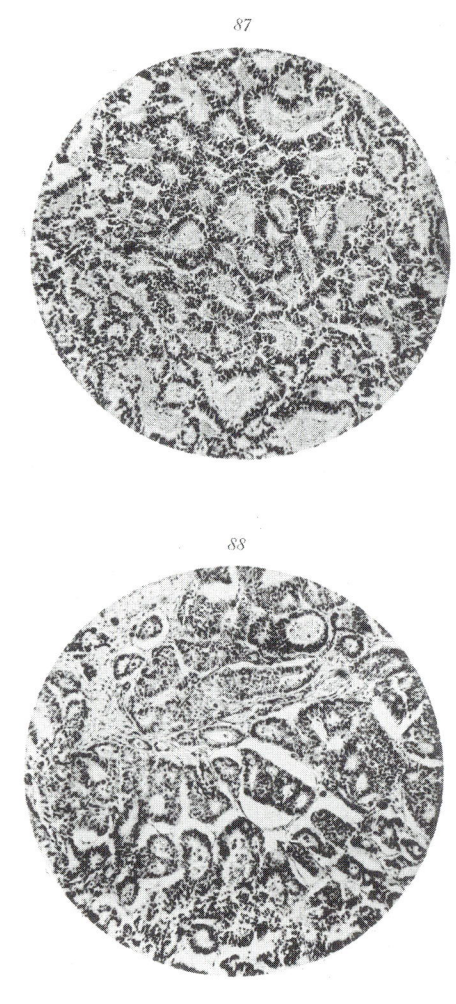

Plate XIII

Plates

Explanation of the illustrations: plates I–XIII

Figs 1–76 were photographed with the Zeiss apochromatic oil immersion 2.0, aperture 1.30, at a tube length of 160 mm, projection eyepiece 2 and a bellows length of 50 cm. Magnification is thereby ca. 600x, as is demonstrated by a scale comparison in Plate VII. This was achieved through photographic recording (under the same conditions) of a Zeiss lens micrometer ($1/100$ mm).

Fig. 77 was taken using the Zeiss a_2 lens, but otherwise the same conditions as previous figures.

Figs 78–88 with Zeiss 16 mm lens, projection eyepiece 2, tube length 160. Bellows extension varied.

Fig. 89 with Zeiss D, otherwise as in Fig. 77.

Figs 1–9 Monospirem stage. Figs 1, 2, 6, 8 and 9 a little bit more advanced than Figs 3, 4, 5 and 7.

Figs 10–18 Stage between monospirem and monaster.

Figs 19–27 Monaster stage as seen from above.

Figs 28–39 Monaster stage in section.

Figs 40–48 Early diaster stage.

Figs 49–57 Late diaster stage.

Figs 58–66 Dispirem with cell cordoning.

Figs 67 and 68 Asymmetric mitoses from carcinomas.

Fig. 69 3-way division, Fig. 40 4-way division from benign epidermis growth on the edge of poor granulations after phlegmon of the finger

Fig. 71 Asymmetric 4-way division from one carcinoma.

Figs 72–74 Cell divisions with scattered atrophic chromosomes.

Figs 75 and 76 Two-part giant forms, Fig. 75 from a benign wart, Fig. 76 from a sarcoma of the adrenal gland.

Figs 1, 10, 19, 28, 40, 49, 58 Epidermis cells.

Figs 2, 11, 20, 29, 41, 50, 59 Sebaceous follicle cells.

Figs 3, 12, 21, 30, 42, 51, 60 Cells from a Molluscum contagiosum.

Figs 4, 13, 22, 31, 43, 52, 61 Hair follicle cells.

Figs 5, 14, 23, 32, 44, 53, 62 Cells from lymph follicles.

Figs 6, 15, 24, 33, 45, 54, 63 Vessel epithelium cells.

Figs 7, 16, 25, 34, 46, 55, 64 Cells from Lieberkühn's follicles.

Figs 8, 17, 26, 35, 47, 56, 65 Cells from an epidermis carcinoma with minor anaplasia (cf. Fig. 77).

Figs 9, 18, 27, 36-39, 48, 57, 66 Cells from an epidermis carcinoma with severe anaplasia (cf. Fig. 79). Fig. 36 a dwarf form.

Fig. 77 Epidermis carcinoma with minor, Fig. 78 same with medium, Fig. 79 same with severe anaplasia.

Fig. 80 Rectum carcinoma with minor, Fig. 81 same with medium, Fig. 82 same with severe anaplasia.

Fig. 83 Oesophagus carcinoma, primary tumour, low anaplasia with multiple well-developed epidermis balls.

Fig. 84 Mediastinal lymph gland metastasis of the above, stronger anaplasia, fewer and poorly developed epidermis balls.

"Studies on the Specificity, the Altruism and the Anaplasia of cells with Special Reference to Tumours"

Fig. 85 Metastasis of the above from an mesenteric gland, severe anaplasia. Epidermoid character absent.

Fig. 86 Stomach carcinoma, primary tumour, low anaplasia. Glandular tubes arranged as in adenoma, epithelium mostly single-layered.

Fig. 87 Carcinomatous thrombus in the portal vein of the previous cancer. Stronger anaplasia.

Fig. 88 Liver metastasis of the above. Stronger anaplasia. Transition from the adenomatous form to the medullar cancer form.

Fig. 89 (Fig. VII) Malignant tumour of the ovary with a cell formed in the anaplastic way and similar to primordial eggs.

N.b. The photomicrogrammes provided in the original are not of sufficient clarity to warrant their reproduction in this book, in view of the reproduction of the drawings in chapters 7 and 8.

Chapter 12

Hansemann's other articles and books on tumours and related topics

Introduction

In addition to the works which are presented in the previous chapters, Hansemann wrote many other articles and a book ("Microscopic Diagnosis..." 1897o, 1902h). There were also chapters dealing with cancer in other books. The topics of these works included responses to published criticisms and misunderstandings of his own work; minor changes to his views on the nature of "anaplasia" and commentaries on developments in cancer research and treatment up to the time of his death in 1920.

Hansemann also published comments and ideas on bacteriology, serology, endocrinology and other topics. These works are of interest because they indicate Hansemann's nature. Unfortunately for Hansemann, his views on several of these topics were occasionally wrong.

This chapter presents summaries, and occasional complete translations of all of Hansemann's relevant works. In particular, articles and parts of books are mentioned in this chapter if they concern Hansemann's ideas of cancer; if they illuminate Virchow's influence on Hansemann; if they demonstrate Hansemann's philosophical tendencies; or if they show Hansemann to have been wrong on a major issue of medicine. The last are included because they show why Hansemann may have been unpopular in some parts of the medical research community in Germany at the time. The vigor of the intellectual climate in Germany of the time can be easily appreciated.

Pathological/anatomical and histological experiences after Koch's treatment (1891b)

This article appeared during the period of conflict between Virchow and Koch (chapter 3). Hansemann appears to have had a capacity for polemic at a young age, because his views are directly in conflict with those of von Leyden, who was a very prominent physician at the Charité at the time (see chapter 6). Hansemann expresses the view that injections of tuberculin (Koch's treatment) is of no help to patients with tuberculosis. There seems to have been confusion in the writing of the article between the values of Koch's preparation ("Tuberculin") for diagnosis and for therapy. Hansemann concludes as follows:

"If I now return to the consequences at the beginning which one presupposes from the condition created by Koch's remedy, then the following can be briefly said:

1. The created pathological condition is *per se* curable.
2. The same can, under conditions which can never be determined beforehand, endanger to the extreme the life of tubercular patients, even those who are in the first stages of tuberculosis.
3. The same does not destroy all tuberculous sites, and even those which it destroys, it does so only in part, and in such a fashion that one can ("not" omitted in original – eds) expect a healing from it."

Von Leyden was apparently one of those using Koch's preparation as a diagnostic test (i.e. the "tuberculin test"). A summary of his views was presented in the same publication (Von Leyden, 1891, p. 64):

"Gentlemen, as a doctor and clinician, I have tried to discuss the question of the diagnostic significance of Koch's remedy, not merely in respect of the scientific significance – which indeed is recognised on all sides – but also with respect to the care which the doctor must take, for whom the greatest foresight and conscientiousness are an absolute duty, and who must take the full responsibility for all results of his therapeutic measures. Here it is not enough to establish the scientific interest and the scientific value but in contrast, it must always be tested most carefully, whether such interventions as diagnostic injection are, in the interest of the client, necessary or desirable, and whether in this, every danger of harmfulness is excluded with certainty."

Pathological/anatomical and histological observations after Koch's treatment (1891g)

In this paper Hansemann provides the case studies in support of his opinion that "Tuberculin" is not an effective treatment for tuberculosis, and, indeed, that the treatment may be dangerous. The conclusion is very similar to the one provided in (1891b) above.

Von Leyden (above) has an article in the same issue of the journal (pp 33-66) in which his clinical cases are presented in detail.

Cell division in the human epidermis (1891h)

This is an account of mitoses in the human epidermis. Under normal conditions, mitoses are relatively sparse and almost always located in the basal layer of the epidermis. In atrophic conditions of the epidermis, there are fewer mitoses, and in inflammatory and hyperplastic diseases the numbers of mitoses increase, and they can occur in levels above the basal layer. The morphology of the mitoses is generally similar to mitoses in other tissues.

There is a discussion of whether the mitoses in the epidermis under normal conditions should be considered "pathological" in the sense of being continuously provoked by the exposure of the uppermost epidermis to harmful environmental influences. Then Hansemann discusses the role of nutritional mechanisms and leukocytes in hyperplastic increases in numbers of mitoses, and also the nature of differentiation and "physiological cell death" in the fate of epidermal cells. The summary (p. 12 of original) is straightforward:

"If we now briefly summarise the above observations, the following are the results:

1. The mitoses, which are always present in the epidermis, are the expression of a pathological process evoked by direct harmful influence of the external world.
2. Cell division leads to a multi-layered quality of the epidermis, and the keratinisation of the cells is conditioned by this.
3. Only the lowermost layer of the rete Malpighi is to be designated as a germinal layer. Under pathological conditions the germinal layer may disappear infrequently – more frequently it is considerably broadened – and this process gives the epidermis its stamp in each case."

The cancer stroma and Grawitz' theory of dormant cells (1893a)

In this article Hansemann criticises an idea put forwards by Grawitz: – that "invisible" dormant cells exist in the stroma of tissues from which cancer cells arise. Hansemann points out that the ingredients of this hypothesis of cancer formation are similar to Virchow's theory of the connective tissue origin of cancers, and Muller's ideas of "*seminum morbii*" (see chapter 4). Hansemann mentions many writings by Thiersch, Waldeyer and others concerning the origin of cancer cells, as is discussed in chapter 4 of this volume, in Wolff (1902) and in Rather (1978).

Critical reflections on the aetiology of carcinomas (1894a)

This is a general review of parasitic theories of cancer, based on the observation that abnormal intracellular – and particularly intranuclear – structures are to be found in cancer cells. Hansemann cites J. Müller (1838) and Virchow (1847) as proponents of this idea. Hansemann effectively demolishes all the "evidence" that these structures are parasites.

The work is notable first for his opinion of "consensus" statements (p. 14 of the original):

"Foa says prettily (*hübsch*):'The opinions manifested by the authors do not all agree with each other at first, and what for the one could bear the significance of cancer parasites, for the other, on the contrary must only be regarded as a histological element of the tumour, of such a sort that it seemed that one might advance without any order in the study of the question. But, in the current of these two last years, accord would seem to have been established at last between the authors; those who describe as parasites the same bodies which do not in effect have anything to do with cancer, to what it seems are the histological and degenerative products of the tumour.*'

Historically, that is on the whole quite correct, but it means, in plain German: initially, all sorts of things were described in confusion, but now however, one has made the decision to see certain structures as parasites. One type of discussion (*Konferenz*) has decided in definitive way on these forms. The carcinoma parasite has not been discovered, it has been decreed (*beschlossen*)**."

Second, the work is notable for its summary and conclusion (p. 15 of original):

Hansemann stated that after examining all his own slides and those of other authors, there are seven objects which have been interpreted as parasites. This analysis could not be improved on today:

1. Degenerative cellular structures, due to irregular keratinisation, colloid etc normal secretions.
2. Phagocytic phenomena such as cancer cells eat leukocytes or other cells.
3. Invagination, characterised by processes of one cell protruding into another.
4. Abortive or pathological mitoses especially in hyperchromatic cells.
5. Specific organelles e.g. paranucleus.
6. Extracellular droplets and shapes.
7. Cancer cells themselves.

And the last paragraph (p. 15 of original) is worth quoting.

"Virchow once stated in his seminar when asked to highlight how dogmas come about: 'First is the supposition, then the assertion, then the faith (*Glaube*)***, and finally the fanaticism'. This pronouncement can nowhere be better applied than to the judgement of the so-called carcinoma parasites. After Thoma (36), Sv. Huekelom (37), and the work from Lukjanow's laboratory (38, 39) the phase of supposition developed into that of the assertion, within which most of the works are to be included. From the inclusion of the assertions in textbooks by Ziegler (40), L. Pfeiffer (41), Salomonsen (42) and Langerhans (43), it is obvious that we are already in the stage of faith. Let us hope that contrary works will preserve us from fanaticism in this area."

*   This sentence is obscure in the original, and is probably missing a verb (eds).
** The word (*der Beschluss*) had been used for oppressive decrees at least since the infamous Carlsbad Decrees of 1819.
*** Goethe: Faust (Second Study Room Scene) "I certainly hear the message but I lack the faith (*…allein mir fehlt der Glaube*).

On the specificity of the division of cells (1894i)

The studies reported in this paper concern the tissue-specific differences in the appearances of mitoses in *Salamandra maculosa*. The paper enlarges somewhat the findings of Hansemann in the section on "Specificity" in "Studies…" (1893c – chapter 11). Hansemann studied three cell types – the epithelia of the mylohyoid plate, the connective tissue cells of the gill plates and the red blood cells which are mainly found in the lung, but also any other organ of the body. He used either Flemming's or Hermann's solution for fixation, in variable concentrations. Tissue-specific differences were found. The text includes rebuttals of comments by Ribbert. The paper concludes with experimental data to assess effects of toxins administered systemically as follows:

"There are no transitional forms of specific mitoses, in fact they are generally extremely consistent. I have treated the larvae of salamander with a variety of protoplasmic poisons, quinine, chloral hydrate, aconit, apomorphine, and alcohol. These poisons were effective after a short time in concentrated form, and after a long time in diluted form. The poisonings were always carried out until the animal lost consciousness. The animals were examined either immediately, after some hours, or even days later. I had animals frozen and many continued to live after thawing, and were examined at different time points. I also kept some in lukewarm water for days. None of these manipulations achieved changes in the character of the mitoses. Even if one injures the gill plates or the mylohyoid plates (which is very easy to do) the character of the mitoses remained unchanged. Only very occasionally, I have seen tripartite divisions with these injuries, which by the way, I have found once in the lung of a seemingly normal animal."

On the so-called interstitial cells of the testis and their significance in pathological conditions (1895b)

This is an interesting summary of studies of this type of cell to 1895. The idea of their being the source of masculinising hormones apparently was not considered then.

The last paragraph seems to suggest that tumours which are now recognised as chorio-carcinomas of the testis are not of interstitial origin but of vascular origin (actually they are from germinal cells of the testicular germinal cells).

"It was Waldeyer who drew attention to the fact that tumours can arise from these cells, which he called plexiform angiosarcomas. Meanwhile I believe that the group of these tumours of Waldeyer's has been set too widely, and one must restrict them to the type of tumour previously described. The close relationship which Waldeyer perceives the cells to take up *vis à vis* the vessels, has caused him to give to the tumours (a nature) of angiosarcomas, and, I believe, include forms here which allow us to recognise a closer genetic relationship to the vessels than the interstitial cells actually have in reality."

Pathological anatomy and bacteriology (1895d)

This article discusses these two issues in the context of the conflict between Virchow and the bacteriologists, especially Koch (see Hansemann 1891b and chapter 6). Hansemann cannot deny bacterial causation of disease, but is determined to support the role of anatomical pathologists in the study of disease. First Hansemann discusses "disposition and disease", without taking any position on their respective importance in bacterial diseases. Then there is a long flattering discussion of Virchow's contributions to medical science. Braatz is said to have stated that "Cellular Pathology" had killed "Humoural Pathology", but now Bacteriology would kill "Cellular Pathology".

Hansemann continues to be highly flattering of Virchow's "scientific method" and "rigour", and emphasises Virchow's role in exposing the lack of benefit of Koch's tuberculin therapy for patients with tuberculosis. Hansemann is then even handed, and says that Virchow is a true authority on the methods of fact and the science, although some of his theories (such as the connective tissue origin of tumour cells) have been disproved by even his close admirers. Hansemann states that of course, anatomical pathology still has its dogmas, and has delivered little of use to therapy or aetiology; but Hansemann asserts that anatomical pathology guides all surgery, and has illuminated the aetiology of a few diseases, such as thrombosis.

The remainder of the article is rather insulting to bacteriology. He refers to it as a "botanical science", which, despite the large numbers of researchers producing many data, must come to terms with the facts of anatomy and physiology, if it wants to enter medicine. Hansemann then continues in a highly polemical way, criticising bacteriologists for having among other things too few theories. Hansemann, however, fully supports Koch's Postulates as essential for assessing the aetiological role of particular bacteria. After that, Hansemann attacks von Behring's use of convalescent serum in the treatment of diphtheria, and criticises bacteriology for being only interested in aetiology. He insists, without providing persuasive reasons, that the pathogeneses of bacterial diseases are as important as their aetiology and therapy.

Hansemann would probably not have gained support from bacteriologists and immunologists in Berlin by publishing this article.

The diagnosis of malignant tumours: a clinical lecture delivered at the University of Berlin (1895i)

This article illuminates the state of histopathology as a diagnostic tool in Germany at the time. That Hansemann was chosen to give the lecture is an indication of his status as a pathologist. The article begins with statements pointing out that accurate diagnosis is important for the treatment of the patient. The greatest difficulties are with tumours of:

> "... various bones of the body, of the upper portion of the respiratory and digestive tracts, of the anus, the vagina, and the vaginal portion of the uterus. Hereto must be added another class not subject to any particular localization, – namely, certain kinds of syphilitic tumours".

Examples are given of the value of biopsy in the management of cases of a firm lesion of the mouth, of a nasal polyp, and of a lesion of the vaginal portion of the uterus, rectal lesions, syphilitic tumours, and tuberculomas.

Histological techniques are mentioned and bichloride of mercury is recommended for fixation. General principles for diagnosis of sarcoma and carcinoma are given. Karyokinetic figures are mentioned, and the statement is made:

> "If, then, you proceed to examine the karyokinetic figures and find them deviating to any considerable degree from the normal epidermoid type, or differing greatly from each other, many of them with the chromatin irregularly distributed, and fully if they are asymmetrical, then the diagnosis 'carcinoma' is quite assured."

On cure and curability (1897g)

This article seems to be a general "caution" against cancer "cures". There are accounts of many pathological states, such as pneumonia, heart valves, diphtheria etc, and the healing responses of the body to the lesions.

In the last paragraph, Hansemann states that only surgical excision helps malignant tumours, and may prolong or save the life, but it is not a cure, in the sense of correcting the abnormal tissue, in the way that the lung tissue is corrected after pneumonia. No therapy known at that time can stop malignant growth once it has begun.

"The Diagnosis of Malignant Tumours" (1897o) (second edition, 1902h)

This is Hansemann's great contribution to the practice of diagnosing malignant tumours by histopathology. When he wrote the first edition, such diagnoses were mainly based on Virchow's insistence that only invasive lesions could be called malignant. (If Virchow accepted otherwise, then Virchow's own theory of tumours, based on their origin from cells in the connective tissue, would have been unsustainable). Hansemann, however, proposed correctly that malignancy could be diagnosed, in most cases, on the basis of the abnormalities of the tumour cells themselves, especially if the degrees of chromosomal and mitotic abnormalities (being large parts of "anaplastic change", or changes which indicate the degree of underlying anaplasia, see chapter 5) are taken into consideration. Thus Hansemann described the features of malignant cells as they are now understood, and therefore was the original author of the modern criteria for the diagnosis of malignancy in histopathological sections, and the actual founder of the entire discipline of cytopathology.

The section on chorion-epithelioma (chorio-carcinoma) is presented in translation at the end of this section. The ideas here are important because they show that the principles of "anaplasia" apply to germ cells as much as to somatic cells. The theoretical significance is that "embryonic reversion" is not relevant to tumour morphology if the one concept ("anaplasia") can accommodate tumours from cells which produce embryos.

Hansemann's other articles and books on tumours and related topics

Table of Contents (first edition)

Introduction .... p. 1

Importance of histological knowledge of tumours for the biological studies of cells and for the practical assessment of tumours. Dangers of schematisation. Limits of histological diagnosis.

Chapter 1 General classification of tumours: .... p. 5

Difficulty of definition. Necessity of classification. Morphological classifications of the older anatomists. Cruvelhier's classification. The histological basis of Johannes Müller and Virchow. Virchow's anatomical-genetic classification. Homeoplasia and heteroplasia. Virchow's definition of sarcomas and carcinomas. Waldeyer's histogenetic classification. Classification on embryological basis. Importance of the word epithelium. The most recent views of Kölliker and His on 'epithelium'. Difficulties of histogenetic studies. The histogenetic classification cannot be carried through. Physiological classification principle. Aetiological classification principle. Fundamental differences of malignant tumours from infective tumours. Practical necessity for a morphological classification.

Chapter 2: Comparison of the morphology of malignant tumours with the tissue of origin: .... p. 18

Constituted from stroma and parenchyma. Gluge's corpuscles with tails. The cancer cell. Sarcomas as organoid tumours. Relationship between carcinoma and sarcoma. Classification of carcinomas according to the form of their cells and the constitution of the stroma. Cancroids. Cylindrical cell cancers. Medullary cancer. Scirrhous tumors. Colloid cancer. Fungus haematoides. Psammocarcinomas. Classification of carcinomas according to the origin of their cells. Classification of carcinomas according to the origin of their parenchyma. Nomenclature of carcinomas. Tumour-forming organs. Direct and indirect genesis. Metaplasia and variation. Comparison of tumour parenchyma with the mother tissue in carcinomas of the epidermis, of the rectum, of the stomach, of the mammary gland, of the salivary gland, of the kidney, of the liver, of the epidermoidal mucous membranes, of the thyroid, of the urinary bladder. The same comparison in sarcomas of the cartilage, of the bones, of the glia, of the pia mater, of the smooth muscles, of the adenoid tissue, of the endothelia, of the pigmented tissue, of the pigment cells. Combination tumours. Papillary tumours. Malignant cystomas. Malignant teratomata.

Chapter 3: Karyokinetic processes in malignant tumours: .... p. 62

Physiological and pathological mitoses. Classification of pathological forms. Hyperchromasia. Hypochromasia. Reduction division. Asymmetric mitoses. Scattered chromosomes. Physiological mitoses of malignant tumours. Constancy of forms in normal tissue. Changes in tumours. Loss of unified character. Arrangement of mitoses in tissue. Germinal layers.

Chapter 4: Degenerative processes in the parenchyma of malignant tumours: .... p. 74

Historical. Fat metamorphosis. Caseation. Colloid metamorphosis. Chromatolysis. Hyaline inclusions. Glycogen. Mucin. Parenchymal giant cells. Free nuclei. Degenerative processes in comparison with the tendency of the mother tissue towards the same. Causes of degeneration.

Chapter 5: Relationship of metastases and recurrent lesions to the primary tumours .... p. 87

Definition of metastasis. Simultaneous occurrence of several malignant tumours. Disposition of the organs. Small primary tumours with large metastases. Types of (mechanisms of) metastasis. Infection and transplantation theory. Origin of the parenchyma of the metastases. Accord of the parenchyma of the metastases with that of the primary tumours. Deviations of the same. Increase of anaplasia in the metastases and recidivistic lesions.

"The Diagnosis of Malignant Tumours" (1897o) (second edition, 1902h)

Chapter 6: On the stroma of malignant tumours: .... p. 104

Stroma of sarcomas. Hyaline changes. Cylindromas. Metaplastic changes of the stroma. Stroma of carcinomas. Soft cancer. Scirrhus. Vessels. Regressive metamorphoses. Fat metamorphosis. Hyaline change. Amyloid. Small celled infiltration. Giant cells. Amyloid bodies. Calcification. Development of the stroma. Origin of the stroma. Relationship between parenchyma and stroma.

Chapter 7: Behaviour of malignant tumours towards the organ parenchyma: .... p. 123

Distinction of primary tumour and metastasis through the structure, through the age, through the behaviour of the neighbouring tissue. Primary tissue and mother tissue. Collateral hyperplasia. Sharp delimitation of the metastases. Breakthrough of elastic membranes and smooth muscle tissue. Concentric compression. Consumption. Cross-striated musculature. Lung tissue. Infiltration.

Chapter 8: On the function of tumour cells: .... p. 138

Morphological expression of function. The cells of malignant tumours have a function. Secretion. Geotropism. Altruistic function. Decrease and change in the function with increasing anaplasia. Increased capability for independent existence. The concept of anaplasia. Anaplasia as primary condition. Ribbert's theory. Anaplasia and proliferation stimulus. Manoeuvrability. Phagocytosis. Poisonous effect of the tumour cells.

Chapter 9: On the histogenesis of malignant tumours: .... p. 153

Historical. Difficulty in histogenetic recognition. Closely-demarcated development. Diffuse development. The histogenetic theories of Thiersch, Cohnheim, Ribbert. Importance of inflammation. Importance of choked-off cells. Anaplastic change in cells. Development out of previously pathologically changed cells, from benign tumours, from congenital tumours, from heterotopias. Tissues from which malignant tumours develop. Ganglion cells. Striated musculature. Endothelia. Cystic tumours. Histogenesis of metastasis.

Chapter 10: On the aetiology of malignant tumours: .... p. 171

Theory of Thiersch, of Cohnheim, of Ribbert. Statistics. Heredity. Parasites. Infectivity and transplantation. Endemic carcinoma. Increase of carcinomas. Causes of the increase. Increase of nourishment. Traumas, acute, chronic. Chronic stimuli in the oesophagus, stomach, gut, mouth, larynx and bronchi, gall bladder, uterus. Scar formation. Chronic inflammation. Disposition.

Chapter 11: On the importance of the findings for diagnosis: .... p. 183

Forms of examination. Trial excision. Total extirpation. Cadaveric finding. Anamnesis. Localisation. Age of the patient. Clinical course. Status. Technical observations. Differential diagnosis of the *tumor inflammatorius*, of atypical epithelial proliferation, tuberculosis, actinomycosis, plague, typhus-related proliferations, leukaemia, pseudo leukaemia, syphilis. Proof of heteroplasia. Proof of anaplasia. Diagnosis of the malignancy of complicated tumours is a pure matter of experience. Different grades of malignancy.

In comparing the second edition with the first:

– The Introduction, and Chapters 1 are little unchanged.

– Chapters 2 (carcinomas) and 3 (sarcomas) of the second edition are derived from Chapter 2 of the original without change of length.

- Chapter 4 in the second edition is new and discusses the entity of the now-disproved entity of "endothelioma" (see Wolff, 1907 p. 200 ff).
- Chapters 5 and 6 are new to the second edition. The discussion of chorion-epithelioma (a translation of which is presented here) is important, because it is possible to identify anaplasia in tumours of this earliest embryonal cell, and hence anaplasia does not equate with embryonic reversion.
- Chapter 7 of the second edition is an expansion (by 3 pages) of chapter 3 of the first edition.
- Chapters 7–15 of the second edition correspond to chapters 3–11 of the first edition, each being expansions with more tumour types or examples.

Discussion of chorion-epithelioma (chorio-carcinoma), p. 90, second paragraph (2nd edn)

"If now, as I have done in the case of carcinomas and sarcomas, one compares the chorion-epitheliomas with their mother tissue, then it is beyond doubt that those which Marchant denotes as typical are more similar to the mother tissue than the atypical ones. The latter have lost the normal ability to form syncytia and to secrete glycogen. They no longer show the regular cells of the cell layer, but irregular polymorphous cells. This is not without influence even on the degree of malignancy. Because of its importance, I include Marchant's own words here, whose correctness I can completely confirm: 'In any case, the form of the tumour appears to be not without influence on the kind of further spread in the body. Both forms appear to be of approximately similar malignancy. Whilst in the typical cases, the possibility of a dragging along of larger connected parts via the blood stream is present, from which then even larger masses situated in a blood space – very soft complexes of characteristic constitution – can proceed; there takes place in the atypical tissue, an ever further-developing infiltration of the entire tissue with destruction and disintegration penetration under the epithelium, and finally penetration into the lumen of the vessels with correspondingly less dragging around of the isolated, even if multi-nuclear elements. This kind of spreading conditions a predominantly destructive character of the new formation which may be prognostically more unfavourable to the extent that any demarcation between the infiltrating parts from the neighbouring tissue can be scarcely achieved'.

Thus one sees the typical form behaves, *vis à vis* the chorion epithelium, just as the chancroid to the epidermis or the adenoma destruens to the gland epithelium; the atypical form stands in a similar relationship to the chorion epithelium as medullary cancer to a mother tissue. I should thus express myself like this: that anaplasia in the tumour cells can increase and that between the least and strongest form of the same, in the chorion epithelium too, there are, again, all transitions."

On the term "anaplasia" and its essential nature (1900b)

This article corrects assertions made by Beneke (Virchow's Arch. 161: 70–114) that "anaplasia" can mean either a capacity to undergo metaplasia, or a dedifferentiation to embryonal types of cells. This Beneke (son of R. Beneke – see chapter 6 – eds) was at this time trying to introduce a term "kataplasia", which von Hansemann considers is very similar to his (Hansemann's) "anaplasia". The last section is worth quoting:

"It is outright false when Beneke on p. 100 says, 'Of course, Hansemann does not want to place anaplastic cells on the same level as embryonal cells ...

However, despite this statement which is probably based on the difficulty of attempting to create a genuine basis for this hypothesis, it becomes undoubtedly apparent from his train of thought that anaplasia is at least a state close to the physiological embryonal state.'

The truth is that I have never tried to build a foundation for my hypothesis because someone does not build a roof in mid air and then push the house underneath, but the opposite is true, that I made factual observations and build up my hypothesis on anaplasia on those. If such a conclusion as Beneke claims I have made, had occurred to me, I would not have expressed it. Such conclusion is not contained in my work, and it is not logical, as anyone can see who follows my works and writings on the topic and how the term ANAPLASIA has evolved gradually. Beneke's demand on p. 105 that research be conducted into which functional abilities and which morphological characteristics the various cells lose while they undergo blastomatosis, and which remain with them has already been the basis of my studies, and through which I came to the conclusion that those cells (undergoing 'blastomatosis' – eds) lose differentiation and gain autonomy. That phenomenon, for many reasons I do not want to expand on at this moment, I called ANAPLASIA. It does not really matter whether this process now would be called CATAPLASIA according to Beneke's proposal, as long as one knows what I meant the term should stand for when I coined it. In my opinion, the word ANAPLASIA describes the situation better. I can see another error when Beneke on p. 108 calls the dedifferentiation of cells and their individuality an unstoppable slide to the way of prosoplasia, because prosoplasia means further differentiation and, thus, an increase in cell individuality.

I am unable to agree with Beneke in his theoretical considerations but I do agree with him and Wilms in the interpretation of this particular case. Let me prove this to you. When I described a malignant mixed tumour of the kidney a few years ago, I interpreted this in agreement with previous investigators of similar tumours as embryonal in origin and said it was likely that different cell types develop their specific anaplastic versions of cells, which means roughly the same as Beneke says on p. 110. "It rather appears that each form of connective tissue in the tumour formed its own malignant type." O. Israel made a similar mistake as Beneke when in a recent article, Berlin Clinical Bot.... 1900, Volume 28, he writes on the histogenesis of pathological tumours and touches upon my hypothesis with the words: "There is no anaplasia in the sense of cytogenetic atavism". Thus, Israel too, like Beneke, seems to assume that in the processes of anaplasia, cells regress in exactly the same way that they went forward when they went in prosoplasia. The other many differences in opinion that went on from there, between Israel and me, I will come back to on another occasion. Let me now repeat what I have said before on a similar occasion. The theory of ANAPLASIA is a hypothesis. A hypothesis is justified when it is able to explain many phenomena. However, it is only transitory and might disappear due to acquisition of further knowledge, but not through its misinterpretation by others. I am prepared to give up the entire theory of ANAPLASIA anytime as soon as there are new hypotheses which explain the genesis of tumours better than anaplasia does. I would have to insist that the term ANAPLASIA is not being distorted in the meantime."

On nuclear division figures of malignant tumours: addendum to the short communication of Messrs Farmer, Moore and Walker (1904c)

This article deals with the matter of the relationship between chromosomal numbers and malignancy. The translation is complete except for the seventeen references (on p. 191 of the original) already given in other publications.

189 In number 1 of this Central Journal, vol. 24, there is a communication from Messrs Farmer, Moore and Walker. This is an excerpt from a lecture which was given to the Royal Society in London this year. Simultaneously, similar excerpts appeared in the British Medical Journal and in the Lancet. In their investigations, the authors have entered into an area which I have been investigating for more than 20 years, and which, already in 1890, led me to similar results. Here we are dealing with

190 a change in the nuclear division figures in tumours, in contrast with those in normal tissues, and the central point of this publication by the three gentlemen named is that compared with normal tissue, the number of chromosomes becomes less, and that the chromosomes themselves undergo changes of form. At that time, I advanced the assertion that the changed biological properties of the cancer cells do indeed find their morphological expression in the change of nuclear division figures compared with normal ones. Certainly on the other hand, these changes are not yet exhausted with the two facts set down above, but it was at that time necessary, in addition, to study the normal karyokinesis of the entire human body. While doing this it became clear that the cell figures are absolutely characteristic and specific for the individual tissue types, and that one is able to recognise some cell types solely from the form of their karyokinesis. Further investigation has led me now to conclude that this specificity of cell divisions gets lost in carcinomas and often, too, in sarcomas, so that not only do mitoses arise which deviate from the norm, but also the different cell division figures can develop in very different ways in one and the same tumour. Thereby, they reach a further stage of the pathological mitoses observed earlier by Arnold and others and one could prove that such mitoses are to be found in part also in benign tumours, and in inflammatory proliferations, but that they pile themselves up quite particularly in malignancies and that in these latter they take on forms which are distinguished by a reduction in chromosomes. I am not of the opinion of the authors named, that the mitoses in malignant tumours agree with what (as far as I know) Flemming first described as heterotypical mitosis in the testis of salamandra. Certainly, I admit, that in malignant tumours, but occasionally also elsewhere, nuclear division figures can emerge, which possess a certain similarity with a heterotypical mitosis. But it is not these which lead to reduction division, but on the contrary, the reduction of chromosomes takes place, as I have already explained, during this process: firstly through asymmetric mitoses and secondly by the perishing of individual chromosomes, without, for the rest, the vitality of the cells being reduced thereby. Through the fact that the chromosomes later double, multiply, and so on, cells can arise which do indeed contain more chromosomes than normal cells, but in reality, proceed from cells which had lessened numbers of chromosomes. Thus, for the classification of pathological mitoses, the principle of the number of chromosomes resulted, and one could thus distinguish

191 hypochromatic, normochromatic and hypochromatic mitoses. At that time already, moreover, I described the different forms of chromosomes which have now been reported again by the authors named.

Why these changed mitoses can be brought together into one context (*Zusammenhang*) and, in my opinion, must be brought together with the malignancy of tumours and with that quality which I have denoted as anaplasia, I have argued extensively in a substantial number of articles. The word anaplasia has passed almost generally into the nomenclature. I have all the less cause, however, to go more closely into these points here, because my works, the numerous discussions associated with them and further investigations from other sides, have appeared everywhere in accessible journals, and in addition to this, an extensive paper was reprinted in this Central Journal which originated with Hauser.

Below, I list only relevant papers on the subject which are particularly important, without going into numerous communications which are sometimes to be found in works on tumours, regeneration and cell proliferations. The literature not cited here is extensively quoted especially in "Studies on Specificity, Altruism and Anaplasia" as also in "Diagnosis of Malignant Tumours." (17 articles cited here but not translated – eds)

As the gentlemen named did not mention me in their communication, neither in the English journals, nor in this Central Journal, and thereby apparently gave the impression that this literature was unknown to them, I saw cause to have a short notice published in English journals. Thereupon, in the Lancet, the authors named gave a retort that my works were completely familiar to them, but that in their investigations they see a completely different matter, which deviated in principle from my results. I cannot accept that at all, and as these gentlemen, as they say, know my works, it would surely have been necessary to emphasise particularly the differences from my investigations. They only do this, however, in the afore-mentioned retort in the Lancet, and from this it is clear that they see the main difference between our findings in the fact that I have found a reduction division which is brought about by a particular form of the pathological process in the cell, whilst they maintain that a reduction division occurs which seems to be analogous to the heterotypical mitosis at the maturation of the sex cells. That is specifically, for which I have given the fundamental reasons in detail, why it is not accurate. Specifically the differences between the reduction division in tumours and those in the maturation of the egg and in (*in**) the spermatozoa, I have repeatedly argued. And if the authors confirm an approximate similarity between some forms of mitosis in tumours, and maturing sex cells in animals and plants, then I can certainly acknowledge that I cannot accept the identity of these processes in any way at all. Moreover, the essential aspect it seems to me, does not even lie in the way in which the reduction division comes about, but in contrast, that a reduction division occurs at all, and that it is able to explain the anaplastic qualities of the tumour cells. For this, however, I must claim priority *vis a vis* the aforementioned gentlemen, and without this conclusion as to the malignant tumours, the findings of those authors too would certainly have no significance for the explanation of tumours. Therefore I cannot conclude that the investigations of these gentlemen are so different from mine that they make a citation of my works unnecessary and it is understandable that I was compelled to conclude from this that the authors were not familiar with my works and the discussion following upon it.

* "both cases" may be implied (eds)

Malignant growths and normal reproductive tissues (1904q)

This article and the one following represent Hansemann's attempt to clarify the relationship between nuclear size and malignancy. In our view, the overall effect of the article is obscure because Hansemann seems to be unwilling to state that his idea of anaplasia was originally related (although by an unclear mechanism) to oogenesis, but that he still had had the idea originally (see chapter 5).

"SIRS, — In your issue of Dec. 26th, 1903, p. 1830, there is an abstract of some observations by Professor J. B. Farmer, Mr. J. E. S. Moore, and Mr. C. E. Walker. They have been investigating karyokinetic processes in malignant tumours, a field of investigation in which I, too, worked extensively some years ago. Since my observations do not seem to be familiar to these authors, who are, I believe, botanists by profession, I should be glad if you would give me space in your journal for the following remarks. These authors have found that in the cell development of malignant tumours the mitotic figures exhibit certain definite differences from those occurring in normal tissues. The essential alteration lies in the fact that the cells undergo a reductive division, similar to that occurring in the formation of sexual cells, whereby germinal tissue is formed. The authors state explicitly that the cells do not become embryonic, in fact, differ from these through the small number of their chromosomes. In addition, the chromosomes are also changed in shape. These observations coincide more or less with those described some time ago in various publications – e.g., Virchow's Archiv. vol. cxix., 1890, p. 299; *Archiv für mikroskopische Anatomie,* vol. xliii.; the *Festschrift für Virchow* in 1891; and in the *Verhandlungen der Anatomischen Gesellschaft* in 1891, p. 255, and elsewhere. I have given a connected account of these processes in my monograph, entitled, *Studien über die Spezifizität, den Altruismus und die Anaplasie der Zellen* (Berlin, 1893), and reverted to the subject in my book on *Die Mikroskopische Diagnose der Bösartigen Geschwülste* (second edition, Berlin, 1902) on p. 91 ff.

According to my investigations it is not a question of a reduction to exactly one-half the normal number of chromosomes nor does the reductive division occur in the manner seen in the maturation of ova and spermatozoa. According to my observations the reduction is effected in a two-fold manner – either by asymmetrical nuclear division or by a destruction of individual chromosomes without destruction of all the nuclear substance. The first result by either of these two processes is cells with a smaller number of chromosomes than normal. I have called these cells HYPOCHROMATIC. In the further stages of development these chromosomes may be doubled, quadrupled, sextupled, and so on, so that from hypochromatic cells, hyperchromatic ones may arise but always with a smaller than the normal number of chromosomes of human cells. I have sought to correlate with these observations the peculiar characters which the cells of malignant growths possess, especially their greater power of independent existence and their loss of differentiation as compared with the normal tissue cells. The combination of these two properties I have termed ANAPLASIA, an expression now very generally employed in the scientific world even by those investigators who do not altogether agree with the details of my observations on the cell processes. I have also given a detailed account of the change of form of the chromosomes and have shown how extraordinarily manifold their form may be in malignant tumours which, in nearly all cases differ not only from normal tissues but also amongst each other, so that not only in different cancers but in one and the same the most varied forms of chromosomes may be found.

Since these investigations are, perhaps, but little known in England I am naturally anxious in reference to the investigations of Professor Farmer, Mr. Moore, and Mr. Walker to guard my priority of observations in this field.

I am, Sirs, yours faithfully,

Berlin, Jan. 16th, 1904. PROFESSOR D v. HANSEMANN.

Editors' (of the Lancet) *comment.*

We include the response of Farmer, Moore and Walker. See also chapter 5 of this volume.

To the Editors of THE LANCET.

SIRS, — The letter of Professor v. Hansemann, a proof of which you have allowed us to see, contains a number of misleading statements some of which call for comment. Incidentally we may remark that only one of us is a botanist, although two of us have been frequently associated in work on vegetable, as well as on animal, cytology.

We are at a loss to understand why Professor v. Hansemann should assume that we are unaware of his investigations. As a matter of fact we are perfectly familiar with them, and as a consequence with the circumstance that our own conclusions respecting the meaning of the cytological phenomena in question are in all essential features at variance with those arrived at by him. It is perfectly clear both from his letter and still more so from a study of his work of 1902, cited by him, that he has either entirely misapprehended the facts connected with the "reducing" divisions characteristic of sexually reproductive tissue or that he has not succeeded in tracing the similarity that exists between the processes in them and in malignant growths respectively.

Professor v. Hansemann's statement that the occurrence of an odd number of chromosomes in any cell of any animal is necessarily due to either an asymmetrical division or to degeneration (or elimination) is not in accordance with known facts. There is no *a priori* reason why a cell that has undergone reduction should not possess an odd number of chromosomes, and, indeed, some animals *do* exhibit such numbers. It is only the SOMATIC cells that normally must contain an even number and this is due to the fact that ovum and sperm each possess identical (even or odd) numbers before their union in fertilisation.

No one who has examined the dividing nuclei of malignant tissue has doubted the occurrence of abnormalities, but no one, so far as we are aware, and certainly not Professor v. Hansemann, had previously suggested those resemblances between reproductive and malignant tissues that are involved in the recognition, in each, of the existence of the heterotype mitosis. Indeed, we have so far failed to identify these special points in our own communication for the discovery of which Professor v. Hansemann is so anxious to guard his priority. For whilst, in common with others who have worked at this subject, we have naturally recognised the frequent occurrences of irregular nuclear divisions, the conclusions we have reached, as well as the interpretation we have put on the facts, are, as Professor v. Hansemann admits in his letter, widely divergent from those to which he has himself been led.

We are, Sirs, yours faithfully,

J. BRETLAND FARMER.
J. E. S. MOORE.
CHARLES WALKER.

*⁎*In the circumstances we decided to give Professor Farmer, Mr. Moore, and Mr. Walker an opportunity of replying to Professor v. Hansemann in the same issue of THE LANCET in which Professor v. Hansemann's letter appears. — ED. L.

On the functional abilities of cancer cells. A discussion – observation on Beneke's position paper on physiological and pathological growth (1905c)

This is a short note rather than a paper and corrects statements by Beneke in articles in Nos 36 and 37 of the same journal. Here is Hansemann's note in full.

"In nos. 36 and 37 of this weekly Beneke published a lecture which he gave in Königsberg on physiological and pathological growth. In this lecture he is also much concerned with my theory of anaplasia, and at one point (p. 1187) with my view on the function capability of cancer cells. This latter point gives me cause for a short discussion. Certainly, in the coming year in Lisbon, at the request of the Conference Directorate there, I will have the opportunity to speak in detail on the function of cancer cells, but I should not like to wait so long in order to correct a misunderstanding which is to be found in Beneke's essay. He says in the place quoted here: "It is more difficult to prove that the functional achievements of the tumour cells are disturbed. Specifically on this point, the opinions of the authors differ strongly, and even those who speak of a small differentiation of the tumour cells, do not, like for example von Hansemann, avoid the contradiction of simultaneously recognising the specific function capability of cells even in malignant tumours." I must confess that I do not properly understand how Beneke quotes me in this sense, because what is presented more extensively in the following, is exactly what I have mentioned in the same sense in the most various places. To this end, I refer to my "Studies in Specificity, Altruism and Anaplasia of Cells" (Berlin, August Hirschwald) and to the "Diagnosis of Malignant Tumours" (1st edn, 1897; 2nd edn, Berlin, 1902). Also in a sequence of special articles I have gone into detail on these thoughts. Everywhere I have expressly formulated my opinion in the sense that tumour cells with little anaplasia develop a function which is very similar to normal mother cells, in certain circumstances so much that one cannot discover any difference, but that this function, with increasing anaplasia becomes less, and changes, and that cells of tumours with strongest anaplasia show such a deviant function that one can often no longer find any similarity to that of the mother cells. The change in function, indeed, proceeds completely in conformity with the de-differentiation, and therefore, in this respect, I agree completely with Beneke's view, and I do not believe that he can find anything in my contemplations for quoting me on this point as one of his opponents. As far as his nomenclature, with the word "kataplasia" for what I call "anaplasia" is concerned, I have already said earlier that the name is not important to me and that if "kataplasia" should be found better than "anaplasia", I have nothing against this usage. I am solely concerned with the concept, and since for this concept, as Beneke himself states, the word anaplasia has found wide circulation, I do not see the necessity to invent a second, additional word, and I believe therefore that it would be better in practice, to leave the word "anaplasia" to denote the aforesaid cell changes".

Critical contemplations on the tumour theory (1905f)

Hansemann was editor of this journal at this time, and this article is one of several which are to be found in its early volumes. The beginning of the article consists of attacks on authors who do not review the literature of their topics thoroughly, and publish old ideas under new names. He then attacks Ribbert, on this occasion concerning the controversy of "unicentricity" versus "pluricentricity" of the origins of cancers.

We note his comments on multi-focal verus unifocal origins of tumours (p. 561–2, beginning para 4 of the original), because they represent an early account of "field theory" which is not well documented in the English language (c.f. Willis, 1948).

"As far as the first point is concerned, it is undoubtedly to Ribbert's credit that with great energy and exact investigations, he has established that many carcinomata have a single point of origin and that they grow out, out from themselves (*und dass sie aus sich herauswachsen*). Now Ribbert always presents it as if earlier, one had quite generally assumed that a carcinomatous nodule did not grow out of itself at all and only enlarged because the neighbouring cells likewise turned into cancer cells themselves and the growth was thus to a certain extent appositional. I do not know whether this view has ever really predominated anywhere in this fashion. I myself can only say that I have never accepted such a mode of growth. I have never doubted that once a cancer has originated from some point, it can grow out of itself, but I have always been of the opinion, and I stand by it, that there are cancers which do not originate out of themselves in one place, but come into being either simultaneously, or in succession, in different sites, independently of each other, and I believe this view is shared by many other authors, and therefore one distinguishes between "unicentric" and "pluricentric" carcinoma. Now I certainly, like most other authors, was earlier of the opinion that the majority of cancers are pluricentric. Certainly, this view has been substantially altered by the works of Ribbert and Borrmann and later by Peterson's and Borst's examinations. I acknowledge that very many if not most cancers

562 are monocentric, but in no way can I join the exclusive view of Ribbert which he has just reiterated in his latest paper, that this is the only mode of cancer formation, and I believe that Ribbert will have to admit that the investigations such as Rindfleish has just carried out again and just published in the *Verhandlungen der Phys./ Med. Gesellschaft, zu Würzburg*, vol. 37, are reflecting the actual processes. After all, similar cases are not rare indeed, and it would have to be a remarkable chance if Ribbert had not seen one."

Hansemann then follows on with a personal attack on Ribbert, in which he says:

"In reality I believe that the cause of his opposition has yet another reason which is more a psychological one. The fact that cancers can arise monocentrically probably made such an impression on him at the start that he is inclined to interpret all pictures which he sees in his sense".

The article continues with a ranging discussion of many issues in cancer research, including the "dedifferentiation", the parasitic theory, transplantation, hereditary factors, and so on. However, at the end of the article Hansemann makes a point which presages "two-hit" models of cancer in the following (p. 577, second para):

"Now in order to explain malignant tumours, there is still something else. The simple reactive proliferation after defects have once appeared or following customary inflammations, is not sufficient to bring about such a malignant tumour formation, and it is there where the main difference between Ribbert's views on the one hand and on the other, mine and those of many others, is based. A transformation in principle of the character of the cell must happen in order to produce a malignant tumour formation. The cell must become anaplastic. Now the objection has often been made to me that this state of anaplasia does not explain the proliferation capability of the cell. Certainly this cell change does not explain the cause of the proliferation but a particular external stimulus as such is always necessary. But that anaplastic cells, meaning less differentiated ones, are more capable of proliferation than more strongly differentiated ones is clear, from the contemplations which I initiated in my earlier investigations on this object, and which I have briefly repeated here. Thus it seems to me that there is a thorough congruence between anaplasia and proliferation capacity. The proliferation CAPABILITY, however, does not yet involve THE NECESSITY OF A PROLIFERATION. This is only produced by the external stimulus, and after everything which experience teaches, a chronic stimulation is more suitable for this than an acute one-off stimulus. And thus the sequence of thought seems to be completely closed in the context of the origin of tumours with the facts of regeneration and of anaplasia."

In the final sentence (p578), however, Hansemann makes a statement over which those who might seek to enhance his memory might well despair. He reverts to *Virchowismus*, by discussing inflammation-and-cancer ideas, so well publicised by Virchow, and which before him can be traced backwards through Boerhaave to the Ancients (Wolff, 1907).

"Also the question of the separation of benign and malignant tumours which, as Virchow has already emphasised, is not a biological postulate, but solely a practical one, allows a much sharper answer, because thereby it is shown that in reality, there is no sharp delineation between benign and malignant, just as little as between genuine tumours and inflammatory new formations."

Talks by Prof von Hansemann and *Geheimrat* von Leyden on "The Aetiology of Cancers" at the Berlin Society of Medicine 8th March 1905 (1905k)

Von Leyden was a prominent physician (*Geheimer Med-Rat* – see chapter 1), and chairman of the Committee for Cancer Research in Berlin. Hansemann was Secretary of the same Committee.

This article is quoted in full, because any summary would not do it justice.

"The attendance at this session was even greater than that at the one of March 1st. Many clearly anticipated an exaggeration of the dramatic action of the "conflict". In addition, it was of special interest to many to hear Herr von Leyden speak, and see him stand at the podium of the Berlin Medical Society once again after more than two decades. So it happened that not only the lecture theatre of Langenbeck House was full, but also the atrium and gallery were overcrowded and the number of attendees is estimated to have been just under 1,000.

Before the day's programme, there were two short demonstrations, on which we will report on in the next supplement to this publication. Herr von Hansemann then proceeded to give a one hour discourse on the topic "What do we know of the aetiology of cancers?" His insightful (*lichtvollen*), and at times sharply pointed comments, which were delivered in excellent form and with a lively temperament, generated massive applause at the end. The content of the lecture we will reproduce here according to a summary most kindly given to us by von Hansemann himself.

In his introduction the speaker points out that through the enormous growth of the literature, it has virtually become impossible for a single person to tell truth from falsehood, and that this almost requires a specialised study.

There are three main theories which have to be discussed which attempt to explain the aetiology of cancers: That is the infection theory, the heredity theory and the traumatic theory. The INFECTION THEORY is to be proven by transmission of cancers, by the proof of transmission from human to human, through the assertion that cancer is an ever-increasing disease, and finally through proving the existence of cancer parasites. The speaker made clear that transmissions from human beings to animals has never been achieved so far, and that transmission from animal to animal does not have the significance of an inoculation, and thus offers nothing to explain the aetiology of malignant tumours. As far as the so-called epidemics of cancer are concerned, including *cancer à deux*, this is merely coincidence, which is further evidenced by the fact that there are non-infectious diseases which cluster in certain places and also appear occasionally in married people who are unrelated by blood. It would certainly be miraculous if the cancer disease were to be so transmitted and occur to the same extent everywhere. The increase in cases of cancer is a concept challenged by the speaker, in unison with many other authors and above all, he is in agreement with the excellent statistical work by de Bovis which suggests that the increase is spurious and merely due to improved diagnostic abilities. Finally, as far as the proof of parasites is concerned, the speaker is convinced that all the structures indicated as such so far, are not parasites. He even doubts the possibility that such parasites can cause cancer at all, because all parasites known so far in plants and animals only cause diseases which have nothing in common with malignant tumours. He warns against giving the infection theory any publicity in the general population, because this would be, to say the least premature, because this would cause cancer sufferers to acquire the label "infectious", which will only worsen their lot.

Next, the speaker presents evidence that there is little in favour of the HEREDITY THEORY either. This is mainly based on the frequently very unreliable statements by the patients or their relatives, and on the coincidental clustering of tumours in one family, which can be explained in the same way as the clustering in certain places or certain houses.

The speaker tends to favour the TRAUMATIC THEORY*. But here in particular, acute injuries, those which could come under the law of accident, seem to have no aetiological weight. At most, they may worsen an already-existing tumour. In contrast, chronic trauma in the widest sense, meaning mechanical, chemical and thermal irritation, would be in theory well able to cause malignant tumours. The speaker develops the concept that the genesis of malignant tumours springs from an interplay between disposition and external stimulus. In this regard, he emphasises, as he has done many times before, that these external stimuli can be of the most various kinds, and that it may be perverse to believe in the concept of a single aetiology of cancer, but that one must consider multiple different causes, for multiple different malignant tumours.

At an advanced hour, in an atmosphere of increasing tension, the Grand Master of German internal medicine, Herr von Leyden, took the stage for his lecture entitled "On the parasitic theory of the aetiology of cancer". The views of von Leyden have been aired frequently through the proceedings

What do we know of the origin of malignant tumours? (1905l)

of our Committee of Cancer Research in our weekly journal. GEHEIMRAT von Leyden did not present any new data during his speech, but summarised his views in very clear form. Compelling evidence for his view on the parasitic origin of cancers could not, in fact be delivered, but the experiments done by von Leyden recently with astonishing vigour to clarify this important question and make progress, will surely meet with general approval. To deliver a short summary of the talk, von Leyden emphasised, opposite to the position of the pathological anatomists, the standpoint of the clinicians. Of the doctors, on the basis of their practical observations, many believed in the infectiousness of cancer and have done so for a long time. The main reason for imagining the parasitic nature of the illness is its malignancy. The origin of the process in hitherto healthy and blooming bodies, followed by a rapid progressive consumption of bodily strength, implies the action of a parasite and is hard to explain in any other way. The traumatic theory and the heredity theory are untenable. As far as especially trauma is concerned, it has its effect in the origin of the cancer only as the coincidental event**, as also with other infections. Cancer does not originate from the juices of the bodies but springs up locally; thus a very specific stimulus must have had its influence here. This is the reason why it mainly occurs in places accessible to EXTERNAL influences, like skin, stomach and intestines, whereas cancers in other places are much less frequent. Although cancer occurs in animals, these are almost exclusively in domesticated animals, which thus have direct contact with humans. Further in favour of infectiousness of cancers, apart from epidemics and *cancer à deux*, is the development of cancer in puncture sites after the needling of malignant exudates, the infection of an upper lip by a lower lip cancer, and the familiar transfers of cancer by Hanau and E. Hahn. If the pathological anatomists call those last-named results transplantation rather than infection, they would have to admit that they are not able to make any distinction between the two terms in this situation. Certainly, it has only been possible so far to transfer cancer by cancer cells; but it should be considered here that, along with the cancer cells, the entire malignant disease has been transplanted into the other individual. Of special relevance here are the transmissions of cancer in mice by Jensen and L. Michaelis; these latter have been successful already up to the fifth generation. Isolating parasites has failed so far but von Leyden adheres firmly to the view that those bird's eye-like inclusion bodies which he discovered are to be seen as responsible for the origin of the cancer. (These latter, together with closer examinations, are demonstrated with the epidiascope). At the end, von Leyden informed us that in his own cancer ward, Blumenthal and others had recently discovered special chemical and fermentative components in cancers. Discussion on the three talks was adjourned, but it can hardly be expected that it will bring forth anything of substance to clarify this argument."

* This is clear Virchowism. Hansemann here commits one of his rare scientific errors, and it is a continuation of Virchow's theory of chronic irritation as a cause of tumours. (eds).
** of the inoculation of the parasite (eds).

What do we know of the origin of malignant tumours? (1905l)

This is Hansemann's only article in this journal (a weekly medical paper, published in Vienna). It begins with the statement that the answer to the question in the title of the article might best be "nothing yet", and that authors who state particular opinions in the press may be causing public mischief. Next there are complimentary remarks about the Berlin Committee for Cancer Research, from which Hansemann states that he gains valuable insights into the work of other authors. He says that the hope that great discoveries would flow from the formation of the committee is over-optimistic, because great discoveries are not made by committees but by specially gifted people.

The rest of the article concerns the aetiology of cancer, in terms of the three main theories at the time: parasitic, hereditary and traumatic. What follows is a repetition of the ideas in 1905k, etc. His summary, however, can be quoted in full:

"Everything which happens in tumour pathology comes into existence by the reciprocal effect of irritation and irritability. That is the old teaching of Virchow, which, however frequently it has been attacked, and however much, too, the concept of irritation and irritability has changed over the years, has repeatedly been victorious. The irritability of human tissues is variable, and I imagine that there are people who are totally susceptible to cancer formation, and in whom some slight, otherwise trivial irritation is sufficient to cause cancer. We have examples of such a process. The clearest is that of xeroderma pigmentosum. In such people, simple exposure of places in the skin to light is enough to cause a type of eczema which later on leads to cancer. The next stage of irritability is found in those people in whom eczemas and carcinomas can arise by the effect of soot, paraffin, arsenic or, as has been recently proven through X-ray radiation. To this would then be added those cases in which carcinoma comes into existence through chronic mechanical irritations, e.g. oesophageal cancers; gall bladder cancer with formation of gall stones; cancer in undescended testes; and many others. From these considerations, we see to start with that in all these cases, in the sequence which I have listed, irritability decreases and the irritation necessary to produce the same effect must increase. It is wrong to speak of *one* single aetiology of tumours, but I am convinced that if we ever arrive at all at finding the cause of tumours, that then perhaps, we will be able to prove other causes for every single group of tumours."

On the function of tumour cells (1906c)

This is one of Hansemann's most detailed and perceptive discussions of this topic. It is derived from a lecture given at an International Congress in Lisbon in the same year. In preliminary remarks, Hansemann mentions that Bashford (London) and Gaylord (Buffalo) had, despite previously submitting an abstract, failed to appear at the Congress.

In the substantial part of the article, he begins by stating that the functions to be discussed are "secretion" in a wide sense; "geotropism" – the tendency to grow on surfaces and in mutually-adhesive clusters of tumour cells; motility; and finally phagocytosis.

First, Hansemann pointed out that benign tumours most obviously retain the functions of the cell-type of origin (*Mutterzelle*) and that many malignant tumours do so, but to lesser degrees. Then he raises the issue that many malignant tumours exhibit *more* functionality than their original cell type. The first is that carcinomas of non-keratinising epithelium (e.g. oesophagus, bronchus) may show keratinisation – i.e. seem to have acquired the function of keratin-production as part of the neoplastic change. This he ascribes to "metaplasia", similar to that seen in the keratinisation associated with squamous metaplasia of mucus-secreting epithelium, for example in bronchiectatic cavities.

He then mentions the general rule that secretory functions manifest in degree inversely with anaplasia, and discusses this in relation to tumours of the pancreas adrenal and thyroid.

Geotropism is discussed as manifest by a primary peritoneal carcinoma spreading across the whole peritoneal cavity and especially omentum, keeping the properties of mesothelium, although also being metastatic to the lung.

As far as mobility is concerned, Hansemann believes that this occurs only in recently-formed cells just after mitosis. He believes that this is not a characteristic just of tumour cells, and also thinks that motility disappears with increasing anaplasia.

Hansemann describes many situations where tumour cells appear to have ingested other structures, and this is not be be confused with fertilisation in any way (Klebs, Farmer et al). There is then a brief discussion of "increased capacity for independent existence".

Next, there is a discussion of cachexia of cancer. Hansemann states that he recently became converted to the view that such a thing as a specific cachexia produced by secretions of cancer cells does not exist.

The last paragraph reads:

"If, finally, we summarise the results of these considerations, we can briefly say the following. The cells of malignant tumours possess a function and in general, a physiological existence which follows on in every way from that of the normal tissue from which the tumours emanate. With increasing anaplasia of the cells, the function changes initially quantitiatively, and then also qualitatively. Whether the function of the cells ceases completely every time, in the case of strongest anaplasia, it has not for that reason, been possible to establish hitherto, because its morphological expression is so far reduced that it can no longer be recognised in the usual way. Yet from the form of the cells, and from the structure of such tumours, with strongest anaplasia, it is virtually certain that the cells, finally, have no further function than is necessary for their preservation and for their multiplication".

A few remarks on the anaplasia of tumour cells (1907c)

This is largely a correction of assertions by Blumenthal concerning the nature of anaplasia. Being interested in the chemical basis of cancer, Blumenthal apparently asserted that anaplasia is a preliminary event affecting all exposed cells, and that cancer develops in these predisposed cells. This is an early version of the concept of "field theory" (see above). Von Hansemann's response is worth quoting as it seems, in the tradition of excessive *Streitkultur*, overly pedantic.

"If the carcinoma would develop in the liver and no liver cells in the neighbourhood of such a carcinoma display altered chemical properties as Mr Blumenthal states he has found, these liver cells would still lack all properties justifying the term ANAPLASTIC. They neither have assumed lesser differentiation nor have they demonstrated greater autonomy. Using the word ANAPLASIA simply to describe an altered chemical status of collateral liver cells would not only be a wrong use of the word but an utter disfigurement of the term which regrettably occurs all too often in medicine. This is like calling riverbanks STREAMS because someone discovers the presence of water within their soil. Some one coins the term to describe a special state and this word is used by others completely wrongly and gets used for the wrong things. This not only waters down such a term but renders the term unusable and worse. There are some researchers making accusations directed towards the original initiator of the term whereas he bears no guilt concerning the common state of confusion."

On the nomenclature of epithelial neoplasms (1908d)

This short note addresses the use of the word "adenoma" by Orth (Centralblatt f. allgem. Path. u. path. Anat. 15th June, vol. 11, 1908,) and asserts the modern view that all invasive lesions should be considered malignant (those of epithelium, therefore are carcinomas) irrespective of their cytological features. Those with "well differentiated" cytology should not be called "adenoma malignum" or "invasive adenoma" or any similar term. Here it is in full.

"In vol. 11 of the Central Publication for General Pathology and Pathological Anatomy 15th June 08, J Orth, has published an article carrying this title. Thankfully, the author discusses the common causes of misunderstanding which has become especially prevalent of late in relation to use of the word adenoma. This is no more obvious than with those authors working in experimental oncology. The author makes clear that the adenomata of these researchers are carcinomata, and furthermore he advocates the restructuring of the nomenclature in the following way. To distinguish the tumours into cancroid, adenoma malignum and cancer, all of these three being carcinomata. The author points out that there can be all sorts of transitions between these tumours; every expert will have to agree with Mr Orth. In contrast, it is by no means flattering for those individuals in question because of whom Orth has to write this that such a rebuke by an authority was necessary in the first place. It highlights that the individuals in question display a complete lack of knowledge of the cancer literature which should really be the prerequisite for anyone working in cancer research. It has been known for a very long time that destructive adenomata belong to the carcinomata. The discussion back then was as comprehensive as the one even much longer ago about the cancroids belonging to the carcinomata. The results of that discussion have since entered all textbooks and other teaching literature. Thus one would not even need lengthy historical studies to orient oneself in this matter. The new researchers, and especially the young ones amongst them, have to bear the accusation that they display insufficient consideration of known facts. Unfortunately this is not limited to cancer research, but is prevalent in all fields of scientific medicine. There would be a great saving of time and paper if the gentlemen in question would at least consider the landmark papers relevant to their studies and would stop believing that they had carried out a literature review by flicking through a few articles from the last five years."

What is anaplasia? (1909a)

This is a brief and self-explanatory note. The complete translation is as follows:

"In a short article in number 39 of this weekly journal, 'Epithelial heterotopia and metaplasia' Dr Münter writes on p. 1706: 'By anaplasia one understands, as is well known, a phase of incomplete formation in which the characteristics of the completed cell type have not yet been fully expressed.'

As the concept of anaplasia was introduced into the terminology by me, I may perhaps be regarded as an expert for what should be understood by anaplasia, and I can give the assurance that Dr Münter's definition does not correspond at all to what I denoted as anaplasia, and what pathologists who use this term today understand by it and also, according to my definition, must understand by it. (This is fist on the table – eds). I first used the word in an article in Virchow's Arch vol. 119, p. 321, and gave it immediately at that time, the definition which has in essence persisted. The matter is presented in detail in my ('Studies of the Specificity, Altruism and Anaplasia of Cells', Berlin, August Hirschwald, 1893). In various other publications, I have occasionally referred to this topic, in more detail moreover in my 'Diagnosis of Malignant Tumours'. Herr Münter is not alone in his failure to understand the concept, and I have repeatedly found it necessary to establish the concept of anaplasia. As now this concept of mine has been quite clearly become the norm, I can

"Origin and Pathology. Studies and Thoughts in Comparative Biology" (1909f)

only assume that these authors who achieve such erroneous use of the word have not read my works at all. If one looks at the exact expression, any misunderstanding is actually scarcely possible, and as proof, I therefore quote what I said on p. 82 of my 'Studies etc'. There verbatim, is the following: 'After what was said in the previous chapter about altruism, it is a logical consequence that such cells with less altruism and greater independence are less differentiated than the somatic cell from which they proceeded. Thus a "de-differentiation" has taken place. For this process I have proposed the name "anaplasia". Thus anaplasia means a change in the cells in the sense that these are less differentiated than their mother cells, and this lesser differentiation expresses itself in the reduction of altruism and the intensification of capacity for independent existence. This condition is most completely attained in the germinal cells

in which altruism ceases completely and de-differentiation is complete'. From this, it is thus clear that the word "anaplasia", does not, as Münter would like it, mean a phase of incomplete formation, in which the cell type has NOT YET reached full expression, but that it is a matter of a retrogression of already differentiated cells which with this regression in degree of differentiation, simultaneously increase in independent capacity for independent existence. I have already had repeatedly to observe *vis à vis* Ribbert, that it is not simply and solely a matter of a de-differentiation, because only the germinal cell is really de-differentiated; but that it is a matter of a lesser differentiation which does not need to go back via the path of normal differentiation, but can go its own ways. Then, in the following section on p. 82, I have explained that the anaplastic cell is not to be confused with the embryonal cell. Indeed it is the eternal mistake which is made with endless frequency, that young cells or anaplastic cells are described and understood as embryonal cells. After, in earlier times, Virchow and Rabl had already energetically opposed this view, and after I had repeatedly argued the error of this idea, one should really finally retreat from the notion of cells which have already been differentiated once and which now change in some way, whether by anaplasia or by cell division or by metaplasia, of regarding them as embryonal. Embryonal cells are only those which, in development, stand between egg cell and complete body cell; thus those which are in the phase of prosoplasia. What Münter incorrectly understands by anaplasia, is the embryonal cell, and too, what he understands by prosoplasia, is in consequence completely erroneous. I recommend all those gentlemen who wish to concern themselves with these things, really to follow up the original works and not limit themselves to quotations of papers in other places.

1851

"Origin and Pathology. Studies and Thoughts in Comparative Biology" (1909f)

This volume of approximately 500 pages deals with Darwinism in relation to pathology (1909 was the centenary of Darwin's birth). Here we present translations of the Contents pages, and sections dealing with tumours. Hansemann's thinking is more complex than in previous works.

Contents

Foreword
Chapter 1 Introduction
Chapter 2 Concerning Preformation
Chapter 3 Types and Varieties
Chapter 4 Variability
Chapter 5 Preconditions for Constancy
Chapter 6 Altruism
Chapter 7 Fitness (*Zweckmässigkeit*) and Orthogenesis
Chapter 8 Lamarkism
Chapter 9 Functional Adaptations
Chapter 10 Epidemics
Chapter 11 Physiological Death
Chapter 12 Concluding Remarks
Name Index
Subject Index

The following is a translation from the section on Preconditions

168 "Rosa distinguishes namely between phylogenetic variations, which Scott calls "mutations" and non-phylogenetic variations which he would like to call "Darwinian variations" and which Scott calls

[1] Variations and Mutations, American Journal of Science, 1884, vol. 48.

169 individual variations. In chapter 3 already we drew attention to the fact that this distinction cannot be comprehensively recognised.

Now in fact, we do see the same thing during the development of a single metazoan from the egg cell. Hereto, the differentiation arises by division of work with loss of certain properties, so that the special capabilities of the cell are thrust into the foreground. By way of this too, we see that a regression to the less differentiated embryonal form is not possible. In the text-books, there has indeed been much talk of such an embryonal change, for example, the inflammation of tumour formation and of regeneration. Virchow, already, objected energetically to this view, and presented the proof that one must not mistake young cells, that is to say, those which have just emerged from a cell division, with embryonal cells.

It has been postulated by various authors that during the regeneration of some lower animals, e.g. lumbriculus, lumbricus, planaria, tubellaria among others, indifferent cells pile up at the point of regeneration, from which then, the individual differentiated body divisions develop anew. Here we cannot go more closely into these complicated circumstances, but in contrast, it should only be noted that by this, it is not a matter of the re-emergence of embryonal cells, but only of cells which according to their form are indifferent. These authors demonstrate expressly that regeneration here does not proceed like the formation of the same organs during embryonal development. From this alone, it is already clear that the apparently indifferent cells, which provide the matrix for the new formation, cannot be body cells which have become embryonal*.

Especially during tumour formation and later at the development of malignant tumours, the assertion has been made that because the cells became embryonal they could take on properties possessed by the cells of malignant tumours. In my "Studies of Cells"[1]

[1] Berlin, 1893
* i.e. regeneration is not embryonic recapitulation (eds).

"Origin and Pathology. Studies and Thoughts in Comparative Biology" (1909f)

I tried to show that this view too is incorrect, and that what I have termed anaplasia of the cells, does indeed mean a dedifferentiation, but not a return to embryonal properties. If one wished to compare that with phylogenetic phenomena, one could take as examples the neotenic (*neotenische*) forms, and if one wished, call these tumour cells neotenic. But never ever are they embryonal cells. The neotenic forms too, as Rosa[1] observes quite correctly, are

"less differentiated, but in no case do they regain the breath of variability, the phylogenetic force, which are peculiar to the originally indifferent forms. Grawitz[2] stated that in leukemia, the blood takes on embryonal form. Grawitz proceeds from the erroneous premise that the blood, as has often been expressed earlier, is a tissue with liquid intercellular substance. That is not the case, for the blood is the product of the metabolism of all cells in the body, and thus not at all something with an independent existence, but rather a result which is much more comparable to a secretion than to a tissue. Comparison of leukemic blood with embryonal blood can thus be only a purely morphological comparison, which stands in no relationship to the physiological circumstances.

Thus, indeed, I am of the opinion that the processes during ontogenesis can also in this point, be compared with those of phylogenesis, and that the biogenetic basic law retains its significance in this direction too. Rosa says on p. 87:

"Therefore, between the phylogenetic and ontogenetic development there is the fundamental difference that during the former, the idioplasma is formed slowly, and in this way, evokes the reformation of the types, whilst in the course of the latter, it retains its specific character unchanged."

Doubtless, this fundamental difference is to be acknowledged, but it plays no part in the line of thought here,

[1] same citation, p. 73
[2] Lecture to the Berlin Medical Soc. 20th May 1908.

because ontogenesis proceeds from the germinal plasma, which has already been differentiated in a definite direction, whilst phylogenesis proceeds from the substance which follows only certain physical laws, but is for the rest, however, limitlessly variable living substance.

The following deals with "differentiation":

In differentiation, the origin of bisexuality is also to be sought. Differentiation led first to two very similar, but not very like individuals, who came via a process of dedifferentiation, into a dependency relationship. Copulation of two such dedifferentiated individuals, results again in a generation of daughter individuals. The general spread of sexual propagation does not indicate a necessity of it, but of its phylogenetically long age, just as every other organic arrangement, which has a certain spread in the animal kingdom, e.g. the eyes, the central nervous system, the liver, or still more the ciliated movement and mitotic cell division.

......

We also see indeed in certain malformations of the human being, the so-called hirsute individuals, whose lanugo hairs acquire such a special fully developed form, that quite specific defects of the teeth emerge.

The following deals with ageing and cancer

....

"In this sense one can say that one human being has aged earlier than the other, which Cassalis, dressed up as "a man is only as old as his ages". There is thus a particular disease of the vessels, arteriosclerosis, which except in certain circumstances is a disease of old age, and there is an old age involution of the vessels, which is assigned among the old age phenomena. The latter, unlike atherosclerosis, do not cause changes in other organs, and it would be incorrect to consider all age changes to arteriosclerosis, as Demange tries to do. The phenomena of old age are co-ordinated with arteriosclerosis, not subordinated to it.

The question whether tumour formations too belong to the phenomena of age is of great significance. The detailed statistics which have been developed in recent years have demonstrated sufficiently that specifically the malignant tumours are actually not illnesses of advanced age. Sarcomas, even, come to apply quite pronouncedly to youthful ages. Carcinomas do indeed appear in their greatest number at a greater age, but such cases in people over 70 years are actually rather seldom. Apparently, people who are disposed to carcinoma formations have died off before this time. If, however, a carcinoma once develops in a very old person, it can be observed, almost without exception, that it takes an unusually benign course. Indeed, some of these carcinomas are found at the autopsies of very old people, without them having appeared clinically in any way at all. They remain relatively small, grow very slowly, and have only a slight tendency to make metastases. The great number of cancer cases lies between 40 and 60 years."

"Atlas of Malignant Tumours" (1910k)

This volume was apparently commissioned by the Committee for Cancer Research, specifically as a diagnostic handbook. It was not intended to deal with theory to any great extent. The book has an introductory section on methods of seven pages and a general section (pages 8–17) which includes an account of "anaplasia" in relation to descriptive terminology. There is no significant discussion of chromosomes, nor any detailed account of overall theories of tumours. The following is a translation of the contents and the section on anaplasia.

Contents

	Page
Methods of Examination	
Diagnosis	1
1. General Part	8
2. Special Part	17
A. Carcinoma	19
B. Sarcoma	36
C. Carcinoma sarcomatoides	41
D. Malignant teratoma	41
E. Papillary cystoma	43
F. Endothelial tumours	45
G. Chorion-epithelioma	49

"Atlas of Malignant Tumours" (1910k)

This translation concerns "anaplasia".

[p. 18, second paragraph] "The malignancy of a tumour is characterised physiologically by the lesser differentiation of the cells and the intensified capacity for independent existence, that is to say, by that condition which has been called ANAPLASIA. This anaplasia is also expressed in all tissues, cells which are sufficiently specialised histologically, thus, for example, in the majority of epithelia, particularly in the outer epidermis, in the goblet cells of the gut and in many other sites. They are expressed to a lesser extent in the usual connective tissue and in endothelia. But this anaplasia may reveal a very variable worsening of degree. It may be so slight that it cannot be recognised histologically. To this belong all those cases which cause considerable difficulty for diagnosis and whose character is only apparent by their later course. Fortunately these are the less frequent. Much more frequently does it happen that the dedifferentiation of the cells has made further progress and that for this reason it can be also histologically recognised. That presupposes exact knowledge of the normal structure of the tissues and of their benign proliferations. If the dedifferentiation has proceeded even further then it can also be recognised histologically with little difficulty, and if it has reached a high degree then the tumour cells approach the most indifferent form, that of a sphere. Also in high grade examples of anaplasia, very marked differences in the final form of individual cells occurs, so that the cells vary greatly in form and size, for which reason the latter have been termed POLYMORPHOUS. The deviation from normal tissue which is the expression of this anaplasia can be the same within one and the same tumour, it can, however, reveal itself very differently at different sites. It can accord completely with the metastases and the regressing phases with the mother tumour or in metastases or regressing phases, it may become more pronounced. Between the various grades of anaplasia, all possible transitions occur, so that clearly-demarcated borders between them can be drawn just as little as between the smallest grades of anaplasia and of atypical growths.

Two things arise from this: that the different tissues in different types of tissue may have a very different appearance that, for example, the carcinomas of the outer skin may not always be similarly formed, just as little as those which proceed from the mucous membranes and that the sarcomata, which for example develop from cartilage or from the lymph nodes or from connective tissues exhibit a very different structure. Secondly, arising from this, the tumours showing strongest anaplasia in all tissues strive towards a unified type, namely, that of the most powerful anaplasia, so that polymorphous-celled or round-celled carcinoma may originate as much from the skin, as from the mucous membranes, or from some internal nodal organ. From this it can be recognised that the origin of the tumour can only be recognised from the histological appearances of the tumour in those tumours where cells still exhibit certain specialised character. That is to say, anaplastic only to a small degree, whilst in a markedly anaplastic tumour one can no longer see from the microscopic picture, from which tissue it has developed.

From this standpoint we should approach individual tumours the demonstration of which we shall now go into... ...."

And again, p. 9 beginning approximately line 10.

"This comparison is particularly significant because it has been shown that in malignant tumours the cells develop certain differences which, compared with the mother tissue, indicate a lesser differentiation. The anaplasia of tumour cells is, of course, only provable morphologically in those cases where the mother cells themselves have characteristic forms and where the anaplasia is sufficiently clearly developed. There will always be borderline cases, in which diagnosis is uncertain or remains impossible. But that is the same in every area of medicine. At no point are the borders between the various phenomena so clearly drawn that one could establish them with absolute certainty. Thus, we see that often difficulties arise which even the most practised cannot overcome, which become ever less, the more practised the investigator is in these things. Therefore, particularly, difficulties arise in the demarcation between benign warts and mucous membrane tumours compared with carcinomas, fibromas, myomas, osteomas, chondromas, etc, compared with sarcomata."

Pathological anatomy and the diagnosis of cancer (1910l)

This article is mainly about the terminology and diagnostic criteria of cancer. Hansemann quotes Virchow (p. 35 of original) but discounts Virchow's idea of "alveolar cells" as a diagnostic feature. He states that the number of mitoses in a section of a tumour means usually rapid growth, but has no other significance. There are several diagnostic points which are relevant even today (2006). On p. 40 of the original, there is a discussion of "collateral growth" of adjacent cells. At the end of the article, Hansemann stresses the need for accurate diagnosis, and laments that experimental cancer research has so far offered few helpful insights to the understanding of aetiology and therapy of cancer.

Experimental chemotherapy of animals with tumours (1912a) (with v. Wassermann)

This article describes the treatment of experimental tumours in mice with selenium and eosin. The agent is toxic, and many mice die during the treatment. Of the survivors, some die because of factors which are not discovered at autopsy. In those mice which survive, recurrences occur, although sometimes after some months. Hansemann concludes (pp 9–10):

"The question is now very obvious, and everyone with whom we have discussed this matter, has directed this question to us: is the means which we have used here for tumourous mice to be regarded as a cancer-remedy or can it become such? Von Wassermann has already expressly emphasised that there can be no question of this, but in contrast we can only say that this method of injecting and then spreading out from the blood circulation has effect on mice tumours, and in point of fact on quite specific types of such tumours. In order to counter any misinterpretations, I feel it my duty to confirm expressly yet again, and I should like here to stand up for my view quite particularly, the standpoint which I have had for a long time. Unfortunately it has become generally the practice to regard these mouse tumours as mouse cancers. Virtually throughout the world, they are called this. Wherever I could, I have contradicted this. I am firmly convinced that they are not carcinomas. I cannot repeat all the reasons for this here. They have been widely published. Above all, however, the mouse tumours behave biologically quite differently from cancers in human beings, as far as their mode of growth, their process of spreading, their formation of metastases is concerned. It is thus quite unjustified to have the idea that what is possible here in these mouse tumours can be applied to the human being. Anyone who knows what a human tumour is, and who has at the same time concerned himself with these mouse tumours, can recognise the extensive biological difference between these two diseases, which is so much a difference in principle, that I am not in a position to draw any kind of parallel, and therefore, I would like to conclude with the express warning against regarding the means used here successfully in mice as a method of healing cancer. That would summon up, not only amongst doctors but also amongst the public at large, quite incorrect ideas and hopes whose fulfilment cannot be a prospect in any way at all. Here, as von Wassermann has already emphasised, a fundamental fact has been established, the possibility of which has certainly been disputed hitherto, that through suitable chemical means, proceeding from the blood stream, on can reach the nuclei of tumour cells and by destroying the same, can therapeutically influence tumours."

Discussion (of Experimental chemotherapy of animals with tumours) (1912b)

This is a report of discussions of the general topic. Hansemann was the secretary of the meeting, and only one of many speakers. He reiterated his view that the "mouse tumours being studied have nothing to do with human carcinomas" and provided the pathological reasons for his view. Sticker referred to Hansemann's ideas as "esoteric", and as being shared by very few researchers. It was suggested that Hansemann's beliefs would spell the end of modern experimental cancer research.

Thus Hansemann possibly made himself unpopular with another group of medical research workers.

Experimental chemotherapy of animals with tumours (1912c)
(with v. Wassermann)

This article is very similar to Hansemann (1912a).

On altruistic diseases: A talk delivered to the Society for Doctors' Continuing Education in Görlitz, 13th January, 1912 (1912d)

This article in fact contains material relevant to early endocrinology. Hansemann, however, demonstrates his "Professorial" style of expression, and also his continuing belief in this abstruse philosophical application of "Altruism" to cell biology. Only translation of pages 433 and 434 is presented (below). The remaining pages deal with the thyroid, the pituitary (he documents empty sella syndrome), the pathology of acromegaly, diabetes, cretinism, Basedow's disease, also Addison's and tetany after removal of the parathyroid glands, adrenalin excess not due to disease of the adrenal cortex; hypoplasia of bone marrow as another altruistic disease; small adrenal glands in anencephaly, although the babies are not necessarily small; hypogonadism in man and animals. Hansemann then states that psychoses, polysarcia, cardiac arrhythmias, and arthritis deformans are all manifestations of postmenopausal life. "Altruistic" diseases of the kidney, lungs, liver and spleen are considered, but not clearly defined.

It begins:

"A good deal has been written over many years on the topic which I should like to deal with today so that the facts are well-known. But the details of this matter have been considered from very different standpoints, and therefore have not been gathered together in a unified way, such as I would like to present to you here.

You will remember that by the expression "altruism in the animal body" one understands the reciprocal activities between one unified group of the cells and the rest of the body, in such a fashion moreover that every cell group takes on a certain activity for the body, and in return receives from the body, in a certain way, metabolic products. This expression which has meanwhile been generally accepted, was in its time, derived from philosophical considerations of Herbert Spencer, who invented the expression "altruism" for the reciprocal activities of certain human beings in relation to mankind.

My investigations on altruism were founded first and foremost on two important events in physiology, namely such that the cells of the body possess an inner secretion i.e. they release metabolic products of a specific nature into the body. Secondly, my views were based on the fact that as the body develops, types of cell arise which are of essentially specific nature i.e. the various types of cell cannot fill in for other cells, and that a metaplasia of the cells is only possible between closely related cell types: i.e. I proceeded from the presumption of a far reaching specificity of cells. On both points, there are today many different opinions.

As far now as the specificity of cells is concerned, one was actually in earlier years convinced of the opposite, i.e. it was thought that cell types can turn into other cell types willy-nilly. Virchow still regarded connective tissue as the matrix of numerous other tissues, especially too, the epithelia, the epidermis and the gland cells. He believed too that the parenchymal cells of carcinomas originated from connective tissue. Later it was maintained, especially by Ziegler that the leukocytes are undifferentiated cells, from which all possible types of tissue can proceed.

Only gradually and after many investigations, has it been established that all these observations are wrong, and that finally, extraordinarily little has been left of the large field of metaplasia. In fact, today, we only know one true metaplasia between two closely related tissues, between cartilage and bone, and between connective tissue and bone, and so also between closely related epithelia, e.g. between sebaceous gland epidermis. For the rest, however, nothing is known of a metaplasia, and if lately it is claimed from several sides that epidermis can arise from connective tissue or vice-versa, connective tissue can arise from epidermis, only based on histological slides, this proof is not compelling and only likely to reintroduce fresh confusion into an already-clarified area.

Secondly, as far as internal secretion is concerned, many authors have still not made it clear that such inner secretion is appropriate for all cell types. On the contrary, one has always had much more the presupposition that only certain types of cell possess an internal secretion, e.g. the cells of the pancreas, the adrenal, the thyroid, the parathyroid epithelial bodylets, or of the hypophysis cerebri. That the remaining types of cell have an inner secretion must be firmly maintained. The gland cells too do not secrete their entire metabolic product into the lumina of the gland, but a part of their metabolic products returns to the circulation. I have in the past particularly proved this in the case of the lung and the liver. But the same can also be maintained of the remaining gland cells. That all types of tissue which are not of a secretory nature, as for example connective tissue, musculature, brain, spinal cord substance, adipose tissue and so on, all deliver their products of their metabolism into the circulation, is self evident. Thus one can quite generally classify tissues into those which possess only an inner secretion, and those which simultaneously have an internal and an external secretion. There are none which exclusively possess only an external secretion.

A further consideration is directly associated with this. One has frequently comprehended the blood as a liquid tissue, and I believe that this idea originally goes back to Virchow. Even in more recent works, for example by Grawitz in his well-known book on disorders of the blood, blood is described as liquid tissue, whereby the liquidity of the blood is designated as an intercellular substance. This idea is now incorrect. The blood cannot be equated with connective tissue, with cartilage or another tissue which consists of cells and intercellular substance, but instead, the blood is a resultant product. It is the result of the metabolic products of all cell types of the body. All metabolic products of any cell group at all get into the blood, and are distributed by the blood to all the other cell types. Only thereby is it possible that every type of cell produces the specific product of secretion, whether externally or internally, which is peculiar to this type of cell. Thereby, however, a close connection exists between the individual types of cell and it is self-explanatory that if one of these cell types becomes diseased, and secretes too much, too little, or a wrong product, then the blood mixture will become a wrong one and the remaining cell types will not be able anymore to deliver the specific product, but only in some modification or other.

You will clearly see from this, gentlemen, that out of these considerations the old concept of "dyscrasia", which was despised after the introduction of Cellular Pathology but which more recently has begun to be resume its old glory finds its explanation and becomes accessible to scientific investigation. Thus in the final instance, the concept of dyscrasia is based on altruism of cell functions as I have presented it in detail.

Now the significance for the rest of the body of an inner secretion of an organ is very various, so that it (the significance) is not solely dependent on the size of the organ. A tiny organ can secrete a very important substance; a large organ a relatively unimportant substance, but even large organs can deliver important products. We see for example that the lungs bring oxygen into the body. One could speak specifically of a secretion of oxygen into the body, and more recently, it has become clearer and clearer, that in point of fact, the oxygen of the lung does not only reach the red corpuscles by diapedesis, but is facilitated by the activity of the alveolar epithelium. We know from the liver that its activity apart from secreting bile, consists in the fact that it synthesises glycogen, and that it participates in the production of urea. On the other hand, we know relatively little of the internal secretory activity of such large organs as the kidneys, although the fact of it has been proved. This latter, however, obviously plays an only very small part in diseases of the kidney. On the other hand, we know very small organs, which deliver very important secretory products into the interior of the body, as for example the adrenal, pituitary, thyroid, parathyroid epithelial bodylets. We also know the same quite particularly of the cells of the gonads. Concerning the significance of the secretion for the rest of the body, it will essentially depend on the nature of the illness which develops as a change in any organ. But not only on the significance of the secretion, but also, on the circumstance whether the inner secretion increases or decreases, or finally, whether, along with the inner secretion, the organ also possesses an outer secretion. I would now like to discuss this in several particular examples.

It has long been known that the pancreas is particularly suited to demonstrate these relationships, because we know the significance of the inner secretion as also of the outer secretion for intestinal digestion. Now there are diseases of the pancreas which only affect the external secretion, there are such which only affect the inner secretion, and some which affect both. From what has been said so far, it is clear that if only the external secretion of the pancreas is changed, leading indeed to certain disturbances, that the resulting illness cannot, however, be termed altruistic, but that much more, the altruistic disease, whose cause is a disease of the pancreas must be attributed to the inner secretory activity of the organ. We will not consider more closely those diseases which come about through change of external secretion. As far now as the inner secretion of the pancreas is concerned, it has been indicated in various places that it is exclusively the cells of Langerhans Islets which provide this inner secretion. I consider this view as wrong, based on reasons that I cannot elaborate on here, but which I should like to do so in more detail elsewhere. I am much more of the opinion that in this, the entirety of the pancreatic cells have to be considered in terms of internal secretion. Now we know quite specifically what happens when the inner secretion of pancreatic cells is reduced. Regardless of what causes the reduction of internal secretion, whether it is an inflammation which destroyed the pancreas totally or whether it was a particular disease which I have called granular atrophy of the pancreas, or lipomatosis of the pancreas, or finally through tumour formation: in all cases we recognise that thereby a common resultant metabolic disturbance arises which we call by the name diabetes. Thus we know that with a reduction of the inner secretion of the pancreas, an altruistic illness arises.

In contrast, we do not know of a single case where the inner secretion of the pancreas was increased, and whether through this increase of production, a more general metabolic disturbance is produced too. That such cases are also possible is proven by observations in other organs. The best example for this, as is well known, is the thyroid gland. This organ can become diseased in two directions. One group of illnesses leads to a reduction in thyroid secretion, the other group results in an increase. If the thyroid secretion is reduced, then the group of illnesses arise which, according to the type of disease has been called, cretinism, myxoedema, or cachexia strumi-prava, a disease which, as is well known, can be ameliorated or cured by feeding thyroid substance. Naturally, such relief of the illness only lasts for so long as the body is supplemented with thyroid substance. If one ceases supply, then the body will return to its previous cretinous state. If however, the thyroid gland produces too much, we encounter a different form of disease namely the so-called Basedow's disease. To a certain extent, Basedow's illness presents the opposite of cretinism. In cretinism, the metabolism is slowed down, but in Basedow's illness, it is increased. In cretinism, a strong increase of fat occurs, and in Basedow's it is reduced." (end p. 434 of original).

"On Conditional Thinking in Medicine and its Importance for Practice" (1912f)

This book essentially considers the multifactorial nature of causation of disease. Hansemann is reluctant to accept "aetiology" as a definite part of the scientific basis of medicine. However, Hansemann no longer quotes Virchow, and does not defend the philosophy of "Cellular Pathology". Chapter 6 of the book is devoted to tumours and consists of a rambling series of ideas on aetiological factors, cell-type related phenomena and the manifestations of anaplasia, most of which is covered in previous articles in this chapter. Here we present the Foreword, the Contents, Chapter 1 and the "Final Points".

"Foreword"

The recognition principle, which is detailed in the following pages, does not, as is well known, originate with me. On the contrary it has been gradually prepared and has been more or less clearly delineated by numerous authors. It would be difficult to nominate any one inventor because even those researchers such as Roux, Mach, and particularly also Verborn, and others were already able, when establishing this same principle, to call on earlier authors. I have tested and thought through this recognition principle for some considerable time, and have applied it to the most various areas of medicine, and have consistently found it to be wholly practical. At no single point have I encountered anything which might hinder or contradict the application of this principle. On the other side, the causal mode of thought in medicine has seemed to me ever more unpractical and contradictory. In hardly any branch of medicine has it satisfied me. Many errors and failures which have emerged in recent years, in spite of the enormous progress which medicine can claim, are more or less connected with this causal mode of thought. Anyone concerning himself more deeply with these questions will recognise without difficulty that the causal principle of recognition does not correspond to the strict rules of logic and science. Thus as Verborn particularly has emphasised, it is not merely unnecessary but in contrast is unequivocally harmful.

The aim of the following lines is to argue this both theoretically and practically. I do not imagine that the medical world will steer directly into this mode of thought in full sail, but I do have the hope that this writing will perhaps stimulate research workers and practising doctors to wean themselves away gradually from the harmful causal mode of thought and adopt the useful conditional one.

"On Conditional Thinking in Medicine and its Importance for Practice" (1912f)

Contents

Foreword

Chapter 1. Introduction

Chapter 2. Traumatic illness and poisonings
          a. Traumatic illnesses
          b. Poisonings

Chapter 3. Tuberculosis

Chapter 4. Other infectious diseases

Chapter 5. Non-infectious illnesses

Chapter 6. Tumours

Chapter 7. Preconditions for illness which result from prognosis

Chapter 8. Epidemics
Final points

Chapter 1
Introduction

For more than twenty-five years, medicine had found itself in the aetiological age, and it is justifiably proud of this, because these so-called aetiological studies have brought forth such a full range of valuable and pioneering knowledge, that views have been completely transformed not merely in medicine, but also, in many respects, in the total field of biology. And what is of essential significance here is the fact that this change in views establishes its validity not merely in theoretical science but also in the area of therapy and very particularly that of prophylaxis.

Since the principle of aetiological research was introduced into science and has meanwhile now been worked with for twenty-five years, we are justified in looking back for a moment and asking ourselves not only what has been achieved thereby, but quite especially whether the expectations which have been attached to it have been fulfilled, and if they have not been fulfilled, where the reasons for these failures are to be sought.

Viewed from the philosophical standpoint, aetiology means the theory of causes and effects, but I should like to believe that, just as the concept has developed in medicine, aetiology is not completely covered by the concept of the theory of cause and effect, although in the majority of cases, aetiology and cause are used, linguistically, to mean the same thing. For almost no area of medicine is there such a strict relationship between cause and effect as is logically demanded by the use of these words, so that the word aetiology, as it is used in

medicine, is covered more by the concept of the theory of causative conditions than by the concept of the theory of causes. However, this somewhat hair-splitting distinction which has gradually been formed through practice, is known to the fewest people; yes indeed, it is even said the aetiology of an illness is this and that, e.g. a bacterium, and thus the theory of the cause is used linguistically as synonymous with the cause itself.

Mach[1] says: "In the more highly developed natural sciences, the misuse of the concepts of cause and effects becomes ever more limited, and ever less frequent".

Therewith he expresses a fact, but one would have to ask oneself whether it is here only a matter of habit or whether it is a necessary matter of progress in the natural sciences. Undoubtedly, the latter is the case. By "a more highly developed natural science", we should understand one which as far as possible approaches an exact science. Now, as is well-known, there is only one single exact science, and it has acquired this name because, proceeding from the most simple basic, and not further to be proven, principles one can, by correct conclusions advance to the most difficult problems without making a mistake. This science is mathematics alone, and it earns the name exactly because it proceeds only from known conditions, that is to say, because it creates for itself exclusively, the conditions for its problems.

This view has been the customary one for quite a long time, because David Hume, already ("Concerning Understanding" Lipps, Leipzig, 1904, p. 96) says: "Finally algebra and arithmetic appear as the sole sciences in which a chain of conclusions right up to any complicated degree at all, is possible, without complete exactness and certainty being lost in the process"). The more a science approaches mathematics and its method of work, the more is it to be denoted as "exact". But already those disciplines closest to mathematics, namely, mechanics and physics, are not completely exact, and thus not so highly developed as mathematics, because they work with problems which come at them from outside, whose conditions they do not create themselves, but must first investigate, empirically in part,

[1] "Recognition and Error", Leipzig, 1906, 2nd edn, p. 278.

3   and the result of this is that already here, with simple logical continuation of the conclusions, the result is not necessarily accurate, but can be erroneous and incorrect. The more a science depends on empiricism, the less it is able completely to discover and to recognise the conditions for its problems. It will always have to be satisfied with some conditions, and the absence of knowledge of a part of the conditions leads, in simply logical continuation of the thought process to the extreme, finally to error, as, from conclusion to conclusion, the defects (which have arisen in the absence of knowledge of individual conditions) must accumulate.*

As, now, in the majority of the natural sciences, conclusions can never be gained by purely theoretical contemplation, or from the mere conceptualisation of the objects, one is exclusively dependent on empiricism, and empiricism also leads to the relationships between cause and effects. Hereto I should like to quote a sentence from Hume (ibid, p. 94): "There is no effect, even if it be the most simple, which from the properties of the objects, as they present themselves to us, is comprehensible without further ado, or without the aid of memory, could be predicted by calculation". As however, one may not be satisfied with simple experiences and the collection of them, and reaches errors, differently from mathematics, by theoretical conclusion, one has recourse to the causal association of phenomena. "Now the only association or relationship of objects, which can lead us beyond our recognition of the direct impressions of memory and the senses, is the causal one, as it is the only one on the basis of which we can draw a correct conclusion from one object to the other. The idea of cause and effect stems from experience; in so far as the latter teaches us that certain objects in all earlier cases have consistently been associated with each other" (Hume, ibid, p. 120). From all this, it is apparent that Mach's pronouncement that a natural science is the more highly developed the more the misuse of the concepts "cause and effects" is limited is not a simple experiential fact, but emerges of necessity from the nature of things.

* This reminds one of the "Student's Scene" in Goethe, *Faust I* (eds).

4   But then it is also permissible to turn this sentence of Mach's around and to say: "The more use of the concepts of cause and effect which is made in a science, the less highly developed it is", and according to this one would have to come to the conclusion that medical science is still in the first initial stages of its development, because in no other is more use made of the concepts of cause and effect.

That is not a reproach made which is made of the research method in medicine or of the standpoint at which medicine finds itself at the moment. Therewith, we do not intend to maintain that medical research is on the wrong track. On the contrary, the recognition that medicine is still at the initial stages of its research seems to me to offer some consolation *vis à vis* the obviously incorrect idea that because of the enormous discoveries in the last eighty years of medicine, we have already reached a closing off point, that the innumerable gaps, the numberless failures in medicine will not be permanent, that the gaps can be filled, and that in place of failures, successes will emerge. Only

"On Conditional Thinking in Medicine and its Importance for Practice" (1912f)

from this standpoint can we understand Dubois-Reymond* *Ignoramus et Ignorabimus*, if we admit the *Ignoramus* and at the same time, limit in the time sense, the *Ignorabimus*.

Whenever new pioneering discoveries are made, they like to capture the spirit so completely, that frequently, everything which hitherto seemed useful and advantageous, is forgotten or pushed aside as useless. This mistake has been made for as long as scientific research has existed, but remarkably, this experience has never made a school for itself, but at every new discovery, the same happens again and again. When, in its time, however, the microscope was introduced into research, it was believed that we could neglect the macroscopic of contemplation and it was hoped, by microscopic investigation of diseased parts, to be able to prove specific phenomena for every diseased change. Virchow, campaigned most energetically against the specifists (*Spezifiker*) and the specificity of the disease products, and, along with microscopic examination,

* Dubois (see also chapter 5) also exhibited the exultation, élan and pride of Sciencism, and was himself a peak of achievement, created by Science in Germany (eds).

he taught and practised most intensively the macroscopic mode of contemplating things. But today there are still many anatomists who can see macroscopically only imperfectly and they believe that they can advance in their mode of contemplation if initially they first examine every disease change microscopically. This view leads to a serious error because there are indeed many questions in pathologically anatomy which cannot be solved microscopically at all and can only be solved by the macroscopic mode of contemplation. Thus microscopic examination does not replace the macroscopic mode of contemplation but only completes it and takes it further wherever it has reached the limit of its possibility.

When then, further, more refined histological methods of examination were introduced, especially staining technique, then one fell into a similar logical error. One believed examination of tissues in unfixed and unstained conditions to be superfluous, and once again an evil habit entered the issue, namely, of throwing without ado all tissues which were to be examined into fixative, without submitting them beforehand to examination (of the tissue) fresh. Because of this, it has happened that some pathological changes, as for example, fatty conditions, and the cloudy swelling were neglected for a long time, the latter indeed quite specifically denied, and only in recent times has one turned again to examinations of fresh objects and has realised that these more refined methods of examinations too, do not substitute for the original coarser ones and only complete them. Perhaps here I may recall an example which happened only recently (Proceeding of the German Pathological Society, Leipzig, 1909). By more refined examination of bones, it was believed that one could draw a sharper distinction between rickets and osteomalacia. It became clear, however, that these differences are thereby quite specifically unclear, and thus one arrived at the remarkable result, which seemed because of the preceding investigations to be unbelievable that osteomalacia and rickets are the same disease, whilst the clinical, coarsely anatomical mode of contemplation teaches that here it is a matter of two completely different events. Virchow often used to say that there are certain things which one can see better at a distance than when

one gets up close, and he pointed to the shape of clouds, which one also only recognises if one does not directly enter the cloud itself.

When bacteriology was in its first beginnings, and made a mighty impression through its extraordinary discoveries, one fell again into the same error, and believed that bacteriological examination was sufficient to establish certain diseases, as for example, tuberculosis of the lung by the proof of tubercle bacilli. Only further experiences taught that this proof of bacilli is in many respects of greatest significance, but that it is certainly not in a position to exclude auscultation and percussion, but that only together with these latter do good results eventuate.

Although one might well believe that by this and similar experiences doctors would have been on the look-out for this problem, one has, on the contrary, initially fallen into the same error in X-ray examinations, believing them to be the only method of salvation in investigation. Thereby the value of this inestimably valuable method has been significantly discredited and indeed, quite unnecessarily. Because if one had drawn the correct conclusion from earlier experience, one would not have put X-ray examination in place of other examinations, but one would have, on the contrary, right from the very beginning seen it as a complement.

The most modern science is chemical and biological reactions at the sick bed, and here too, the same thing in principle has happened again."

Final Points

1. The firm and unchangeable relationship between cause and effect is a philosophical and purely theoretical problem which does not occur in practice.
2. The more exact a science is, the less one speaks within it of "cause and effect", and all the more of preconditions (*Bedingungen*).
3. Hitherto the causal mode of contemplation has in practice mostly been used in the purely empirical sciences, which are burdened with most sources of error.
4. Every occurrence cannot be traced back to one cause, but to a sum of preconditions.
5. The number of these preconditions is in reality incalculably large, but the significances of these preconditions are not of equal value for the emergence of the event. More distant ones are in general of less importance than those lying closer. But simultaneous preconditions too are quantitatively and qualitatively distinguished from each other in their effects.
6. There are necessary preconditions without which the event never takes place, and there are preconditions which can be substituted with others, substitution preconditions or replacement preconditions of lesser quality (*Ersatz*), which can apply for each other.
7. In individual cases, the replacement preconditions of lesser quality can become necessary preconditions.
8. For many events, there is not one necessary precondition, but in contrast, two or more. Under no circumstances does the event take place if one of these preconditions is absent. The event can never be produced by one of these preconditions alone. In such a case the event can be prevented (*verhindert*) if one of these preconditions, irrespective of which, is removed (*aufgehoben*).
9. If two or more necessary preconditions for an event are present, and one of these preconditions is always present, whilst the other only appears sometimes, then the precondition appearing sometimes is of greater significance insofar as in practice, it becomes relevant particularly when what is involved is the prevention of the event.
10. Therefore, it is not necessary in practice, neither would it be possible to take every existing precondition into account. It is sufficient, much more, that one limits oneself to the necessary preconditions and to a number of the substitution preconditions. General data concerning this cannot be adduced; here much more, judgment is to be made from case to case.
11. In many cases, more distantly lying preconditions can also be necessary, which demonstrate more closely situated *Ersatz* preconditions.
12. The conditional mode of contemplation makes it possible to establish sources of error in the observation, to make the formulation of the question more precise, and it avoids one-sidedness in the mode of contemplation. All these errors are always present in the causal mode of contemplation and are under all circumstances, greater than in the conditional mode of contemplation.

On precancerous conditions (1913e)

13. The conditional mode of contemplation is not merely of theoretical significance in the purely scientific sense, but on the contrary, it is also of practical significance and has direct influence on how one proceeds in the individual case.

14. The conditional mode of contemplation makes it possible to penetrate further into recognition than the causal mode of contemplation, and thereby, in addition still, provides an aetiological enlightenment for such events, in which the causal mode of contemplation fails completely."

On precancerous conditions (1913e)

This long article seems to be directed at general medical practitioners. It reviews the general idea of predispositions to cancer, both hereditary, and by local chronic lesions, including ulcers, and the effects of irritations (recognising that this is an old concept). He warns against single traumatic episodes as a cause of cancer and quotes (p158) a medico-legal case as follows:

"From these considerations one could easily draw the conclusion that many forms of cancer belong to the traumatic diseases and that they therefore are subject to accident legislation. Doubtless one could construct such a connection in various types of cancer. If for example a person acquires burn scars on the lower extremities and a cancer develops there decades later, then according to all our experience, it can be asserted with certainty that this carcinoma would not have developed if the burn had not occurred previously, i.e. amongst the aetiological factors for the cancer, the burn is a necessary precondition. But in many cases, one has in practice simply gone much too far in this respect. Thus, for example, a case appears repeatedly in the literature and has often been quoted in learned opinions, in which a man's belly collided with an axle and he later developed a gastric carcinoma. An outstanding expert drew the following deduction from this:

'The collision (the exact locality of which, by the way, was not known at all) created a shuddering in the stomach. The stomach shaking led to haemorrhages. An ulcer developed from the haemorrhages, and a cancer originated from the ulcer. Not only in this case was the accident insurance sum paid out to the heirs, but as well, the opinion became a precedent and has been applied to many other cases, and yet it can clearly be seen without further ado that each individual stage in this sequence is fantasy and to be most extremely doubted'. These two examples may be sufficient to show that here too, no general data can be given and that we cannot warn urgently enough against generalisation. Every case is to be analysed critically, and any conclusion which is not really based on actual observations must be most sternly avoided. Thus one cannot say for instance, that carcinomas are of traumatic origin, and one can no longer assert that for individual cases of cancer, traumatic conditions for the aetiology of cancers occur."

There is no mention of cytologically atypical "in situ" lesions as precancerous.

Demonstration of slides produced by Herr Fibiger concerning the artificial induction of cancer (1913g)

This is a report from the proceedings of Medical Society, 7th May 1913, with Herr Orth in the Chair. Fibiger has reported that a parasite in a cockroach can transmit cancers of the stomach from mouse to mouse in an experimental study. Fibiger described his experiments in this meeting. The cockroach is the large, light brown

American type, and the intermediate host for the nematode. Von Hansemann's role is to confirm that the lesions of the mouse are in fact, carcinomata.

C. Lewin is reported as commenting that perhaps the effect of the nematode is through an invisible virus because Peyton Rous has just managed to cause a fowl sarcoma, and another of osteosarcoma character, by the inoculation of transmissable agents.

(Fibiger achieved considerable fame at the time and was awarded the Nobel Prize for Medicine in 1924. However, Fibiger's rats were inbred, and it was later realised that his discovery was only of an inherited susceptibility to tumour formation under the influence apparently, of a specific irritant. See Shimkin, 1977).

A working hypothesis for research on Leukemia (1914a)

This note does not address tumour theory to any great extent, but outlines how epidemiological investigations might be carried out.

On changes in the tissues and tumours after ray treatment: Demonstration lecture before the Hufeland Society 19th March 1914 (1914b)

This is a short paper describing extensive radionecrosis of the pelvic organs of two women treated with radiotherapy (20,000 mg-hours of thorium) for carcinoma of the cervix. At the autopsies, he states that he found "extensive exuberantly growing cancer tissue" in excrescences lining the pelvic cavity. Von Hansemann ended the article as follows:

"These two cases prove, which is not surprising, that clinically-healed cases can relapse. They prove further that it is not the exudations which have arisen through the burning which cause the later extensive ulcerations. Yet it seems to me, that in these two cases, the ulcerations developed more quickly than is usually the case, and in both cases, I am of the opinion that through the radium treatment, an irritation/stimulus (*Reiz* – see Notes on Translation) has arisen which has accelerated the proliferation of the cancer. Thereby, one is led to the question whether it is advantageous to treat with such large doses and thereby to hasten the destruction of very extensive tumours to the greatest depth. Furthermore, I draw attention to my data in the *Z. f. Krebsforschung* vol. 14 (1) where I proposed a fractionated method of treatment with small doses, which is particularly based on the experiences detailed above, that the older cells are more easily destroyed than the younger ones, and that one must first allow the young ones to become old, in order to annihilate them entirely."

On the cancer problem (1914d)

This article divides the periods of cancer research into histological, aetiological, experimental and therapeutic. The histological period has seen great progress in that diagnosis can be made on small pieces, but blood tests are still not specific enough for diagnosis. In the aetiological period, he believes that there is much unsound literature relating to infectious agents. Only Fibiger's work, according to Hansemann, is reliable. In his account of the experimental work, he refers to the work of Hanau and Jensen, but believes that many so-called mouse tumours are not true carcinomas. Finally, in the account of the "therapeutic" period, he discusses surgery, radiotherapy, arsenic, and some other methods. His overall point is that cancer therapies do not reverse the cancerous process in cells, and therefore, according to him, are not true healing of the illness, but merely an ablation of the lesion by various methods.

Cancer therapeutics in theory and practice (1914i)

This article begins with a review of cancer therapy, and especially the use of arsenic and other metals, as well as cantharides, selenium, and immune sera. He then discusses radiotherapy and its adverse effects (radionecrosis of normal tissues). He suggests fractionation of dosage of radiotherapy, but has the idea that a moderate irradiation could kill all the older cells, leaving the young ones. After a break of 24 hours to several days (to let the young cells ripen), it is suggested that repeated doses could be given.

(This is presumably so that the young ones would be finally exhausted – eds).

He suggests that resistance of some tumour cells to X-ray damage is not only a function of how much radiation is given, but is also influenced by variable vascularisation, some parts of tumour being better nourished than other, and that perhaps the stroma plays a role.

This article is of interest in that fractionation of dosage was already popular among French radiotherapists, but not uniformly agreed as optimum in Germany (Heilmann, 1996; Tubiana et al 1996). Von Hansemann is giving an opinion on a topic which is perhaps beyond his expertise, because no specific protocols are suggested, and he does not refer to any of the considerable literature which had already accumulated concerning fractionation by this time.

The problem of cancer malignancy (1920a)

Early in this article, Hansemann included a 5 point summary of his position on cancer pathogenesis as follows.

"1. There is *per se* no single characteristic property of a cancer cell, BUT ONLY IN COMPARISON WITH THE MOTHER TISSUE. Thus it is necessary to compare the parenchyma of every type of cancer with its mother cells. Only thereby can one arrive at an opinion as to what changes take place in cancer cells in comparison with normal cells.

2. It was established that such changes are both morphological and physiological. The morphological changes are expressed in a different degree of differentiation, which in many cases can progress to complete spherical forms of the cell. Physiologically, it is established that the cells primarily acquire greater capacity for independent existence.

3. These different degrees of dedifferentiation together with the increased capacity for independent existence, I termed ANAPLASIA, a name which in this sense has now entered medical nomenclature,

and which has led only a few times to misunderstanding, which latter I have corrected each time in the literature.

4. In my first works, I thought it necessary to trace the origin of anaplasia back to asymmetric cell division, in that my particular point of departure was that the cancer cells lost those inheritable parts which signified their intrinsic specificity. It will become established later *(im weiteren)* if this view was correct or false.

5. The loss of hereditary components in the cell, i.e. of chromosomes or parts of chromosomes, can arise not only by asymmetrical cell division, but also by degenerative phenomena of individual chromosomes or in parts of chromosomes, which I described earlier in 1891."

In the remainder of the paper, von Hansemann discusses Boveri's theory (see chapter 6 of this vol – eds); then he notes a mistake by Benda that Hansemann's theory involves excess growth by way of embryonal reversion; and then reviews a chemical theory of the cancerous lesions (Orth). Next, Hansemann defends his idea of "altruism". Hansemann then addresses the question of growth in cancers in relation to his own theories, and the aetiological agents which have been established. He discusses "chemical" mechanisms at the end of the article, and indicates that cellular chemistry, physiology, abnormal physiology (as seen microscopically), and abnormal cell morphology (as also seen microscopically) are all important aspects of the investigation of tumours. Criticisms of Ribbert's and Lubarsch's ideas are included in the text at various points.

Appendix A
Hansemann's early *curriculum vitae*; letters

Copies of approximately thirty of Hansemann's letters were obtained by courtesy of the Manuscript Department (*Handschriftenabteilung*) of the *Staatsbibliothek* in Berlin; approximately five from the *Referat Handschriften-Rara* of the *Staats- und Universitätsbibliothek* Bremen; and one from the *Bayerische Staatsbibliothek,* Munich.

Translations of two letters from the collection of the *Staatsbibliothek* in Berlin are presented below. The letter held in the collection in Bremen concerns the Anti-Ultramontane movement. The other letters relate to administrative matters concerning pathological specimens, anthropological specimens, the Committee for Cancer Research, the University and some other minor issues.

This is an early *curriculum vitae*. The person to whom the letter was sent is not known to the present authors. The dates marked with an asterisk seem to be incorrect.

"15th May 1885*
Curriculum Vitae of D v H

B 1858, Eupen, my father owned a factory. Until aged 16, I was tutored privately in the spirit of a *Realschule* to prepare me to join the merchant class. When I then decided to study natural sciences, I went to the Gymnasium Charlottenburg, which was later renamed Friedrich-Wilhelm Gymnasium, and at Easter 1886*, I attempted the Certificate of Maturity (matriculation). Of my undergraduate studies, I spent 3 semesters in Berlin, one in Kiel and 3 in Leipzig. In the latter University, I did an elective during the long summer holidays, in 1883, with Professor Cohnheim, and in the subsequent semester, did a special assignment under Prof Weigert. In Spring 1885, I passed the State Exam, and the Doctoral Exam. My military duties I fulfilled in Berlin, at the Second Guard Regiment, partly as a one-year volunteer (Summer 1882) and in Kiel as a one-year volunteer doctor at the first Naval Division, 15th June to 14th December 1885. Furthermore, I did a voluntary 6-week military exercise and finally for the 10th Royal Saxon Infantry Regiment (No 134) from 11th April to 12th May this year.

After obtaining medical registration, in parallel to my position as army doctor, I was assistant to Prof Petersen, in the Surgical Children's Hospital, under the Red Cross at Kiel. It was there that I completed the enclosed work which was originally presented to the Leipzig faculty as a Doctoral Thesis. It has been re-worked and added-to, and published this Spring in the Archives of Pathological Anatomy and Physiology and Clinical Medicine. Since the 18th Dec 1885, I have been married to the daughter of Imperial Post Director Walter in Leipzig.

Since the beginning of January of this year, I have been working in the Institute of Pathology, in Berlin.

(Signed) David Hansemann".

Appendix A: Hansemann's early *Curriculum vitae*; letters

The following letter is apparently either to or from von Leyden; the addressee is not indicated. It may have been meant for a Committee. It shows that Hansemann was interested in the Virchow Chair, which ultimately went to Orth. Several of the bibliographic statements are incorrect.

There may have been a first page, which we have not seen. The part we have reads:

"According to a notice, there is a Faculty meeting. The Minister himself has ordered me on holidays. On the Agenda I see the decision on the successor to Virchow. As one of his oldest pupils, I would like my opinion expressed to the Faculty, even if I am not an anatomical pathologist. Of those who are famous and known to me, I would like to recommend Professor Dr von Hansemann, as the foremost candidate for the position.

Firstly to his personality, I have got to know him very well, 44 years old, Virchow's assistant for 9 years, did his Dr habil in 1890. Since 1890, chief Prosector at the Friedrichshain. Have been able to observe the degree of energy and professionalism which he exhibits in his field. In addition, in matters transcending his specialty, he has proven himself able to complete anything which he has tackled. Pathological anatomy nowadays is a broadened area influenced by advances in other disciplines, and it has thus become a necessity for the pathological anatomists to consider these. A good example would be bacteriology. All members of the Faculty should know that Professor von Hansemann does not only use modern technology but works in the spirit of new methods. He encompassed bacteriology, as well as medical chemistry, the importance of which for pathological anatomy was already recognised by Virchow. From his publications it becomes clear that he successfully nurtured these disciplines and knew how to utilise them for pathological anatomy.

I do not wish to omit to point out that his whole working style to see, the results of his work from his careful collection is done with great skill. Anyone who takes the trouble to visit the Institute in Friedrichshain which he has created out of nothing will recognise the exemplary order and system of his on-going studies and the important slides.

Faculty should also know that despite the pre-eminent character of the Charité, Professor von Hansemann has been successful in his role as a teacher. He reads common and special Pathological Anatomy, and hold seminars, prosections and demonstrations at the Virchow Institute. Another index of his success as a teacher are the numerous publications by his pupils. I felt obliged to tell you all of this and I would like to take the liberty to nominate Professor von Hansemann as the number one candidate for Virchow's Chair. I would like to point out that the fashionable argument contra, that he has previously only taught here, and not worked here, should not be allowed to prevent him being nominated. I would like to remark that Professor von Hansemann had already been offered a Chair at Leiden."

Unsigned.

Appendix B

Supplementary index entries to "The Science of Cancerous Disease from Earliest Times to the Present" (Wolff, 1907)

Wolff's book is a very thorough compendium of cancer research to that date. It has less analysis than would be possible in such a book today, owing to greater current knowledge.

To assist any reader who wishes to consult it, Table 1 shows on what pages the relevant Notes appear for each section. Table 2 lists citations of Hansemann (whose name is absent from the list of persons). Table 3 provides some additional supplementary index entries.

Table 1

Book section	Text pages	Pages for Relevant Notes
Preface	xv–xvii	591
Black bile theory	3–45	591–597
The lymphatic theory	49–98	597–604
The blastema theory/histological period	99–180	604–614
Cellular pathology and its significance for cancer	181–270	614–628
The embryonal theories	271–338	628–639
Cell theories	339–430	639–652
Theories of parasitism	431–590	652–673

Table 2

Subject matter	Page
– Hansemann's theory	xlix, 1
– histogenetic principle	257
– on endothelioma	258–9
– chorionepithelioma derived from embryonal tissue	298–9
said to be principal advocate of Klebs' fertilisation theory in Germany, referring to 1890 article, and Arch f anat and Physiol (which is not listed either in Index Med or the Obituary list)	361

Appendix B: Supplementary index entries

– on amoeboid movements of tumour cells	370
– amoeboid movements of embryonal cells	371
– phagocytic features of cancer cells	371
– other features of cancer cells (no reference)	371
– and function of cancer cells	372
– and why ca pancreas must be able to continue to produce the anti-diabetic agent	372
– report of bile secretion by ca liver cells	374
– functions of tumour cells similar to those of mother cells	374
– and in a "specially equipped site" i.e. capacity for independent existence	375
– and fat in tumour cells	376
– and the colloid or hyaline process	378
– and nuclear disintegration	379
– and caseous product	379
– and calcification	380
– cornification, hyaline drops, in carcinoma cells	380
– the cancer cell is not particularly frail	383
– theories of asymmetric karyokinesis	389–397
– supporters and opponents of Hansemann's theory (Stroebe, Müller, Beneke especially)	397–405
– (Beneke opposed reactivation of embryonal genes)	403
– on metaplasia	412
(Lubarsch supports Virchow)	413
– classification of tumours by morphology	418
– opposes Grawitz	422–423
– responsibility for proliferation of altruistic relations	443
(embryonal theories and Kelling)	452
– on vacuoles in cells thought to be parasitic in origin	582
– inclusions possibly parasitic	583

(In the Notes)
– wrong on Müller as first to use "stroma"	605 (n 17)
– referred to	626 (ns 395, 397, 398)
	663 n 164
	643 (ns 120, 121-6, 129, 134)
	645 n 213
	646 n 247 and following

Appendix B: Supplementary index entries

Table 3

Thiersch	188 ff,
(ejusdem)	191
According, above and contrary are pre-Galenic?	10
Laennec distinguished homologous and heterologous tumours	76
Broca's familial breast cancer, and hereditary influence	300–301
Virchow's error on growth (not from within themselves, but by recruitment)	321
Growth by transformation	327
Schleicher introduced "karyokinesis"	344
"Central bodies", centrosomes or polar bodies – "directly next to the nuclear membrane, opinions of significance varied"	349
Embryonal cell and "neoplastic" cell are not identical – Bard	352
Fertilisation theory in England: Simon in 1878; Stattock and Ballance, Creighton	360–361
Schleich has hypothesis that carcinoma can be compared only to the development of the fertilized egg	364
As an enlargement of Recklinghausen's theory	367
von Leyden described parasites in tumour cells	566

Appendix C
Published obituaries

These are all presented in full, but with footnotes added at the relevant places.

1920. Centralbl. f. allg. Path. u. path. Anat., Jena, 31: 113
David von Hansemann
Original Communications

In these days of early deaths in nature we got news that also a human life had ended prematurely. A life rich in work and success; David von Hansemann, Privy Counsellor of Medicine and Ordinary Professor of the University of Berlin, Prosector of the Rudolf Virchow Hospital has died on 28 August, aged only 62 years. It was a twist of fate that he had to die of just that disease he had dedicated most of his life to researching and fighting.

It is impossible to evaluate the scientific role of von Hansemann properly in such a short obituary. However, there is hardly a problem in the field of pathology he has not commented on, based on his own experience and research. Thus, we owe him a great many contributions to current knowledge and he has fertilised our thinking. He was gifted with a sharp mind, inherited from his father and grandfather, especially the latter, who was a famous merchant and had made a name for himself as a Minister of Finance who was viewed as one of the most important men of his time. Von Hansemann emerged out of the school of Rudolf Virchow under whom he served as an assistant for 9 years between 1886 and 1895. He was also Prosector of Berlin's largest hospitals providing a rich and diverse spectrum of sections. Von Hansemann viewed pathological anatomy, his greatest passion, as an exact science in the framework of science as a whole. A plethora of single observations always led him to question their role in the greater picture and this gift inevitably led him far beyond the field of pathology to get involved with biology, anthropology, embryology, paleontology and philosophy. It was the latter in which he immersed himself, with great passion in the last years of his life, very much like his own father did.

Von Hansemann's busy research activities were crowned by immense success. Even in his younger years, he made a name for himself with his work on the specificity, the altruism and anaplasia of cells, which later on became the basis and the beginning of his research activities and views on the origin of malignant tumours. The important law of the close relationship between cells in the body via secretion has even been touched upon in this early work. In addition, Von Hansemann became famous for emphasising the role of constitution and disposition on the pathogenesis of disease. His last major work he wrote on the condition of thinking in medicine.

Unfortunately, the lack of space here prohibits an in depth evaluation of von Hansemann's large body of work. So we conclude with the assessment that he made everlasting contributions which will forever link his name with our beautiful science, Pathology. He would have continued enriching us with the fruits of his research and thinking as evidenced by the nearly completed manuscript on basic pathology, which was discovered as part of his estate. He worked on this for many years and often referred to this as his scientific legacy. Hopefully, we will achieve the printing of this work as soon as possible. That will give him one last opportunity to speak to us and we all will feel how his work will reach far beyond his death.

With joy and pride, we want to state and feel that he was one of us.

C HART
Of Berlin

1920 Virchow's Arch. 227: v.

On the 28th of August, David Von Hansemann, who had served as Editor of the journal for a short time (from Volume 215 onwards), died at almost 62 years old. His passing is a great loss for medical science, especially for those parts of Medicine to which this Journal is mainly dedicated. As a disciple of Rudolf Virchow, whom he served for 9 years as an assistant, until he became Prosector at the Hospital Friedrichshain, von Hansemann published a significant body of his scientific work in this very Journal. The hallmark of his papers was that he always emphasised basic principles and his tendency, even with dealing with specific single problems, always to put them in their context within science. He has contributed significantly to the biggest and difficult problems in pathological morphology and biology, such as normal versus pathological growth, tuberculosis and other infectious diseases and has also contributed to the treatment of these conditions. One of his greatest achievements has to be that he stood firm against the excesses of a new emerging school of thought, the one-sided dogmatic proponents of bacteriology who threatened to confuse the minds, especially in Berlin. His gift of always seeing the greater picture protected him from becoming lost in overspecialisation, and furthermore led him towards other common biological anthropological and phylogenetic questions. As a University teacher and counsellor of medical doctors as a whole, as well as through his scientific work and his friendly personality he gained a much revered position in the medical scene of Berlin. He became so much a part of this city that he declined calls to leave and even rejected a professorship Ordinarius. He will be forever remembered and held in high esteem.

O Lubarsch

1937 Proceedings of the German Pathological Society. 29th Conference, Breslau 27–29, 1936, Gustav Fischer, Jena, pp 370–378.

(Editor's note. This biography was written in a period when the policy of the German government of the time was to produce apparently "normal" biographies of past national figures to support the government's attitudes and policies. Many implications concerning Hansemann in this biography may not be correct (see chapter 1) The biographer (Ostertag) was involved in studies of the brains of individuals who had been euthanased for incurable diseases, and was a member of the National Socialist Party – Kater, 1998).

David von Hansemann
5 11 1858- 28 8 1920

Sixteen years ago, – on the 28th August 1920 – at the age of 62, David von Hansemann died: first director of the Pathological Institute at what was at that time the Friedrichshain Hospital, today's Horst Wessel Hospital, and later the first holder of the Office of Prosector at the largest hospital in Berlin, the Rudolf-Virchow-Hospital.

It is difficult for the present writer, after such a time span, to set up a monument to his great predecessor in office, as is usual in this publication, a monument, the erection of which was overlooked at the time of Germany's greatest suffering. If, in spite of it, this can now happen, the undersigned may owe it to the circumstance that a lively picture of this excellent teacher still stands visible before him, to whom specifically the ex-service students of medicine, in their examination semester, felt particularly attracted. Certainly, however, the institute in the Rudolf-Virchow-Hospital has changed its aspect following the present author's assumption of the post; from Hansemann's time only two colleagues remained and as a monument of permanent memory the basis of an excellent collection. From David von Hansemann's family, his memoirs were placed at our disposal, which Hansemann had written during the war, in the evenings while he was in the field, under the title "Personal development and self criticism"[1].

David von Hansemann's external life developed in a straight line. Born on the 5th November 1858, at Eupen, in the border country (*Grenzland*)*, he was able to live through a carefree childhood and also a financially comfortable life. Quite early he became familiar with problems of "Germanness" (*Deutschtum*). His grandfather was the well-known finance politician, sometime Prussian Finance Minister, and founder of the Discount Company. His son Gustav, a well-known expert in business and economics, was able in later years to devote himself exclusively to academic interests and in this, mainly to problems of physics and philosophy. The son, David von Hansemann, had originally been destined for

Appendix C: Published obituaries

the career of a businessman, returned to school however, because this profession did not allow for personal influence in wider circles, studied medicine in Berlin, Kiel and Leipzig, completed the state examination there in 1885, and gained the doctoral degree, under Cohnheim's direction, with a dissertation on "Tuberculosis of the mucous membranes of the mouth".

After completing his second half year's service in the Navy, he entered the Berlin Pathological Institute, as a pupil of Virchow on the recommendation of Cohnheim and Weigert, and remained there for fully nine years, until the 31st March, 1895. On the 25th July 1890, his Doctor habil, on "Cell divisions in the human epidermis" was accepted. A large number of works made him, who had already concerned himself early on with the problem of growth, and already then had offered opposition in his struggle against the

[1] I wish especially to thank the family for this; these pages which were written straightforwardly in the field, give a clear picture of the man, who was at pains to give account responsibly for his life, of what he did, and what he neglected to do. Long or short interruptions and repetitions do indeed disturb one a little, but it is specifically these which allow us to recognise what problems, medical, scientific and philosophical, drew this clever man into their magic circle time and time again.
* in 1858 part of Germany, but in 1937, a part of Belgium (eds).

over-valuation of bacteriological results, widely known. Thus, on the first of April 1895 he was chosen for the position of Prosector at the Friedrichshain Hospital. Rudolf Virchow, who at that time was the decisive city delegate in the Health Commission, had expressed himself against the establishment of further appointments of Prosectors in Berlin. The establishment of a Pathological Institute in the Friedrichshain Hospital was determined by the Berlin city deputies during Virchow's absence in Egypt. Once the establishment of the Prosectorship was made, even Virchow could not change anything, and with a reference which appropriately evaluated the scientific achievements of the young David von Hanseman, he recommended him for this post.

Here, an extraordinarily fruitful period began. Ever more voluntary collaborators arrived, and particularly from the turn of the century, the number of his pupils constantly increased. In particular, his student at that time, Carl Hart, distinguished himself with a sequence of fine works. In March 1897, he became Extraordinary Professor at the University. In 1904, because of the poor circumstances in the Institute there, he rejected the leadership of the Pathological Institute at the Moabit Hospital, transferred, however, on the 1st October 1906 to the newly-built Rudolf-Virchow Hospital. What could be achieved against the, at that time, all-powerful city *Baumeister* (Town planner) Ludwig Hoffman, David von Hansemann achieved through persistent struggle.

Up to the year 1934, the Institute remained essentially unchanged. Measures, which have today to be undertaken towards improvement, coincide completely with the plans of the late first Prosector.

Nomination as medical privy Councillor was followed in December 1914 by appointment as Honorary full Professor of the University. In the same year, he was called up for war service; on 1st July 1916, as Army Pathologist of the Eight Army he went to the Eastern Front and only returned home after the collapse. His merits, along with other distinctions, were recognised by the conferring of the Iron Cross First Class.

The external humiliation of his much-loved people was a heavy burden for him, who had from his youth onwards, concerned himself with the pressing questions of the German Fatherland, and who had, far-sightedly, been anxious about his Fatherland. His concerns applied equally to the shameless emergence of its internal oppressors and thus it was actually automatic that it was precisely returned ex-servicemen who thronged into his lectures and courses, whilst others saw in them (the courses) only the burdensome overcrowding of their lecture theatres and took it very badly when the ex-servicemen took up their weapons again to save society from the Red Terror. He thanked these ex-service students with his full understanding, and with infinite patience, took the greatest pains to introduce them to pathology, and to further their knowledge, above all to educate them as doctors. Many a one who listened to his words at that time, and whom I questioned in this regard, retains little of what he heard, but all of them still acknowledge Hansemann's efforts for the future medical generation.

In the year 1920, already early in the year, a serious illness sent him to his invalid's bed, a carcinoma to which he, for a long time still full of optimism, succumbed in late summer.

From his entry into the Virchow Institute, he dedicated himself uninterruptedly with constant industry to fertile research activity. He had at his disposal a large collections of the Charité, later that of the large Berlin Hospitals. It is scarcely possible today, within the framework of these few lines, to give an overview of David Hansemann's works, and

to bring his work once more before the eyes of our contemporaries. A glance at his own numerous writings and those of his pupils reveals the enormous versatility with which he was always at pains, to approach questions on the broadest foundation, and to take a position *vis à vis* almost every problem of pathology on the basis of daily careful observations. In addition, von Hansemann's scientific persona (*wissenschaftliche Persoenlichkeit*) has been firmly established historically long since. In the year 1893, his book appeared: "The Specificity, Altruism and Anaplasia of Cells" (*sic*), which in spite of many fundamental and heuristically valuable view points is today regarded as almost only of historical value, but it was, all the same, the first work in which the influence of cells of the most various tissues and organs, were clearly distinguished from each other, and in which were indicated the reciprocal relationships of the inner secretion appropriate in like fashion to all cells of the organism.

In an article "Milestones of cancer research" A Dietrich writes, "If Hansemann in 1890 saw the loss of individuality in favour of more powerful capability for proliferation (as "anaplasia"), in asymmetric nuclear division, and thus with sacrifice of the chromosome complement, such a change could in no way be confirmed as essential precondition of atypical transformation. In spite of this, Hansemann's work remains a milestone of tumour research in that it contributed to a deepening of formal understanding even if it was not able to clarify the origin of tumours, or above all, the essence of malignancy.

The concept of anaplasia remains as nothing other than a rearrangement (*Umschichtung*) of the formal tissue changes and the retroconclusion as to a change of essence connected therewith. In this, Hansemann was first to establish clearly "THE FAILING PARTICIPATION IN THE RECIPROCAL RELATIONSHIP (ALTRUISM) OF TISSUES and the intensification of independent viability". The problem of the origin and of the essence of malignant growths remains the great question to which David von Hansemann repeatedly turned. It finds expression in his works on the "Microscopic Diagnosis of Malignant Tumours" (1903) (*sic*) and in the "Atlas of Malignant Tumours" (1910). Alongside these, as the bibliography indicates, is a number of small works in which he returns to this problem repeatedly.

It was David von Hansemann above all, who, on the basis of his observations of the arising of diseases, attributed considerable significance to the construction and function of the human body, and repeatedly he emphasised the importance of the constitution as soon as he had opportunity, on the basis of numerous fundamentally important observations, to take up a position again.

In his lifetime, David von Hansemann was often reproached because in the struggle against the purely bacteriological direction in the theory of infectious diseases, he went too far with his contradiction of Behring's protective inoculation, and against Koch's teaching. If, however, one places oneself back in those times, when bacteriology made claim to explain all disease pictures, and if one takes into account in what way Koch's tuberculin was often used to the detriment of the invalids, then one will understand that the doctor David von Hansemann could not remain silent when he was supposed to witness how business-minded doctors fell onto tuberculin, promised a cure for sufferers and therewith, harmed them. He was in this at pains to achieve the greatest objectivity and only expressed himself in public

at the moment, when he, at the dissecting table, had convinced himself of the effects of this uncritical mode of treatment; it remains his achievement, that he persistently stood up for the importance of the constitution, and of the "accidental predisposition" in the matter of the arising of infectious diseases, and therewith prepared the path for the concept which is today no longer assailable.

In his book "Descent and Pathology" in 1909, he set down comparative biology studies and thought. In 1912 he tried to make a general scientific mode of thought a general principle for doctors; that occurred in his last big work on "Conditional Thinking in Medicine and its Importance for Practice". It is a confession of faith in his biologically oriented world-view, which, considerably deepened, finds expression in his memoirs which exist only in handwritten form.

This striving for conscientious exactness is evident in the numerous normal-anatomic works of David von Hansemann. Not only did he submit cell division in the human epidermis to a normal histological examination, also he studied the interstitial cells of the testes in hibernating animals. In the area of comparative pathology, there are very valuable observations on rickets in domesticated animals, a monograph on dwarfism and we should mention in addition, the examination of the brains of Helmholtz, Bunsen and Menzel. His efforts towards a comparative anatomy as also anthropology and phylogenesis are proved in addition by specimens in the collection of the Rudolph Virchow Hospital. David von Hansemann, well equipped by a favourable destiny, did not need to shun any expense when it was a matter of getting hold of important research material. Pettiness and monstrous short-sightedness on the part of the City of Berlin, led to the fact that he also had to provide the greatest part of his collection from his own pocket, and was able therefore to bequeath it in his will to various significant researchers. It is only with sadness that one can look at these fragments of a once unique and excellent collection.

Hard work, talent, all-embracing knowledge enabled this researcher and scholar to bring valuable enrichment to science and to general medicine. Thus there was no lack of external recognition for him.

Inter alia, this was expressed in the fact that, in 1906, at the International Medical Congress in Lisbon, he, as delegate of the Berlin Medical Society, gave the major keynote address, and that in 1907, he was sent to the Biologists' Congress in Boston, and in 1910 to the International Congress of Cancer in Paris. In like manner, he represented Germany at the first Brussels Cancer Congress. The Berlin Medical world expressed its confidence in von Hansemann when it chose him as member of the Executive Committee of the Central Committee for Further Medical Education, just as he was active as Chairman of the Berlin Lecturers Association and was Secretary for many years of the Berlin Medical Society.

David von Hansemann refused calls to Professorial Chairs once outside Germany, on another occasion to Marburg, and again to Koenigsberg. He had made a beautiful home for himself in Berlin, and probably also did not want to miss the circle of scholars which he had created for himself in Berlin. In addition, his heart belonged very much to the practising doctors whom he looked after in further education lectures,

to whom he gladly devoted numerous articles in the medical press which was accessible to the practising doctor. More than external honours, he was pleased by the trust of his colleagues who summoned him as Executive Secretary of the Berlin Medical Society and against whose degeneration into a platform for self congratulation and advertising he took up arms. A little book on "Superstition in Medicine and its Dangers for Health and Life" was an example of the way in which he always used his science to be useful to the doctors and the people. Already at the beginning of this address, his human side was evident. Uprightness and openness are not only emphasised by Hart in his obituary; also his staff, his collaborators, whom I was still able to get to know in the Institute, particularly praise this unconditional, open gentle calm confidence as soon as one had become closer to him, whilst those less well known to him often had the impression of inaccessibility and of pride. David von Hansemann probably scarcely discussed much with anyone what he set down in his manuscript "Process of Development and Self Criticism", and what may have seemed to the outsider to be overbusiness, as for example his activity in national groups, reveals itself when one reads his manuscript as a necessarily limited practical application to the State of his biological way of looking at things. The population-political section could have just as well have been written recently, and what he says about other forces which were forcibly intruding into the German (ethnically pure) folkness (*Volkstum*), shows his clear insight particularly sharpened by his borderland German origin (*grenzlanddeutsch*). His anxiety for Germany was equalled by his worries about the youth of the nation. In his introduction to the aforesaid manuscript, there is a sentence; "Let the writer therefore write for youth, and therefore comprehensible and inviting for them. If he is successful in that, then he has done his work, which is rewarding and which can bear fruit if the seed falls on good ground." If von Hansemann was permitted to be a scholar blessed with external goods, this never allowed him to forget his duty to the people (*Volk*); he became a doctor, in order, as such, more to have influence on wider circles. If his position *vis à vis* others was in his earlier years determined by a strongly marked civic pride, he grew, with the experiences of the great war wholly into his people. What, and how, he writes about this is amongst the most beautiful aspect of his war-time memoirs.

It was not granted to him, as he had hoped, to continue to work influentially.

B. Ostertag – Berlin.

[A list of Hansemann's publications follows in the original, and these have been made the basis of the list in Appendix D (eds).]

Appendix D
Bibliography of David Paul von Hansemann

The works of Hansemann are in the same order as in the list in the obituary by Ostertag (1937). Additional articles which were found in Index Medicus are included at the end of the sublist for each year.

Page numbers were not included in Ostertag's list. Where a reference is cited in the text of this volume, the article has been consulted and the page numbers have been inserted. Where a work is cited in Index Medicus, those page numbers have been inserted, but not necessarily checked. For works which we have not consulted, and the work has not been found in Index Medicus, the page numbers remain omitted.

The title "Arch. f. path. Anat., etc., Berl.," has been replaced by "Virchow's Arch." consistent with long tradition. The article, "Specificity of cell division" was wrongly dated as "1893" by Ostertag, and has been listed here as 1894i. Articles which are presented in full translation are marked "T"; those with only an abstract provided are marked with "A".

Some works have the same titles. The later-dated articles are usually comments on the original article, as might appear as a "Letter to the Editor" nowadays (2006). Others are probably due to errors by Ostertag or the compilers of Index Medicus. We have found no instances of verbatim duplicate publishing.

1886   Tuberculosis of the mucous membranes of the mouth.
Ueber die Tuberculose der Mundschleimhaut. Inaug.-Diss. (see Virchow's Arch. 103: 264–275).

1887   The pathology of Malpighian bodies in the kidney.
Zur pathologischen Anatomie der Malpighi'schen Körperchen der Niere. Virchow's Arch. 110: 52–80.

1888   A contribution to the mechanism of hydronephrosis, including a few case reports.
Beitrag zur Mechanik der Hydronephrosen, nebst einigen casuistischen Mittheilungen. Virchow's Arch. 112, 539–548.

1889 a)   Extensive paralysis associated with diphtheria (observations in self).
Ausgedehnte Lähmungen nach Diphtherie (an sich selbst beobachtet). Virchow's Arch. 115, 534–547.

    b)   (with Martius). A case of intermittent congenital myotonia.
Ein Fall von Myotonia congenita intermittens. Virchow's Arch. 117: 587–606.

    c)   Comments on the work of H. Lorenz: "Examinations of the brush border and its role in normal and diseased kidneys".
Bemerkungen im Anschluss an die Arbeit von H. Lorenz: Untersuchungen über den Bürstenbesatz und dessen Bedeutung an normalen und pathologischen Nieren. Zschr f.

klin. Med., 15: Hft. 5–6. n.b. Index Medicus follows with "Centralbl. f. klin. Med. Leipz. 10: 313–315", and this reference has not been checked.

d) On Polymastia.
Ueber Polymastie. Verhandl. d. Berl. Gesellsch. f. Anthrop. Berl. (no vol. no.): 434–443.

1890 a) On the asymmetrical cell division in epithelial cancers and its biological significance. (Complete translation in chapter 7).
Ueber asymmetrische Zelltheilung in Epithelkrebsen und deren biologische Bedeutung. Virchow's Arch. 119: 299–326.

b) On primary cancer of the liver.
Ueber den primären Krebs der Leber. Berl. klin. Wschr. 27: 353–356.

1891 a) On pathological mitoses. (Complete translation in chapter 8).
Ueber pathologische Mitosen. Virchow's Arch. 123: 356–370.

b) Pathological/anatomical and histological observations after Koch's method of treatment. (Summary and comments in chapter 12).
Pathologisch-anatomische und histologische Erfahrungen nach der Koch'schen Behandlungsmethode. (Vortrag Hefeland Gesellschaft.). Berl. klin. Wschr. 28: 121–123.

c) Karyokinesis and cellular pathology. (Complete translation in chapter 9).
Karyokinese und Cellularpathologie. Berl. klin. Wschr. 28: 1039–1042.

d) On the origin and multiplication of leukocytes.
Ein Beitrag zur Entstehung und Vermehrung der Leukocyten. Verhandl. d. anat. Gesellsch. (Jena) 5: 255–258.

e) Pathological/anatomical and histological observations after Koch's injection method.
Pathologische-anatomische und histologische Erfahrungen nach der Koch'schen Injectionsmethode. Therap. Monatsh.

f) Historical review of the pathological anatomy of tuberculosis.
Historischer Ueberblick üeber die pathologische Anatomie der Tuberculose. Therap. Monatsh., Berl. 5: 81–84.

g) Pathological/anatomical and histological observations after Koch's treatment. (Comments in Chapter 12).
Pathologisch-anatomische und histologische Erfahrungen nach der Koch'schen Behandlungsmethode. Veröffentl. d. Hufeland. Gesellsch. in Berl. Vortr. pp 14–21.

h) Cell division in the human epidermis. (Summary and comments in chapter 12).
Ueber Zelltheilung in der menschlichen Epidermis. Festschr. Rudolf Virchow. G. Reimer, Berlin pp 1–12.

1892 a) On the Anaplasia of cancer cells and asymmetrical mitosis. (Complete translation in Chapter 10)
Ueber die Anaplasie der Geschwulstzellen und die asymmetrische Mitrose. Virchow's Arch. 129: 436–449.

b) On ochronosis.
Ueber Ochronose. Berl. klin. Wschr., 29: 660–662.

c) On the stereoscopic merging of microscopic photogrammes.
Ueber Stereoskopische Vereinigung mikroskopischer Photogramme. Verhandl. d. Physiol. Gesellschaft, Berl.

1893 a) Cancer stroma and Grawitz's theory of 'dormant' cells. (Summary and comments in chapter 12).

Das Krebsstroma und die Grawitz'sche Theorie der Schlummerzellen. Virchow's Arch. 133: 147–165.

b) Centrosomes and attraction-spheres in resting cells.
Ueber Centrosomen und Attractionssphären in ruhenden Zellen. Anat. Anz., Jena, 1892–3, 8: 57–59.

c) "Studies of the Specificity, Altruism and Anaplasia of Cells with Special Reference to Tumours". (Complete translation in chapter 11).
Studien über die Spezificität, den Altruismus und die Anaplasie der Zellen mit besonderer Berücksichtigung der Geschwülste. A. Hirschwald, Berlin.

1894 a) Critical reflections on the aetiology of cancers. (Summary and comments in chapter 12).
Kritische Bemerkungen über die Aetiologie der Carcinome. Berl. klin. Wschr. 31: 11–16.

b) Trophic disturbances after severing the sciatic nerve.
Ueber trophische Störungen nach Continuitätstrennung des Nervus ischiadicus. Berl. klin. Wschr. 31: 191.

c) Adenomyxosarcoma of the kidney.
Adenomyxosarcom der Niere. Berl. klin. Wschr., 31: 717.

d) Communications on diphtheria and diphtheria convalescent serum.
Mittheilungen über Diphtherie und das Diphtherie-Heilserum. Berl. klin. Wschr. 31: 1127; 1195.

e) Discussions of 1894 d). Therap. Monatsh.

f) Relevance of the pancreas to diabetes.
Die Beziehungen des Pankreas zum Diabetes. Ztschr. f. klin. Med., Berl., 26: 191–224.

g) Diseases of the pancreas in diabetes.
Ueber Pankreaserkrankungen bei Diabetes. Atti d. xi Cong. med. internaz., Roma, 1894, ii, patol. gen. ed anat. patol., 143–148.

h) On "larvirte" (latent) diphtheria.
Über "larvierte" Diphtherie. Dtsch. Med. Wschr

i) The specificity of cell division. (Summary and comments in chapter 12).
Ueber die Specificität der Zelltheilung. Arch. f. mikr. Anat., Bonn, xliii, 244–251, 1 pl.

1895 a) The relationship of Löffler's bacterium to diphtheria.
Ueber die Beziehungen des Löffler'schen Bacillus zur Diphtherie. Virchow's Arch. 139: 353–381.

b) On the so-called interstitial cells of the testis and their relevance in disease. (Summary and comments in chapter 12).
Über die sogenannten Zwischenzellen des Hodens und deren Bedeutung bei pathologischen Veränderngen. Virchow's Arch. 142: 538–546.

c) Communications on diphtheria and diphtheria convalescent serum.
Mittheilungen über Diphtherie und das Diphtherie-Heilserum. Verhandl. d. Berl., med. Gesellsch. (1894–1895), xxv, pt. ii, 185–206. [Discussion], pt. i, 232–284. Discussion, *also*: Communications on diphtheria and diphtheria convalescent serum. Wien. klin. Wschr., 1895, viii, 185; 203; 242. See 1894d and 1894e.

d) Pathological Anatomy and Bacteriology. (Summary and comments in chapter 12).
Pathologische Anatomie und Bacteriologie. Berl. klin. Wschr. 32: 653–658; 680–684.

e) An unusual malformation of a uterus.

Ueber eine eigenthümliche Missbildung des Uterus. Ztschr. f. Geburtsh. u. Gynaek., Stuttg. 32: 315.

f) On some of the rarer tumours of the stomach.
Ueber einige seltenere Geschwülste am Magen. (Vortrag).

g) On the large interstitial cells of the testis.
Ueber die grossen Zwischenzellen des Hodens. (Vortrag.) Verhandl. d. Physiol. Gesellschaft.

h) Alveolar pores in normal lungs.
Ueber die Poren der normalen Lungenalveolen. Sitzungsb. d. k. preuss. Sitzung d. Akad. D. Wissensch. zu Berl., 1895, 999–1001, 1 pl.

i) The diagnosis of malignant tumors. (Summary and comments in chapter 12). Internat. Clin., Phila., 5th series, i, pp 208–215.

1896 a) On the pathogenesis of false diverticula of the intestine.
Ueber die Entstehung falscher Darmdivertikel. Virchow's Arch. 144, 400–405.

b) A commonly occurring epiglottic pathology in syphilis.
Ueber eine häufig bei Syphilis vorkommende Veränderung an der Epiglottis. Berl. klin. Wschr., 1896, xxxiii, 236.

c) A rare case of Addison's disease.
Ein seltener Fall von Morbus Addisonii. Berl. klin. Wschr., 1896, xxxiii, 296. [Discussion], 310.

d) Dissecting aneurysms.
Aneurysma dissecans. Berl. Klin. Wochenschr.

e) Endotheliomas.
Ueber Endotheliome. Dtsche med. Wschr., Leipz. u. Berl., 22: 52.

f) On the nomenclature of malignant tumours.
Über die Benennung der bösartigen Geschwülste. Allg. Med. Zbl.

g) Pyometra from carcinoma. Myomas of the round ligament.
Pyometra bei Carcinom. Myomas ligamenti rotundi. Zschr. f. Gynaecol.

h) Techniques of dissection of the nose and sinuses.
Sectionstechnik zur Untersuchung der Nase und ihrer Nebenhöhlen. Handb. d. Laryngol. u. Rhinol., Wien, , iii, 261–265.

i) A rare case of Addison's disease. Med. Age, Detroit, xiv, 294.

1897 a) On hyaline cells in gastric polyps.
Über hyaline Zellen in Magenpolypen. Virchow's Arch. 148: 349–354, 1 pl.

b) A comment on the functions of cancer cells and altruism.
Einige Bemerkungen über die Functionen der Krebszellen u. den Altruismus. Virchow's Arch. 149: 194–196.

c) Demonstration (of a collection of specimens).
Demonstration (Sammlungspräp). Berl. klin. Wschr.

d) On acromegaly.
Über Akromegalie. Berl. klin. Wschr

e) Demonstration of miscellaneous preparations.
Demonstration verschiedener Präparate. Berl. klin. Wschr.

f) Demonstration of pancreatic changes in diabetes.
Demonstration Pancreasveränderungen bei Diabetes. Berl. klin. Wschr.

g) On cure and curability. (Summary and comments in chapter 12).
Über Heilung und Heilbarkeit. Dtsche Med. Zschr. Berl. 18: 287–289.

h) Techniques for dissection of the larynx and trachea.
Sectionsmethode des Kehlkopfes und der Luftröhre. Handb. d. Laryngol. u. Rhinol. Wien, 1896–7, i: 290–292.

i) On a few fatty conditions in animal bodies.
Über einige fettige Zustände im Tierkörper. Verhandl. d. Physiol. Gesellschaft. (Februar.)

j) Lecture on microscopic slides.
Vortrag über mikroskopische Präparate. Verhandl. d. Physiol. Gesellschaft. (Juni.)

k) On changes in the kidneys from ligation of the ureter.
Über Veränderungen in den Nieren bei Unterbindung des Ureters. Verhandl. D. Physiol. Gesellschaft. (Oktober.)

l) On serous meningitis.
Über seröse Meningitis. Verhandl. D. 15. Kongr. f. Innere Med.

m) Addendum to "A communication on the question the optic chiasma".
Zusatz zu "Ein Beitrag zu der Frage der Kreuzung der Sehnerven." (Hellendall.) Arch. f. Anat. u. Physiol.

n) On fatty infiltrates of the renal epithelium.
Über die Fettinfiltration der Nierenepithelien. Virchow's Arch. cxlviii, 355–365, 1 pl.

o) "The Microscopic Diagnosis of Malignant Tumours". (Summary and comments in chapter 12).
Die Mikroskopische Diagnose der bösartigen Geschwülste. A Hirschwald, Berlin. (for 2nd edn see 1902h).

1898 a) A study of the pathogenesis of gall stones.
Ein Beitrag zur Entstehung der Gallensteine. Virchow's Arch. 154: 380–383.

b) Secondary infection with tuberculous bacilli.
Die secundäre Infection mit Tuberkelbacillen. Berl. klin. Wschr. 35: 233–237. [Discussion], 245: 247.

c) Three case reports of hermaphrodites.
Drei Fälle von Hermaphroditismus. Berl. klin. Wschr. 35: 549.

d) The effect of hibernation on cell division.
Über den Einfluss des Winterschlafes auf die Zelltheilung. Arch. f. Physiol., Leipz., 1898, 262.

e) Congenital anomalies of larynx and trachea.
Missbildung des Kehlkopfes und der Luftröhre. Z. f. Laryngol u. Rhinol.

f) On Acromegaly.
Über Akromegalie. Veröffentl. d. Hufeland. Gesellsch. in Berl. (1897), pt. ii, 30–38.

g) Changes in the kidneys caused by ligation of the ureter.
Ueber Veränderungen in den Nieren bei Unterbindung des Ureters. Arch. f. Physiol., Leipz. 147.

1899 a) On scientific judgment.
Über eine wissenschaftliche Urteilbildung. Virchow's Arch. 156.

b) Investigations on the formation of emphysema of the lung based on specimens of Mr Sudsuki from Tokoyo.

Untersuchungen über die Entstehung des Lungenemphysems nach Präparaten des Herrn Sudsuki aus Tokio. Berl. klin. Wschr.

- c) On anatomical findings in scurvy.
  Über anat. Befunde bei Skorbut. Verhandl. d. D. P. Gesellschaft.
- d) Research into the development of Morgagni's pouches.
  Untersuchungen über die Entwickelung der Morgagni'schen Taschen. Arch. f. Laryngol. u. Rhinol., Berl., ix, 81–85, 1 pl.
- e) The brain of Hermann von Helmholtz.
  Über das Gehirn von Hermann von Helmholtz. Ophth. klin., Stuttg., iii, 43–45.
- f) Demonstration of spermatogenesis in Orang-Utang.
  Demonstration zur Spermatogenese des Orang-Utang. Verhandl. d. Physiol Gesellschaft.
- g) Early diagnosis and therapy of aortic aneurysms.
  Frühdiagnose und Behandlung der Aorten-Aneurysmen. Verhandl. d. XVII Kongr. f. Innere Med.
- h) On Victor von Ebner's doubts about the existence of normal pores between alveoli of the lung.
  Über Victor von Ebners Zweifel an der Existenz normaler Poren zwischen den Lungenalveolen. (no details given – see 1900m)
- i) Rachitic microcephaly in two siblings.
  Rachitische Mikrocephalie bei zwei Geschwistern. Dtsche. med. Wschr., Leipz. u. Berl., 25: Ver.-Beil., 50.

1900 a) The role of malignant adenomata in oncology.
  Über die Stellung des Adenoma malignum in der Onkologie. Virchow's Arch. 162: I, 453–460.
- b) Anaplasia – the term and its essence. (Summary and comments in chapter 12).
  Über den Begriff und das Wesen der Anaplasie. Virchow's Arch. 162: 549–553.
- c) An anatomical specimen illustrating foreign body migration.
  Ein Präparat von Fremdkörperwanderung. Berl. klin. Wschr. 37: 221.
- d) Seventy–second Convention of German scientists and Doctors in Aachen from 16–22 September.
  72. Versammlung deutscher Naturforscher u. Ärtze zu Aachen vom 16–22 Sept. Berl. klin. Wschr
- e) On selected cellular pathology and their role in forming the basis of organ-therapy.
  Einige Zellprobleme und ihre Bedeutung für die wissenschaftliche Begründung der Organtherapie. Berl. klin. Wschr. 37: 901–904; 932–935.
- f) Congenital malformations of the nose.
  Die angeborenen Missbildungen der Nase. Handb. F. Laryngol u. Rhinol.
- g) Experiences on infections in the corpse.
  Erfahrungen über Infektionen an der Leiche. Dtsche Ärzte-Ztg., Berl. II: 500–503; 526–528.
- h) A case presentation on the calcification of the cerebral vessels.
  Ein casuistischer Beitrag zur Verkalkung der Hirngefässe. Verhandl. d. Dtsch. path. Gesellsch., 2 Tag., München, 1899, Berl., 1900, 399–404.
- i) Report on five years at the Pathological-Anatomical Institute of the Friedrichshain Hospital. *Berichte über die 5 Jährige Tätigkeit in der pathol.-anat. Anstalt des Krankenhauses Friedrichshain.* Verlag B. Schuhmacher, Berlin.

- **j)** On selected cellular pathology and their role in forming the basis of organ-therapy.
  Einige Zellprobleme und ihre Bedeutung für die wissenschaftliche Begründung der Organtherapie. Verhandl. d. Gesellschaft dtsch. Naturf. u. Ärzte. Verlag Gg Reimer, Berlin.
- **k)** "Diseases originating from the habits and vices of everyday life".
  Die Krankheiten aus den Gewohnheiten und Missbräuchen des täglichen Lebens. 6 populäre Vorträge. G. Reimer, Berlin.
- **l)** (with Japha). A case of polyarthritis rheumatica (Discussion)
  Ein Fall von Polyarthritis rheumatica. Berl. klin. Wschr. 37: 1161.
- **m)** On Victor von Ebner's doubts concerning the existence of regular pores between alveoli.
  Über Victor von Ebner's Zweifel an der Existenz normaler Poren zwischen den Lungenalveolen. Arch. f. mikr. Anat., Bonn, 60: 337–341. See 1899h
- **n)** Contributions to the knowledge of rickets.
  Beiträge zur Lehre von der Rachitis. Berl. klin. Wschr. XXXVII, 1244 – [Discussion].

1901 a) On the pathological anatomy and histology of carinomas.
  Ueber pathol. Anatomie und Histologie des Carcinoms. Dtsche med Wschr
- **b)** On renal tumours.
  Über Nierengeschwülste. Zschr f. klin. Med.
- **c)** The zoology of intestinal parasites.
  Die Zoologie der Darmparasiten. Ewalds Klin. 111.
- **d)** Investigation of the hibernation organ.
  Untersuchungen über das Winterschlaforgan. Verhandl. d. Physiol, Gesellschaft.
- **e)** On pulmonary syphilis.
  Über Lungensyphylis. Verhandl. d. XIX Kongr. Innere Med.
- **f)** The microscope and advances in histopathological diagnosis.
  Das Mikroskop und die Fortschritte der histologischen Diagnostik. Ausbau i. d. diag. Appar. d. klin. Med., Wiesb., 3–13 11 Abb.
- **g)** "Rickets of the Skull".
  Die Rachitis des Schädels. August Hirschwald, Berlin.
- **h)** Contribution to the prognosis of brain diseases in childhood
  Beitrag zur Prognose der Gehirnkrankheiten im Kindesalter. Berl. klin. Wschr. 38: 177. (Discussion).
- **i)** Contributions to the knowledge of rickets.
  Beiträge zur Lehre von der Rachitis. Berl. klin. Wschr. 38: 85–86.
- **j)** Diseases originating from the habits and vices of everyday life
  Die Krankenhaften aus den Gewohenheiten und Missbräuchen des täglichen Lebens. (Lectures given in October and November 1899). 2nd edn. G. Reimer, Berlin.

1902 a) On parasitic aetiology of cancer.
  Über die parasitäre Ätiologie des Carcinoms. Dtsch. Med.Wschr.
- **b)** On cure and curability of pulmonary tuberculosis.
  Über Heilung und Heilbarkeit der Lungenphthise. Berl. klin. Wschr.
- **c)** True and false diaphragmatic hernias.
  Echte und unechte Zwerchfellhernien. Berl. klin. Wschr.
- **f)** A case of true nanosomia (dwarfism, eds).
  Echte Nanosomie mit Demonstration eines Falles. Berl. klin. Wschr. 39: 1209–1212.

Appendix D: Bibliography of David Paul von Hansemann

- **g)** On the structure and essential meaning of vascular islands of the pancreas.
  Über die Struktur und das Wesen der Gefässinseln des Pankreas. Verhandl. d. D. P. Gesellschaft
- **h)** "The Microscopic Diagnosis of Malignant Tumours (2nd edn)". (Summary in chapter 12).
  Die Mikroskopische Diagnose der bösartigen Geschwülste. A Hirschwald, Berlin. 2nd edn.
- **i)** in the Zeitschr f klin Med, 44

1903 a) Malakoplakia of the urinary bladder.
  Über Malakoplakie der Harnblase. Virchow's Arch. 173: 302–308.
- **b)** On tuberculosis acquired from food. [discussion]
  Über Fütterungstuberculose. Berl. klin. Wschr., 40: 141; 170.
- **c)** Discussion of same (no details given)
- **d)** A skull with bilateral temporo-mandibular joint ankylosis.
  Über einen Schädel mit doppelseitiger Kieferankylose. Berl. klin. Wschr. 40: 633–635.
- **e)** General diagnostic microscopy.
  Die mikroscopische Diagnostik (allgemeines). Lehrb. d., klin. Untersuchungensmethoden
- **f)** The diagnostic microscopy of faeces.
  Die mikroskopischen Untersuchungen Faeces. Lehrb. d. klin. Untersuchungensmethoden
- **g)** The anatomical basis of the dispositions.
  Die anatomischen Grundlagen der Dispositionen. Die Dtsch Klinik.
- **h)** Acid fast bacilli in *Python veticularis.*
  Über säurefeste Bacillen bei Python veticularis. Centralbl. f. Bakteriol. [etc.], 1. Abt., Jena, 34: 212.
- **i)** The anatomy of the laryngeal polyps.
  Die Anatomie der Kehlkopfpolypen. Therap. Monatsh., Berl. 17: 607–611.
- **j)** Studies of the aetiology of epityphylitis (appendicitis – eds).
  Ätiologische Studien über die Epityphlitis. Mitt. a. d. Grenzgeb. d. Med. u. Chir., Jena, 12: 514–531.
- **k)** Miliary tuberculosis of the lungs.
  Über die Miliartuberkulose der Lungen. Verhandl. d. deutsch. path. Gesellsch., Jena, 15: 224–230.
- **l)** (Index Medicus announces a new journal)
  Zeitschrift für Krebsforschung; in Verbindung mit dem klinischen Jahrbuch. Im Auftrage des Comités für Krebsforschung hrsg. von E. von Leyden, M. Kirchner, Dr. Wutzdorff. Redigiert von Prof. von (und) Georg Meyer. v. 1. Jena, 8°.
- **m)** Rickets in non-human primates.
  Über die Rachitis der Affen. Virchow's Arch. 172: 174–178.

1904 a) Multiple primary malignant tumours simultaneously occurring in one individual.
  Das gleichzeitige Vorkommen verschiedenartiger Geschwülste bei derselben Person. Ztschr. f. Krebsforsch., Jena, 1904, i, 183–198.
- **b)** Multiple primary malignant tumours simultaneously occurring in one individual. *Über das gleichzeitige Vorkommen mehrerer primärer Geschwülste bei einem Individuum.* Dtsche med Wschr., Leipz. u. Berl., 30: 119.
- **c)** On nuclear division in malignant tumours. (Complete translation in chapter 12).
  Über Kernteilung in bösartigen Geschwüsten. Biol. Zbl. 24: 189–192.

- **d)** A case of chorion epithelioma in a male patient.
  Fall von Chorionepitheliom beim Manne. Ztschr. f. Geburtsh. u. Gynäk., Stuttg. 51: 400–405.
- **e)** The size of nodules in acute miliary and chronic miliary tuberculosis.
  Die Grösse der Knoten bei akuter und chronischer Miliartuberkulose. Centralbl. f. allg. Path. u. path. Anat., Jena, 15: 257–261.
- **f)** The importance of pathological anatomy in medical teaching and for the general practitioner.
  Die Bedeutung der pathol. Anatomie für den med. Unterricht und den prakt Arzt. Zschr. f. ärztl. Fortbild.
- **g)** Skull pathology in rickets.
  Über die rachitischen Veränderungen des Schädels. Ztschr. f. Ethnol. Berl., 36: 373–383.
- **h)** Appraisal of ancient Patagonian, allegedly syphilitic bones from the Museum at La Plata.
  Beurteilung altpatagonischer, angeblich syphilitischer Knochen aus dem Museum zu La Plata. Zschr. f. Ethnologie.
- **i)** Demonstration of an abnormal rat skull.
  Demonstration über abnormen Rattenschädel. Verhandl. d. Physiol. Gesellschaft. (December 1903).
- **j)** On the influence of pathological processes on mitosis.
  Über die Beeinflussung der Mitosen durch pathol. Prozesse. Verhandl. d. Physiol. Gesellschaft.
- **k)** Demonstration of a few rare specimens.
  Demonstration einiger seltener Präparate. Verhandl. d. D. P. Gesellschaft.
- **l)** Addendum to the previous article on medical studies and quackery.
  Zusatz zu vorstehendem Artikel über med. Studium u. Kurpfuscherei. Zschr. f. ärztl Fortbild.
- **m)** Obituary Rudolf Virchow.
  Virchow, Rudolf, Nachruf. (no details given).
- **n)** "The human skeleton. A brief overview for non-doctors participating in archaeological excavations".
  Das menschliche Skelett. Eine kurze Zusammenstellung für Nichtmediziner zum Gebrauch bei Ausgrabungen. A. Hirschwald, Berlin. 14 p., 6 pl. 8°.
- **o)** On abnormal rat skulls.
  Über abnorme Rattenschädel. Arch. f. Anat. u. Entwcklngsgesch., Leipz., 376.
- **p)** Perforation of an aortic aneurysm through an oesophageal carcinoma.
  Durchbruch eines Aortenaneurysma in einen Oesophaguskrebs. Berl. klin. Wschr. 41: 860.
- **q)** Malignant growths and normal reproductive tissues. (Reprinted in Chapter 12). Lancet, Lond., 1904, i, 251.

1905 a) What do we know about the origin of malignant tumours?
Was wissen wir über die Ursache der bösartigen Geschwülste? Berl. klin. Wschr. 42: 313; 361.
- **b)** Closing speech of the sitting of the Berlin Medical Society.
  Schlusswort auf der Sitzung der Berliner Med. Gesellschaft. Berl. klin. Wschr.
- **c)** The functional capacity of tumour cells; comments on Beneke's dissertation on physiological and pathological growth. (Complete translation in chapter 12).
  Über die funktionellen Leistungen der Geschwulstzellen; eine Diskussionsbemerkung zu Beneke's Aufsatz über physiologisches and pathologisches Wachstum. Berl. klin. Wschr. 42: 1379.

d) Thyroid gland and thymus in Basedow's disease.
Schilddrüse und Thymus bei der Basedow'schen Krankheit. Berl. klin. Wschr. 42: Fest.-Num., 65.

e) The relationships of certain sarcomata to angiomata.
Die Beziehung gewisser Sarkome zu den Angiomen. Ztschr. f. Krebsforsch., Berl. 3: 234–246.

f) Critical contemplations of tumour theory. (Summary and comments in chapter 12).
Kritische Betrachtungen zur Geschwulstlehre. Ztschr f. Krebsforsch., Berl. 3: 560–578.

g) Comments on the alleged heterotypical nature of cell divisions in malignant tumours. *Einige Bemerkungen über die angeblich heterotypen Zellteilungen in bösartigen Geschwülsten.* Biol. Centralbl., Leipz. 25: 151–156.

h) First ever report of yeast-induced brain disease.
Über eine bisher nicht beobachtete Gehirnerkrankung durch Hefen. Verhandl d. deutsche path. Gesellsch. 1905, Jena, pp 21–24.

i) Syphylitic diseases of the cardiovascular system.
Syphylitische Erkrankungen des Zirculationsapparates. Verhandl. d. V. internatl. Dermatol. Kongr.

j) The significance of follicles in the appendix.
Die Bedeutung der Follikel im Processus vermiformis. Beitr. z. wissensch. Med. Festschr. f.. Georg Mayer, Berl. pp 91–100.

k) (with von Leyden) Talks on the aetiology of cancers. (Summary and comments in chapter 12).
Die Ätiologie der Krebse. Dtsche med. Wschr. 31: 430.

l) What do we know about the origin of malignant tumours? (Summary and comments in chapter 12).
Was wissen wir über die Ursache der bösartigen Geschwülste? Med. Bl., Wien. 18: 195–197.

m) "Superstition in medicine and its danger for health and life".
Der Aberglaube in der Medizin und seine Gefahr für Gesundheit und Leben. B. B. Teubner, Leipzig.

1906 a) Rickets, a disease affecting the community at large. Discussion xliii: 1201.
Über Rachitis als Volkskrankheit. Berl. klin. Wschr. 43: 249–254.

b) The influence of domestication on diseases of animals and man.
Der Einfluss der Domestikation auf die Krankheiten der Tiere und der Menschen. Wien. med. Presse, 47: 1130–1132. Also, (Abstr.): Berl. klin. Wschr. 43: 629.

c) The function of tumour cells. (Summary and comments in chapter 12).
Über die Funktion der Geschwulstzellen. Ztschr. f. Krebsforsch. 4: 565–577.

1907 a) Miscellaneous remarks concerning carcinoma of the epidermis.
Einige Bemerkungen über Epidermiscarcinom. Berl. klin. Wschr. 44: 723.

b) Observations on the narrowing of the upper thoracic aperture in relation to pulmonary tuberculosis.
Einige Bemerkungen über die Stenose der oberen Brustapertur und ihre Beziehung zur Lungenphthise. Berl. klin. Wschr., 1907, xliv, 844.

c) A few comments on the anaplasia of tumour cells. (Summary and comments in chapter 12).
Einige Bemerkungen über die Anaplasie der Geschwulstzellen. Ztschr. f. Krebsforsch. 5: 510–515.

- **d)** A case of symbiosis.
  Ein Fall von Symbiose. Sitzungsber. D. Gesellschaft Naturforsch. Freunde.
- **e)** "The brains of Th. Mommsen (Historian), R.W. Bunsen (Chemist) and A. von Menzel (Painter)".
  Ueber Gehirne von Th. Mommsen, Historiker, R.W. Bunsen, Chemiker und Ad. von Menzel, Maler. E. Nägele, Stuttg. 18 p. Forms Hft. 5 Abt. A. of: Biblioth. Med.
- **f)** A case of acute leukaemia.
  Fall akuter Leukämie. Berl. klin. Wschr. 44: 821–823.

1908 a) True megalencephaly.
  Über echte Megalencephalie. Berl. klin. Wschr. 45: 7–11.
- **b)** (with Sonnenburg & Krauss). Aetiology and pathogenesis of epityphlitis (appendicitis – eds).
  Ätiologie und Pathogenese der Epityphlitis. Dtsche med. Wschr., Leipz. u. Berl., 34: 769–772.
- **c)** Formative stimuli and sensitivity to stimuli.
  Formative Reize und Reizbarkeit. Ztschr. f. Krebsforsch., Berl., 1908, vii, 69–79.
- **d)** On the nomenclature of malignant epithelial neoplasms. (Summary and comments in chapter 12).
  Zur Bezeichnung der bösartigen epithelialen Neubildungen. Ztschr f. Krebsforsch. 7: 1.
- **e)** On the asymmetry of the surfaces of the atlanto-occipital joint.
  Über die Asymmetrie der Gelenkflächen des Hinterhaupts. Ztschr. f. Ethnol. 40: 994–997.
- **f)** On the brain of Hermann von Helmholtz.
  Über das Gehirn von Hermann v. Helmholtz. Zschr. f. Psychol. u. Physiol. d. Sinnesorgane.
- **g)** Is cancer catching?
  Ist Krebs ansteckend? (no details given).
- **h)** A case of lupus of the larynx cured by Cantharides.
  Über einen durch Canthariden geheilten Fall von Kehlkopflupus. Berl. klin. Wschr. 45: 1425.

1909 a) What is anaplasia? (Complete translation in chapter 12).
  Was ist Anaplasie? Berl. klin. Wschr. 46: 1850–1.
- **b)** Discussion remarks on a few tumour-related questions.
  Discussionsbemerkungen über einige Geschwulstefragen. Dtsch. Med. Wschr.
- **c)** A method of luxation of the skull at autopsy.
  Die Luxation des Schädels als Sektionsmethode. Centralbl. f. allg. Path. u. path. Anat., Jena, 20: 1.
- **d)** Investigation of cardiac muscle using ultraviolet light.
  Untersuchungen an der Herzmuskulatur im ultravioletten Licht. Verhandl. d. D. P. Gesellschaft.
- **e)** The importance of the mental ossicles for the formation of the chin.
  Die Bedeutung der Ossicula mentalia für die Kinnbildung. Ztschr. f. Ethnol., 41: 714–721.
- **f)** "Origin and Pathology". (Summary and comments in chapter 12).
  Deszendenz und Pathologie. A Hirschwald, Berlin.

1910 a) On macrobiotics.
  Über Makrobiotik. Berl. klin. Wschr. 47: 189–192.
- **b)** Hufeland and the Hufeland Society; Festschrift.
  Hufeland und die Hufelandische Gesellschaft; Festrede. Berl. klin. Wschr. 47: 243–248.

- c) Remarks on the technique of microscopy.
  Einige Bemerkungen zur mikroskopischen Technik. Berl. klin. Wschr. 47: 1766.
- d) Report of another case of osteoblastoma.
  Mitteilung eines weiteren Falles von Osteoblastom. Ztschr. f. Krebsforsch. 7: 529–532.
- e) A contribution to the histological pathogenesis of parotid tumours.
  Beitrag zur Histogenese der Parotistumoren. Ztschr. f. Krebsforsch. 9: 379–382.
- f) The anatomical basis for the indication of Freund's Thoracic operation.
  Die anatomische Grundlage für die Indikation der Freund'schen Thoraxoperationen. Arch. f. klin. Chir., Berl. 92: 988–998.
- g) Cancer phobia and the influence of the doctor on the cultural education of mankind.
  Die Krebsfurcht und der Einfluss des Arztes auf die kulturelle Erziehung des Menschen. Verhagen & Klasings Monathefte.
- h) Demonstration of a tooth from a *Caecharodonzahn* from Spitzbergen.
  Demonstration eines Caecharodonzahnes aus Spitzbergen. Sitzungsber. d. Gesellschaft Naturforsch. Freunde.
- i) Freedom of Science.
  Die Freiheit der Wissenschaft. Die Grenzboten.
- j) On the nomenclature of tumours.
  Über Benennung der Geschwülste. Conf. internat. pour l'etude du cancer.
- k) "Atlas of malignant tumours". (Summary and comments in chapter 12).
  Atlas der bösartigen Geschwülste. A. Hirschwald. Berlin.
- l) Pathological anatomy and diagnosis of cancer. (Summary and comments in chapter 12).
  Pathologische Anatomie und Diagnose des Krebses. Ztschr. f. Krebsforsch., Berl. 10: 34–41.
- m) The Berlin Medical Society and pathological anatomy.
  Die Berliner medzinische Gesellschaft und die pathologische Anatomie. Berl. klin. Wschr. 47: 1961.

1911 a) An unusual case of pulmonary syphilis.
  Ungewöhnlicher Fall von Lungensyphilis. Berl. klin. Wschr. 48: 67.
- b) Typical and atypical pulmonary tuberculosis.
  Über typische und atypische Lungenphthise. Berl. klin. Wschr. 48: 1–5.
- c) The quackery act and demonic illnesses.
  Kurpfuschereigesetz und dämonische Krankenheit. Berl. klin. Wschr.
- d) The fiendishness of ultramontanism against doctors.
  Über ärztefeindlichen Ultramontanismus. Berl klin. Wschr.
- e) A syphilitic skull from South America.
  Demonstration über einen syphilitischen Schädel aus Südamerika. Ztschr. f. Ethnol. 43: 128–130.
- f) Is there inheritance of acquired properties.
  Gibt es eine Vererbung erworbener Eigenschaften. Naturwiss. Wschr.
- g) The nomenclature of tumours.
  Über die Benennung der Geschwülste. Trav. de la 2. confér. internat. pour l'étude du cancer, Par., pp 574–585. [Discussion], 639–646.

- **h)** Communication on the development of crested chickens with special reference to the question of the inheritance of acquired somatic properties.
  Beitrag zur Entwicklung der Haubenhühner mit besonderer Berücksichtigung der Frage über die Vererbung somatische erworbener Eigenschaften. Sitzung d. Gesellschaft Naturforsch. Freunde.

- **i)** On abnormal *Lophiodon* tooth.
  Über einen abnormen Lophiodonzahn. Sitzung. d. Gesellschaft Naturforsch. Freunde.

- **j)** Hygiene and cancer.
  Hygiene und Krebs. Hygieia (Internat. Hygien. Ausstellung Dresden).

1912 a) (with von Wassermann A.) Experimental chemotherapy of animals with tumours. (Summary and comments in chapter 12).
Chemotherapeutische Versuche an tumorkranken Tieren. Berl. klin. Wschr. 49: 4–10.

- **b)** (with various other authors) Discussion (of Experimental chemotherapy of animals with tumours – eds). (Comments in chapter 12).
  Discussion. Berl. klin. Wschr. 49: 222–225.

- **c)** (with von Wassermann A.) Experimental chemotherapy of animals with tumours. (Comment in chapter 12).
  Chemotherapeutische Versuche an tumorkranken Tieren. 49: 2. Teil: 499–518.

- **d)** On altruistic illnesses. (Summary and comments in chapter 12).
  Über altruistische Erkrankungen. Berl. klin. Wschr. 49: 433–436.

- **e)** Changes of the pancreas in diabetes.
  Pankreasveränderungen bei Diabetes. Berl. klin. Wschr.

- **f)** "On the Conditional Thinking in Medicine and its Significance on Practice". (Summary and comments in chapter 12).
  Über das konditionale Denken in der Medizin und seine Bedeutung für die Praxis. A. Hirschwald, Berlin.

- **g)** Comments on the lecture: transplantation of experimentally-induced atypical epithelial proliferations.
  Bemerkungen über einen Vortrag: Transplantationen experimentell erzeugter atypischer Epithelwucherungen. Zschr. f. Krebsforsch.

- **h)** General constitution as the basis of disease.
  Die Konstitution als Grundlage von Krankheiten. Med. Klin., Berl., 8: 933–938.

- **i)** Brief comments on Leydig's interstitial cells of the testis.
  Kurze Bemerkungen über die Leydigschen Zwischenzellen des Hodens. Arch. f. Entwcklngsmechn. d. Organ., Leipz., 34: 475.

- **j)** On the battle of the eggs in the ovaries.
  Über den Kampf der Eier in den Ovarien. Arch. f. Entwcklngsmechn. d. Organ., Leipz., 35: 223–235.

- **k)** Changes in the pancreas in diabetes mellitus.
  Pankreasveränderungen bei Diabetes. Verhandl. d. Berl. med. Gesellsch 43: 2. Teil, 184–193. [Discussion], 1. Teil, 135.

- **l)** Changes in the pancreas in diabetes mellitus.
  Pankreasveränderungen bei Diabetes. Dtsche med. Wschr., Leipz. u. Berl., 38: 729.

1913 a) On the dissolvability of gall stones.
Die Lösungsmöglichkeit der Gallensteine. Virchow's Arch. 222: 139–152.

- **b)** On the nomenclature of tumours.
  Über die Benennung der Geschwülste. Ztschr. f. Krebsforsch. 13: 1–11.
- **c)** Comments on the article of Hess.
  Bemerkungen zu Artikel Hess. Dtsch med. Wschr.
- **d)** The inheritance of disease.
  Die Vererbung von Krankheit. Arch. f. Soziale Hygiene
- **e)** Precancerous states. (Summary and comments in chapter 12).
  Über präkanzeröse Krankheiten. Ztschr. f. Geburtsh. u. Gynäk., Stuttg. 74: 149–160.
- **f)** Chapter, carcinoma, sarcoma, endothelioma etc.
  Kapitel Carcinom, Sarkom, Endotheliom etc. Real-Encyclopädie d. ges. Heilkunde, 4. Aufl.
- **g)** Demonstration of slides generated by Mr Fibiger on the artificial induction of cancer. (Summary and comments in chapter 12).
  Demonstration von Präparaten des Herrn Fibiger zur künstlichen Erzeugung von Krebs. Berl. klin. Wschr, (I), 998.

1914 a) A working hypothesis for the research of leukaemia. (Summary and comments in chapter 12).
  Eine Arbeitshypothese für die Erforschung der Leukämie. Berl. klin. Wschr. 51: 9.
- **b)** Changes in tissues and tumours following radiotherapy. (Summary and comments in chapter 12).
  Über Veränderungen der Gewebe und der Geschwülste nach Strahlenbehandlung. Berl. klin. Wschr., 51: 1064.
- **c)** The incidence of tumours in the tropics.
  Ueber das Vorkommen von Geschwülsten in den Tropen. Ztschr. f. Krebsforsch., Berl., 14: 39–45.
- **d)** On the cancer problem. (Summary and comments in chapter 12).
  Über Krebsprobleme. Dtsche med. Wschr. 40: 1753–1756.
- **e)** On senescence in the *Bacillus Rosii*.
  Über Alterserscheinungen bei Bac. Rosii. Sitzungsber d. Gesellschaft Naturforsch. Freunde.
- **f)** Myxoglobulosis of the appendix.
  Über die Myxoglobulose des Wurmfortsatzes. Verhandl. d. dtsch. path. Gesellsch., Jena, 17: 568–573.
- **g)** Immaturity as a prerequisite for disease.
  Infantilismus als Bedingung für Krankheiten. Ztschr. f. ärztl. Fortbild., Jena, 11: 449–453.
- **h)** "Superstitions in Medicine and their dangers for health and life". (2nd edn).
  Der Aberglaube in der Medizin und seine Gefahr fuer Gesundheit und Leben. Aus Natur und Geisteswelt.
- **i)** Cancer treatments in theory and practice. (Summary and comments in chapter 12).
  Krebsheilmittel in Theorie und Praxis. Ztschr. f. Krebsforsch., Berl. 14:139–150.

1915 a) Chronic pulmonary lymphangitis is a separate disease entity.
  Die Lymphangitis reticularis der Lungen als selbständige Erkrankung. Virchow's Arch. 221: 311–321.
- **b)** Callus formation after bony injuries.
  Ueber die Callusbildung nach Knochenverletzungen. Berl. klin. Wschr. 52: 151.

- c) Lung respiration of the tortoise/turtle.
  Die Lungenatmung der Schildkröten. Sitzungsber. d. Akad. d. Wiss.
- d) Callus formation after bony injuries.
  Kallusbildung nach Knochenverletzungen. Dtsche med. Wschr., Leipz. u. Berl., 41(sic): 175.
- e) Demonstration of an anatomical specimen of total duodenal atresia.
  Demonstration eines Präparates von totaler Atresie des Duodenums. Berl. klin. Wschr., 52: 986.
- f) General reflections on pathogenesis of disease with special emphasis on emphysema of the lung.
  Allgemeine ätiologische Betrachtungen mit besonderer Berücksichtigung des Lungenemphysems. Virchow's Arch. 221(sic): 94–106.
- g) Chronic pulmonary lymphangitis is a separate disease entity.
  Über die Lymphangitis chronica pulmonis als selbständige Krankheit. Berl. klin. Wschr. 52: 987.

1916 a) General reflections on pathogenesis of disease with special emphasis on emphysema of the lung.
  Allgemeine ätiologische Betrachtungen mit besonderer Berücksichtigung des Lungenemphysems. Virchow's Arch. 221. (this reference is the same as listed by Index Medicus for 1915f)
- b) Interstitial emphysema of the thymus as a cause of death.
  Interstitielles Emphysem der Thymusdrüse als Todesursache. Virchow's Arch. 222:
- c) The role of anatomical diagnosis of dysentery/shigellosis.
  Über die Bedeutung der anatomischen Diagnose der Ruhr. Berl. klin. Wschr. 53: 1185–1187.
- d) Does war influence the development or the proliferation of tumours?
  Beeinflusst der Krieg die Entstehung oder das Wachstum von Geschwülsten? Berl. klin. Wschr. Xiii (sic), 265.
- e) Remarks on the relationship of non-autogenicity to transplantation.
  Bemerkungen über die Beziehungen der Bastardierung zur Transplantation. Arch. f. Entwicklungsgesch. der Organismen.
- f) Does war influence the development or the proliferation of tumours?
  Beeinflusst der Krieg die Entstehung oder das Wachstum von Geschwülsten? Med. Klin., Berl. 12: 278.
- g) Does war influence the development or the proliferation of tumours?
  Beeinflusst der Krieg die Entstehung oder das Wachstum von Geschwülsten? Ztschr. f. Krebsforsch., Berl. 14: 492–516.

1917 a) On pneumocephalus.
  Über Pneumocephalus. Virchow's Arch. 224
- b) On the phenomenon of convergence.
  Über Konvergenzerscheinungen. Berl. klin. Wschr.
- c) Perforation of the lamina cribrosa by pressurized air.
  Die Perforation der Lamina cribrosa durch Luftdruck. Berl. klin. Wschr. 54: 430.
- d) Purulent meningitis after head injury.
  Eitrige Meningitis nach Kopfverletzungen. Berl. klin. Wschr. 54: 741–743.
- e) On the so-called: 'long Russian bowel' disease.
  Über den sogenannten langen russischen Darm. Med. Klin. Berl. 13: 957–959.

| | **f)** | The predisposition of the adrenal gland to tuberculosis.
Die Disposition der Nebennieren zur Tuberculose. Zschr. f. Tuberkulose. |
|-------|--------|---|

1918 a) Streptomycosis, Staphylomycosis and Diplomykosis as war-related illnesses.
Strepto-, Staphylo- und Diplomykosen als Kriegskrankheit. Med. Klin., Berl. 14: 531–534.

    b) Freund (Wilhelm Alexander). [–1917.] München. med. Wschr., 65: 190.

    c) Cases of influenza from the epidemic in the last century.
Grippefälle aus der Epidemie im vorigen Jahrhundert. Med. Klin., Berl. 14: 824.

1919 a) Acute leukaemia.
Akute Leukämie. Med. Klin., Berl. 15: 5.

    b) Hypoplasia of the heart and vessels.
Über die Hypoplasie des Herzens und der Gefässe. Med. Klin., Berl. 15: 57–60.

1920 a) The problem of cancer. (Summary and comments in chapter 12).
Das Problem der Krebsmalignität. Ztschr. f. Krebsforsch. 1919–20, 17: 172–191.

    b) On the concept of inflammation with special reference to the fatty degeneration and the cloudy swelling.
Über den Entzündungsbegriff mit besonderer Berücksichtigung der trüben Schwellung und der fettigen Degeneration. Med. Klin., Berl. 16: 247–253.

1921 a) Has war influenced the development of malignant tumours?
Hat der Krieg die Entstehung bösartiger Geschwülste beeinflusst? Handb. d. ärztl. Erfahr. im Weltkr., Leipz. 8: 53–56.

Literature cited

N.b. Each citation of a work in a language other than English starts with our translation of its title, which is followed by the title in the original language, and the citation ends stating the language of the original work.

Citations of previously-published translations of works in languages other than English, start with the English-language title but do not necessarily include the title of the original work which was translated. This is because many of these "English translations" are not verbatim translations of original texts, but "English versions" or even "English adaptations" of original texts.

Ackerknecht E. (1953) "Rudolf Virchow, Doctor, Statesman, Anthropologist". University of Wisconsin Press, Madison, Wisconsin.
Adami J.G. (1908) "Principles of Pathology". vol. 1. Lea and Febiger, Philadelphia.
Adam C. and Tannery P. (eds) (1996) "Works of Descartes" / *Oeuvres de Descartes* Reprinted by Librarie Philosophique, J Vrin, Paris. (In French).
Adams F. (1849) "The Genuine Works of Hippocrates". Translated from the Greek, with a preliminary discourse and annotations, by F. Adams. Sydenham Society, London.
Alison M.R., Poulsom R., Forbes S. and Wright N.A. (2002) An introduction to stem cells. J. Pathol. 197: 419–23.
Allbutt T.C. (1921) "Greek Medicine in Rome". Macmillan, London.
Allen G.E. (1975) "Life Science in the Twentieth century". Wiley, New York.
Andral G. (1836) "Dictionary of Medicine and Practical Surgery" / *Dictionnaire de medecine et de chirurgie pratiques*. Vols 1–15. Gabon, Paris. (In French).
Andree C. (2002) "Rudolph Virchow: Life and Ethos of a Great Doctor" / *Rudolf Virchow: Leben und Ethos eines grossen Arztes*. Langen Müller, München. (In German).
Andreski S. (ed) (1972) "Herbert Spencer: Structure, Function and Evolution". With an introductory essay by Stanislav Andreski. Nelson, London.
Anon (1902) Proceedings of the Committee for Cancer Research (15th May 1902) / *Verhandlungen des Comités für Krebsforschung, Deutsche Medicinische Wochenschrift 1902, 15 Mai*. The document is a supplement (*Vereinsbeilage*) attached to the collection of original papers, together with the "Literature Supplement"(*Literatursupplement*) at the end of the volume of this journal. The meeting was on 21st March 1902, and recorded a controversy about parasitic, Hansemann's and other theories of cancer.
Anon (1927) John George Adami 1862–1926. J. Pathol. Bacteriol. 30: 151–166.
Anon (1980) Rupert Allan Willis. Lancet i: 940.
Arnold J. (1879) Observations on nuclear divisions in the cells of tumours / *Beobachtungen über Kerntheilungen in den Zellen der Geschwülste*. Virchow's Arch. 78: 279–301. (In German).
Attwood H.D. (1980) Rupert Willis. Am. J. Surg. Pathol. 4:511–516.
Audi R. (1999) "Dictionary of Philosophy". 2nd edn, Cambridge University Press, Cambridge, UK.
Austoker J. (1988) "A History of the Imperial Cancer Research Fund 1902–1986". Oxford University Press, Oxford, UK.
Baltzer F. (1967) "Theodor Boveri, Life and Work of a Great Biologist, 1862–1915". Translated by Dorothea Rudnick. University of California Press, Berkley, CA.

Barnes J. (2003) Argument in ancient philosophy. In "Cambridge Companion to Greek and Roman Philosophy". Sedley D.N. (ed) Cambridge University Press, Cambridge, U.K., pp 20–41.

Barnes J. (ed) (2005) "Cambridge Companion to Aristotle". Cambridge University Press, Cambridge, U.K.

Barr A.P. (ed) (1997) "Thomas Henry Huxley's place in science and letters: centenary essays". University of Georgia Press, Athens, Georgia, U.S.A.

Bashford E.F. (1905) Hypotheses explanatory of the nature and origin of cancer reviewed in the light of the results of experimental study. Sci. Rpts on Invest. of the Imp. Cancer Res. Fund, no. 2, Taylor and Francis, London, pp 69–96.

Bashford E.F. (1908) On the occurrence of heterotypical mitoses in cancer. Sci. Rpts on Invest. of the Imp. Cancer Res. Fund, no. 3, Taylor and Francis, London, pp 61–68. (Reprinted from Proc. R. Soc. Lond., B. vol. 77, 1906)

Bauer K.H. (1928) "Mutation Theory in Tumour formation" / *Mutationstheorie der Geschwülst-Entstehung*. Julius Springer, Berlin. (In German).

Bauer K.H. (1949) "The Cancer Problem"/ *Das Krebsproblem*. Springer, Berlin. (2nd edn 1963). (In German).

Beattie J.M. and Dickson W.E.C. (1921). "A Text-book of General Pathology". Heinemann (Medical Books) 2nd edn, London.

Beneke R. (1900) A case of osteo-chondrosarcoma of the bladder, with remarks on metaplasia / *Ein Fall von Osteoid-Chondrosarcom der Harnblase, mit Bemerkungen über Metaplasie*. Virchow's Arch. 161: 70–114.

Bennett J.H. (1849) "On Cancerous and Cancroid Growths". Sutherland and Knox, Edinburgh.

Berenblum I. (1964) The nature of tumour growth. In "General Pathology". Ed. H.W. Florey. Lloyd-Luke Medical Books, London, pp 543–4.

Berenblum I. (1974) "Carcinogenesis as a biological problem". Frontiers of Biology, vol. 34. North-Holland, Amsterdam, pp 275–321.

Bergmann E. v. (1906) Inaugural address at the opening of the Empress-Friedrich House for Medical Further Education / *Festrede bei der Eröffnung des Kaiserin Friedrich-Hauses für das ärztl. Fortbildungswesen*. Z. f. Ärztliche Fortbildung. Issue of 1st March 1906: 129–142. (In German).

Bett W.R. (1955) Sir John Bland-Sutton, Bart.: 1855–1936. Nature 175: 660–661.

Bibel D.M. (1982) Centennial of the rise of cellular immunology: Metchnikoff's discovery at Messina. ASM News 48:558–560.

Bignold L.P. (2002) The mutator phenotype/clonal selection hypothesis can provide a basis for the complex and variable morphological and behavioural features of solid tumour malignancies. Cell. Molec. Life Sci. 59: 950–958.

Bignold L.P. (2003a) The mutator phenotype theory of carcinogenesis and the complex histopathology of tumours: support for the theory from the independent occurrence of nuclear abnormality, loss of specialisation and invasiveness among occasional neoplastic lesions. Cell. Molec. Life Sci. 60: 883–891.

Bignold L.P. (2003b) Pathogenetic mechanisms of nuclear pleomorphism of tumour cells based on the mutator phenotype theory of carcinogenesis. Histol. Histopathol. 18: 657–664.

Bignold L.P. (2003c) Initiation of genetic instability and tumour formation: a review and hypothesis of a nongenotoxic mechanism. Cell. Molec. Life Sci. 60: 1107–1117.

Bignold L.P. (2004) Chaotic genomes make chaotic cells: the mutator phenotype theory of carcinogenesis applied to clinicopathological relationships of solid tumors. Cancer Invest. 22: 338–343.

Bignold L.P. (2005) Embryonic reversions and lineage infidelities in tumour cells: genome-based models and role of genetic instability. Internat. J. Exp. Path. 86:67–79.

Bignold L.P. (2006) Alkylating agents and DNA polymerases. Anticancer Res. 26 (2B): 1327–1336.

Bignold L.P., Coghlan B.L.D. and Jersmann H.P.A. (2006a) Cancer: Cell structures, carcinogens and genetic instability – a background. In "Cancer, Cell Structures, Carcinogens and Genetic Instability." Ed L.P. Bignold, (EXS vol. 96) 1–24. Birkhäuser, Basel, Switzerland.

Literature cited

Bignold L.P., Coghlan B.L.D. and Jersmann H.P.A. (2006b) Hansemann, Boveri, chromosomes and the gametogenesis-related theories of tumours. Cell. Biol. Int. 30: 640–644.
Billroth T. (1924) "Medical Sciences in the German Universities". (Translator not stated). Macmillan, New York.
Bizzozero G. (1894) Growth and Regeneration of the Organism. Lancet i: 728–732.
Bland-Sutton J. (1906) "Tumours Innocent and Malignant". Cassell, London.
Bölsche W. (1906) "Haeckel, his Life and Work". Translation and Introduction by J. McCabe. T.F. Unwin, London.
Bonner T.N. (1963) "American Doctors and German Universities". University of Nebraska Press, Lincoln, Nebraska.
Borst M. (1902) "Textbook of Tumours with a Microscopical Atlas" (2nd edn) / *Die Lehre von den Geschwülsten mit einem Microscopischen Atlas*. J.F. von Bergmann, Weisbaden. (In German).
Borst M. (1923) True Tumours / *Echte Geschwülste (Blastome)*. In Ashoff L. (ed) *Pathologische Anatomie* / "Pathological Anatomy". 6th edn, vol. 1, Gustav Fischer, Jena. (In German).
Boveri T. (1902) On multipolar mitosis as a means of analysis of the cell nucleus. In: "Foundations of Experimental Embryology". Hafner Press, New York, 1974, pp 74–97. Originally published as *Über mephrolige Mitosen* etc. Verhandl. Physik.-medzinische Gesellschaft zu Würzburg. Neue Folge 35: 67–90.
Boveri T. (1914) "On the Question of the Origin of Malignant Tumours" / *Zur Frage der Entstehung der Malignen Tumoren*. G. Fischer, Jena. Translated by M. Boveri, and published as "Origin of Malignant Tumors", 1929, Williams and Wilkins, Baltimore, MD.
Bowler P. (1983) "The Eclipse of Darwinism". The Johns Hopkins University Press, Baltimore, MD.
Boyesen H.H. (1879) The University of Berlin. A brief history. Scribner's Monthly, New York. 18: 205–217.
Boylan M. (1983) "Methods and Practice in Aristotle's Biology". University Press of America, Washington DC.
Bracegirdle B. (1978) "A History of Microtechnique". Cornell University Press, Ithaca, NY.
Bradbury S. (1967) "The Evolution of the Microscope". Permagon Press, Oxford.
Bringmann W.G., Lück H.E., Miller R. and Early C.E. (eds) (1997) "A Pictorial History of Psychology". Quintessence Publishing Co, Carol Stream, IL.
Broman T.H. (1996) "The Transformation of German Academic Medicine 1750–1820". Cambridge University Press, Cambridge, p. 169.
Brophy J.M. (1998) "Capitalism, Politics, and Railroads in Prussia, 1830–1870". Ohio State University Press, Columbus, Ohio.
Browne E.J. (2002) "Charles Darwin". Johnathon Cape, London.
Bruford W.H. (1975) "The German Tradition of Self Cultivation: *Bildung* from Humboldt to Thomas Mann". Cambridge University Press, Cambridge.
Bryant C.G.A. (1985) "Positivism in Social Theory and Research". Houndmills, Hampshire; Macmillan, London.
Büchner T. et al. (ed) (1985) "Tumor Aneuploidy". Springer-Verlag, Berlin and New York.
Buchwald J.Z. (ed) (1996) "Scientific Credibility and Technical Standards in 19th and Early 20th Century Germany and Britain". Springer, Berlin.
Burdette W.J. (1955) The significance of mutation in relation to the origin of tumors. A review. Cancer Res. 15: 201–226.
Byers J.M. (1989) Rudolph Virchow – Father of Cellular Pathology. Amer. J. Clin Pathol. 92: (suppl. 4): S2–8.
Cameron R. (1952). "Pathology of the Cell". Oliver and Boyd, Edinburgh.
Carlson E.A. (2004) "Mendel's Legacy: the Origin of Classical Genetics". Cold Spring Harbor Laboratory Press, Cold Spring Harbor, NY.
Carpenter W.B. (1891) "The Microscope and its Revelations". 7th edn, J. & A. Churchill, London.

Carter R.B. (1983) "Descartes' Medical Philosophy. The Organic Solution to the Mind-Body Problem". The Johns Hopkins University Press, Baltimore, MD.
Carter K.C. (2001) Edwin Klebs' *Grundversuche*. Bull. Hist. Med. 75: 771–781.
Castedo M., Perfettini J.L., Roumier T., Andreau K., Medema R. and Kroemer G. (2004) Cell death by mitotic catastrophe: a molecular definition. Oncogene 23: 2825–2837.
Charle C. (2004) Patterns (chapter 2). In: "A History of the University in Europe". Ed. W. Rüegg, vol. 3, Cambridge University Press, Cambridge, pp 33–82.
Chauvois L. (1966) "Descartes. His Method and Errors of Physiology" / *Descartes. Sa Methode et ses Erreurs en Physiologie.* Editions du Cèdre, Paris. (In French).
Churchill F.B. (1991) The rise of classical descriptive embryology. In: "Developmental Biology, a Comprehensive Synthesis". Ed. S.F. Gilbert, vol. 7. Plenum Press, New York, pp 1–29.
Clapesattle H. (1941) "The Doctors Mayo". University of Minnesota Press, Minneapolis.
Clark C. and Kaiser W. (2003) "Culture Wars: Secular-Catholic Conflict in Nineteenth-Century Europe". Cambridge University Press, Cambridge.
Clark G. and Kasten F.H. (1983) "History of Staining". 3rd edn. Williams and Wilkins, Baltimore, MD.
Classen J. (1908) "Lectures on Modern Natural Philosophy" / *Vorlesungen über moderne Naturphilosophen (Du Bois-Reymond, F.A. Lange, Haeckel, Ostwald, Mach, Helmholtz, Boltzmann, Poincaré und Kant).* C. Boysen, Hamburg. (In German).
Cocks G. and Jarausch K.H. (eds) (1990) "German Professions 1800–1950". Oxford University Press, Oxford.
Cohnheim J. (1882) "Lectures in General Pathology". 2nd edn. Trans A.B. Mckee, 1889, New Sydenham Society, London, section II, pp 746–821.
Cornil R.V. (1886) On the process of indirect nuclear division in epithelial cells / *Sur le procédé de division indirecte des noyaux et des cellules épithéliales dans les tumeurs.* Arch. de physiol. normale et pathol. 8: 310–324. (In French)
Cornil R.V. and Ranvier L. (1882) "Manual of Pathological Histology" / *Manuel d'Histologie Pathologique.* 2nd edn. Translated by A. M. Hart, 1882–1886, Smith Elder, London.
Coser L.A. (1977) "Masters of Sociological Thought". 2nd edn, Harcourt Brace Jovanovich, New York.
Corsi P. (1988) "Lamarck, the founder of evolution: his life and work with translations of his writings on organic revolution". University of California Press, Berkley, CA.
Cottingham J. (1993) "A Descartes Dictionary". Blackwell, Oxford.
Cowdry E.V. (1940) The properties of cancer cells. Arch. Pathol. 30: 1245–1274.
Cremer T. (1985) "From Cell Teaching to Chromosome Theory" / *Von der Zellenlehre zur Chromosomentheorie.* Springer, Berlin. (In German).
Crowther J.G. (1960) "Founders of British science; John Wilkins, Robert Boyle, John Ray, Christopher Wren, Robert Hooke, Isaac Newton". Cresset Press, London.
Cruikshank W. (1790) "The Anatomy of the Absorbing Vessels of the Human Body". 2nd edn, G. Nicol, London. Fascimile edition, Gryphon Editions – Classics of Medicine Library, 1991, AL.
Dabritz W. (1954) "David Hansemann and Adolph von Hansemann: Men of the German Bank and of the Discount Society" / *David Hansemann und Adolph von Hansemann: Männer der Deutschen Bank und der Disconto-Gesellschaft.* Scherpe, Krefeld, Germany. (In German).
Daremberg C. (1870) "History of Medical Sciences" / *Histoire des Sciences Medicale.* J-B Baillière et fils, Paris. (In French).
Darwin C. (1872) "The Origin of Species by Means of Natural Selection, or, the Preservation of Favoured Races in the Struggle for Existence". 6th edn. Mentor Books – New American Library, 1958, New York and London.
Darwin C. (1868) "Variation of Plants and Animals under Domestication". John Murray, London.
Darwin E. (1796) "Zoonomia". J. Johnson, London.
David H. (1988) Rudolph Virchow and modern aspects of tumor pathology. Pathology Res. Pract. 183: 356–364.

Literature cited

Dematteis P.B. and Fosl P.S. (eds) (2002) "British Philosophers 1500–1799". Gale Group, Detroit.
Desmond A. and Moore J. (1992). "Darwin". Penguin, London. pp 538–40 ff.
Dobson J. (1959) John Hunter's views on cancer. Ann. Roy. Coll. Surg. Engl. 25: 176–181.
Dhom G. (2001) "History of Histopathology" / *Geschichte der Histopathologie*. Springer-Verlag, Berlin. (In German).
Dowd N. (ed) (1972) "Hunter's Lectures of Anatomy". Elsevier, Amsterdam.
Driesch H. (1914) "The History and Theory of Vitalism". Translated by C.K. Ogden. Macmillan, London.
Dunn L.C. (1962) "History of Genetics". McGraw-Hill, New York.
Encyclopaedia Britannica (1911) 11th edn, vol. 22, p. 373c.
Epstein C.J. (1986) "The Consequences of Chromosome Imbalance. Principles, Mechanisms, Models". Cambridge University Press, Cambridge.
Ewing J. (1909) Cancer Problems. Harvey Lectures given in 1907–8. Lipincott, Philadelphia.
Ewing J. (1940) "Neoplastic Diseases". 4th edn. W.B. Saunders, Philadelphia.
Farley J. (1982) "Gametes and Spores. Ideas about Sexual Reproduction 1750–1914". The Johns Hopkins University Press, Baltimore, MD.
Farmer J.B., Moore J.E.S. and Walker C.E. (1904) On the resemblances exhibited between the cells of malignant growths in man and those of normal reproductive tissues. Proc. R.Soc. (Lond). 72: 499–504.
Fidler I. (1997) Molecular biology of Cancer: invasion and metastasis. In: "Cancer: Principles and Practice of Oncology". 5th edn. Eds V.T. DeVita, S. Hellman and S.A. Rosenberg. Lippincott-Raven, Philadelphia. pp 135–152.
Fitzgerald P.J. (2000) "From Demons and Evil Spirits to Cancer Genes". Armed Forces Institute of Pathology, Washington DC.
Flemming W. (1878–9) New contributions to the knowledge of the cell and its life phenomena / *Neue Beiträge zur Kenntniss der Zelle und ihre Lebenserscheinungen*. Arch. f. Mikroscop. Anat. 16: 302–435. (In German).
Flemming W. (1880) New contributions to the knowledge of the cell and its life phenomena. Part II / *Neue Beiträge zur Kenntniss der Zelle und ihre Lebenserscheinungen, Theil II* Arch. f. Mikroscop. Anat. 18: 151–259. Translation by L. Piternick (1965), J cell Biol. 25: 1–69. (In German).
Flemming W. (1881) New contributions to the knowledge of the cell and its life phenomena Part III / *Neue Beiträge zur Kenntniss der Zelle und ihre Lebenserscheinungen, Theil III* Arch. f. Mikroscop. Anat. 20: 1–86. (In German).
Flemming W. (1887) New contributions to the knowledge of the cell / *Neue Beiträge zur Kenntniss der Zelle*. Arch. f. Mikroscop. Anat. 29: 89–463. (In German).
Flexner A. (1968) "Universities: American, English, German". With a new introduction by Clark Kerr. Oxford University Press, London. (Originally published 1930).
Forrester J.M. (1994) The homoeomerous parts and their replacement by Bichat's tissues. Med. Hist. 38: 444–458.
Foulds L. (vol. 1, 1969; vol. 2, 1975) "Neoplastic Development". Academic Press, London.
Garrison F.H., annotated by Morton L.T. (1970) "A Medical Bibliography a Check-list of Texts Illustrating the History of Medicine". Andre Deutsch, London.
Gasking E. (1967) "Investigations into Generation 1651–1828". Hutchinson, London.
Gay P. (1968) "Weimar Culture: the Outsider as Insider". Harper and Row, New York.
Gerson L.P. (ed) (1996) "The Cambridge Companion to Plotinus". Cambridge University Press, Cambrige.
Ghislein M.T. and Groeben C. (1997) Elias Metschnikoff, Anton Dohrn and the Metazoan Common Ancestor. J. Hist. Biol. 30: 211–228.
Gilbert S.F. (ed) (1994). "A Conceptual History of Modern Embryology". The Johns Hopkins University Press, Baltimore, MD.

Gilbert S.F. (ed) (2003) "Companion to Developmental Biology". 7th edn. Sinaeur and Assoc. Sutherland, MA.

Glass B., Temkin O. and Straus W.L. (eds) (1959) "Forerunners of Darwin 1745–1859". The Johns Hopkins University Press, Baltimore, MD.

Goodsir J. and Goodsir H.D.S. (1845) "Anatomical and Pathological Observations". Myles McPhail, Edinburgh.

Goodsir J. (1868) "The Anatomical Memoirs of Sir John Goodsir". Ed. W. Turner, with a biographical memoir by H. Lonsdale. A. & C. Black, Edinburgh.

Goschler C. (2002) "Rudolf Virchow: Doctor – Anthropologist – Politician" / *Rudolf Virchow: Mediziner – Anthropologe – Politiker*. Böhlau, Köln, pp 279–394. (In German).

Gotthelf A. and Lennox J.G. (1987) "Philosophical Issues in Aristotle's Biology". Cambridge University Press, Cambridge.

Gunther R.T. (1961). "Micrographia or, Some Physiological Descriptions of Minute Bodies made by Magnifying Glasses, with Observations and Inquiries Thereupon". By Robert Hooke, with a preface by R.T. Gunther. Fascimile edition. Dover Publications, New York.

Haeckel E. (1876) "History of Creation". Translated by E.R. Lankester. Henry S. King and Co, London.

Haeckel E. (1903) "The Confession of Faith of a Man of Science". Translated by J. Gilchrist. Black, London.

Haeckel E. (1907) "The Evolution of Man". Translated by J. McCabe. Watts and Co, London.

Haber F.C. (1959) Fossils and the idea of a process in time in natural history. In: "Forerunners of Darwin 1745–1859". Eds B. Glass, O. Temkin and W.L. Straus. The Johns Hopkins University Press, Baltimore, MD.

Haggard H.W. and Smith G.M. (1938) Johanes Müller and the modern conception of cancer. Yale J. Biol. Med. 10: 419–426.

Hahn H-J. (1998) "Education and Society in Germany". Oxford University Press, Berg.

Hall T.S. (1972) "Descartes, Treatise of Man". With French text and translations and commentary by T.S. Hall. Harvard University Press, Cambridge, MA.

Hall A.R. (1983) "The Revolution in Science, 1500–1750". 3rd edn. Longman, London.

Hansemann David Paul. All works by this author are listed in Appendix E

Harris H. (1995) "The Cells of the Body, A History of Somatic Cell Genetics". Cold Spring Harbor Laboratory Press, Cold Spring Harbor, NY.

Harris H. (1999) "The Birth of the Cell". Yale University Press, New Haven and London.

Harwood J. (1993) "Styles of Scientific Thought. The German Genetics Community 1900–1933". University of Chicago Press, Chicago and London.

Hauptmann S. and Schnalke T. (2001) Rudoph Virchow's view of malignant tumours / *Rudolph Virchows Sicht der malignen Geschwülste*. Pathologe 22: 291–295. (In German).

Hauser G. (1890) Cylindrical epithelial carcinoma of stomach and of the intestine / *Das Cylinderepithel-Carcinom des Magens und des Dickdarms*. Gustav Fisher, Jena. (In German).

Hauser G. (1903) What is the primary epithelial disorder leading to tumour formation? / *Giebt es eine primäre zur Geschwulstbildung führende Epithelerkrankung?* Beitr. z. Path. Anat. 33: 1–31. (In German).

Haviv Y.S. (1999) Figures in the historical dispute over renal function. Part I: from ancient times to the first microscopes. J. Med. Biogr. 7: 211–216.

Heilmann H.-P. (1996) Radiation Oncology: historical development in Germany. Int. J. Radiation Oncol. 35: 207–217.

Henderson W.O. (1984) "The *Zollverein*". 3rd ed. Cass, London.

Henle J. (1853) "A Treatise on General Pathology". Translated by H.C. Preston. Lindsay and Blakiston, Philadelphia.

Hertwig O. (1890) "Textbook of the Embryology of Man and Mammals". Translated by E.L. Mark, 1899, Swan Sonnenschein & Co, London.

Literature cited

Hertwig O. (1892) "The Cell. Outlines of General Anatomy and Physiology". Translated by M. Campbell, 1895, Swan Sonnenschein & Co, London

Hewson W. (1846) "The Works of William Hewson". Ed G. Gulliver. Sydenham Society, London.

Hochstadt S. (1999) "Mobility and Modernity: Migration in Germany 1820–1989". University of Michigan Press, Ann Arbor, MI.

Hodge J. and Radick G. (2003) "Cambridge Companion to Darwin". Cambridge University Press, Cambridge.

Hofmann J. (1981) "The Ministry of Camphausen-Hansemann. On the Politics of the Prussian bourgeoisie in the Revolution of 1848/9 / *Das Ministerium Camphausen-Hansemann. Zur Politik der preußischen Bourgeoisie in der Revolution 1848/49.* Akademie der Wissenschaften der DDR. Schriften des Zentralinstituts für Geschichte; 66), Berlin. (In German).

Home E. (1820) The Croonian Lecture: a farther investigation of the component parts of the blood. Phil. Trans R. Soc. Lond. 110: 1–10.

Horder T.J., Witkowski J.A. and Wylie C.C. (eds) (1986) "A History of Embryology: the Eighth Symposium of the British Society for Developmental Biology". Cambridge University Press, Cambridge.

Hossfeld U. and Olsson L (2003) The road from Haeckel: the Jena tradition in Evolutionary Morphology and the origins of "Evo-Devo". Biology and Philosophy 18: 285–307.

Hughes A.F.W. (1959) "A History of Cytology". Abelard-Schuman, London and New York.

Hun H. (1883) "A Guide to American Medical Students in Europe". William Wood and Co, New York.

Hunter J. (1794) "Experiments on the Blood, Inflammation and Gunshot wounds, in addition to News about the Life of the Author" / *Versuche ueber das Blut, die Entzündung und die Schusswunden, nebst einer Nachricht von dem Leben des Verfassers.* German edition, edited by Everard Home. Classics of Medicine Library, Gryphon Editions, Birmingham, AL, USA.

Hunter J. (1837) "Complete Works". Edited by J.F. Palmer, Sydenham Society, London.

Huvos A.G. (1998) James Ewing: cancer man. Ann. Diagn. Pathol. 2: 146–148.

Israel O. (1902) On Hansemann's anaplasia and the origin of malignant tumours, in particular of carcinoma / *Bermerkungen über die Anaplasie von Hansemann's und die Entstehung bösartiger Geschwülste, insbesondere des Carcinoms.* Virchow's Arch. 167: 533–537. (In German).

Israel O. (1903) Rudolf Virchow. Annual Report of the Smithsonian Institute for the Year 1902. Government Printing Office, Washington DC.

Jacyna L.S. (1983) John Goodsir and the making of cellular reality. J. Hist. Biol. 16: 75–99.

Jarausch K.H. (1982) "Students, Society and Politics in Imperial Germany. The Rise of Academic Illiberalism". Princeton University Press, NJ.

Kainz H.P. (1998) "G. W. F. Hegel: The Philosophical System". Ohio University Press, Athens, OH.

Kater M.H. (1998) "Book Review: Brain research in "Twilight": examples of seducible science from the National Socialist Period: Julius Hallervorden, H-J Scherer, Berthold Ostertag / *Hirnforschung im Zwielicht: Beispiele verführbarer Wissenschaft aus der Zeit des Nationalsozialismus: Julius Hallervorden, H.-J. Scherer, Berthold Ostertag*". Bull. Hist. Med. 72: 358–360.

King-Hele D.G. (1963) "Erasmus Darwin". Macmillan, London.

King-Hele D.G. (1983) Shelley and Erasmus Darwin. In: Ed K. Everest, "Shelley Revalued: Essays from the Gregynog Conference". Barnes and Noble, Totowa, NJ, pp 129–146,

Kirch E. (1937) Gustav Hauser 1856–1935. Verhandl. dtsche. pathol. Gesellschaft 29: 379–381.

Klebs E. (1889) "General Pathology" / *Allgemeine Pathologie.* vol. 2. G Fischer, Jena, pp 519–540.

Koller P.C. (1957) The genetic component of cancer. In: "Cancer". vol. 1, pp 335–403. Ed R.W. Raven. Butterworth & Co, London.

Kölliker A. (1853) "Manual of Human Histology". Translation of *Handbuch der Gewebelehre des Menschen* (1846) by G. Busk and T. Huxley. New Sydenham Soc, London.

Kreitsch P. (1990). The history of the Autopsy Department of the Berlin Charité hospital. 1. Founding of the Autopsy Department and Philipp Phoebus as the first prosector. Zentralbl. Allg. Pathol. 136: 377–387. (In German).

La Berge A. (1994) Medical Microscopy in Paris, 1830–1855. In: A La Berge and M Feingold (eds) "French Culture in the Nineteenth Century". (Wellcome Institute Series). Editions Rodopi BV, Amsterdam, pp 206–326.

Lebert H. (1851) "Practical Treatise of Cancerous Diseases and the Illnesses with which they can be Confused" / *Traité Pratique des Maladies Cancéreuse et des Affections Curables confondues avec le Cancer*. J.B. Ballière, Paris. (In French).

Lanceraux E. (1875) "Treatise of Pathological Anatomy. vol. 1. General Pathological Anatomy" / *Traité d'Anatomie Pathologique. vol. 1. Anatomie Pathologique Génèrale*. Adrien Delahaye, Paris. (In French).

Lee W.R. (ed) (1991) "German industry and German industrialisation: essays in German economic and business history in the nineteenth and twentieth centuries". Routledge, London and New York.

Levine M. (1931) Studies in the cytology of cancer. Am. J. Cancer 15: 144–211; 788–834; 1410–1494.

Lima-de-Faria A. (2003) "One Hundred Years of Chromosome Research, and What Remains To Be Learned". Kluwer, Dordrecht, The Netherlands.

Livesley B. and Pentelow G.M. (1978). The burning of John Hunter's papers: a new explanation. Ann. Roy. Coll. Surg. Engl. 60:79–84.

Lobstein J.F. (1829) "Treatise of Pathological Anatomy" / *Traité D'anatomie Pathologique*. F.G. Levrault, Paris. (In French).

Lockhart-Mummery J.P. (1934) "The Origin of Cancer". J. & A. Churchill, London.

Loeb L. (1945) "The Biological Basis of Individuality". Charles C. Thomas, Springfield, IL.

Loeb L. (1978) Leo Loeb (1869–1959) CA Cancer J. Clin. 28: 367–368.

Loeb L.A. (1996) Many mutations in cancers. Cancer Surv. 28: 329–342.

Loeb L.A. (2001) A mutator phenotype in cancer. Cancer Res. 61: 230–239.

Long E. (1965) "A History of Pathology". (Enlarged and corrected edn). Dover Publications, New York.

Lonsdale H. (1868) Biographical Memoir of John Goodsir. See Goodsir (1868).

Lubarsch O. (1902a) Diagnosis of hypernephroid tumours of the kidneys: remarks on Mr von Hansemann's essay "On tumours of the kidney". *Die Diagnose der hypernephroiden Nierengeschwülste. Bemerkungen zu Herrn von Hansemann's Aufsatz "Ueber Nierengeschwülste"*. Zeitschr. f. klin. Med. (Berlin), 44: 491–495.

Lubarsch O. (1902b) "Pathological Anatomy and Cancer Research" / *Pathologische Anatomie und Krebsforschung*. J. F. Bergmann, Wiesbaden. (In German).

Lubarsch O. (1905) "General Pathology" / *Die Allgemeine Pathologie*. J. F. Bergmann, Weisbaden. (In German).

Lubarsch O. (1921) Virchow' tumour theory and its further development / *Die Virchowsche Geschwulstlehre und ihre Weiterentwicklung*. Virchow's Arch. 235: 235–261. (In German).

Lüder F. (2000) "The Institutionalisation of Pathology at the Metropolitan Hospitals in Berlin 1860–1914 / *Institutionalisierung der Pathologie in den Städtischen Krankenhäusern Berlins 1860–1914* / Inaug. Dissertation, Free University of Berlin. (In German).

Ludewig T. (1986) "Berlin, History of a German Metropolis" / *Berlin, Geschichte einer deutschen Metropole*. Bertelsmann, Munich. (In German).

Ludford R.J. (1925) The general and experimental cytology of cancer. J. Roy. Microsc. Soc. pp 249–292.

Ludford R.J. (1930a) Chromosome formation without spindle development in cancer cells, and its significance. Sci. Rpts Imp. Cancer Res. Fund, no. 9. Taylor and Francis, London, pp 109–119.

Ludford R.J. (1930b) The somatic cell mutation theory of cancer. Sci. Rpts Imp. Cancer Res. Fund, no. 9. Taylor and Francis, London, pp 121–147.

Ludford R.J. (1930c) The chromosomes of transplantable tumour cells. Sci. Rpts Imp. Cancer Res. Fund, no. 9. Taylor and Francis, London, pp 149–153.

Ludford R.J. (1934) Structure and behaviour of the cells in tissue culture of tumours. Sci. Rpts Imp. Cancer Res. Fund no. 11. Taylor and Francis, London, pp 147–169.

Lurie E. (1960) Louis Agassiz: a life in science. University of Chicago Press, Chicago.

McClelland C.R. (1980) "State, Society, and University in Germany 1700–1914". Cambridge University Press, Cambridge.

Magendie F. (1836) "Elementary Summary of Physiology"/ *Précis Élémentaire de Physiologie*. 4th edn. Méquignon-Marvis, Paris. (In French).

Maienschein J. (1986) "Defining Biology: Lectures from the 1890s". Harvard University Press, Cambridge, MA.

Maienschein J. (1991) The origins of *Entwicklungsmechanik*. In: "Developmental Biology, a Comprehensive Synthesis". Ed. S.F. Gilbert, vol. 7. Plenum Press, New York, pp 43–61.

Maienschein J. and Ruse M. (eds) (1999) "Biology and the foundation of ethics". Cambridge University Press, Cambridge.

Malkin H.M. (1984) Julius Cohnheim (1839–1884). His life and contributions to pathology. Ann. Clin. Lab. Sci. 14: 335–342.

Malkin H.M. (1990) Rudolph Virchow and the durability of cellular pathology. Perspect. Biol. Med. 33: 431–443.

Mann T. (1933) Sufferings and Greatness of Richard Wagner. In: "Essays of Three Decades". Translated by H. Lowe-Porter. Secker and Warburg, London.

Mann T. (1939) "The Living Thoughts of Schopenhauer". Translated by R.B. Haldane and J. Kemp. Introductory essay by H.T. Lowe-Porter. Cassel, London.

Marvin F.S. (1936) "Comte, the Founder of Sociology". London, Chapman and Hall.

Martin W.A. (1881) The knowledge of indirect nuclear division / *Zur Kenntniss der indirecten Kerntheilung*. Virchow's Arch. 86: 57–66. (In German).

Martins L.A.-C.P. (1999) Did Sutton and Boveri propose the so-called Sutton-Boveri hypothesis? Genetics Molec. Biol. 22: 261–271.

Mather G.R. (1893) "Two Great Scotsmen, the Brothers William and John Hunter". Macklehose and Sons, Glasgow.

Mauser W. and Sasse G. (eds) (1993) "*Streitkultur*: Lessing's Strategies in the Art of Convincing" / *Streitkultur: Strategien des Überzeugens im Werk Lessing* (Internationale Lessing-Tagung, 1991, Freiburg im Breisgau), Niemeyer, Tübingen. (In German).

Mautner T. (1995) "A Dictionary of Philosophy". Blackwell, Cambridge, MA.

Mayer C.F. (1952) Metaphysical trends in modern pathology. Hist. Med. 26: 71–81.

Meckel J.F. (1837) "Manual of General Anatomy". Translated from German to French by A.J.L. Jourdan and G. Breschet; and from French to English by A.S. Doane. G. Henderson, London.

Metchnikoff O. (1921) "Life of Elie Metchnikoff 1845–1916". Constable, London.

Morgan T.H. (1901) "Regeneration". Macmillan and Co, New York.

Morgan T.H., Sturtevant A.H., Muller H.J. and Bridges C.B. (1915). "The Mechanism of Mendelian Heredity". Constable, London.

Müller J. (1838) "On the Nature and Structural Characteristics of Cancer and those Morbid Growths which may be Confounded with It". G. Reimer, Berlin. Translated by C. West, 1840. Sherwood, Gilbert and Piper, London.

Müller J. (1840) "Elements of Physiology". Translated by W. Balyr. vol. 1. Taylor and Walton, London, p. 26.

Nägeli C. v. (1884) "Mechanical-physiological Theory of Heredity" / *Mechanisch-physiologische Theorie der Abstammungslehre*. R. Oldenbourg, Munich and Leipzig. (In German).

Needham J. (1934) "A History of Embryology". Cambridge University Press, Cambridge.

Neiman S. (1994) "The Unity of Reason: Rereading Kant". Oxford University Press, Oxford.

Newman E. (1976) Life of Richard Wagner. Cambridge University Press, Cambridge.

Nicholson G.W. (1933) Studies in Tumour Formation, Parts XI and XIII. Guy's Hospital Rpts 83: 131–158; 465–496.
Nicholson G.W. (1950) "Studies in Tumour Formation". Butterworths, London.
Nordenskiöld E. (1928) "The History of Biology". Translated by L.B. Eyre. Tudor Publishing, New York.
Nowell P.C. (1976) The clonal evolution of tumor cell populations. Science 194: 23–8
Ober W.B. (1992) Obstetrical events that shaped Western European history. Yale J. Biol. Med. 65: 201–210.
Oberling C. (1952). "The Riddle of Cancer". Translated by W.H. Woglom, Yale University Press, New Haven.
Ohno S. (1971) Ono S. Genetic implication of karyological instability of malignant somatic cells. Physiol. Rev. 51: 496–526.
Oppenheimer J.M. (1946) "New Aspects of John and William Hunter". Henry Schuman, New York.
Oppenheimer J.M. (1967) "Essays in the History of Embryology and Biology". The M.I.T. Press. Cambridge, MA.
Organ T.W. (1949) "An Index to Aristotle". Princeton University Press, Princeton, NJ.
Ospovat D. (1981) "The Development of Darwin's Theory: Natural History, Natural Theology, and Natural Selection, 1838–1859". Cambridge University Press, New York.
Ostertag B. (1937) see translation in Appendix D. (In German).
Pagel W. (1944) "The religious and philosophical aspects of van Helmont's science and medicine". The Johns Hopkins University Press, Baltimore. Supplement No 2 to the Bulletin of the History of Medicine.
Pagel W. (1953) The reaction to Aristotle in seventeenth-century biological thought. In: "Science, Medicine and History". Ed E.A. Underwood. Geoffrey Cumberlege, vol. 1. Oxford University Press, Oxford, pp 489–510.
Pagel W. (1982) "Joan Baptista van Helmont. Reformer of Science and Medicine". Cambridge University Press, Cambridge.
Paget J. (1853) "Lectures on Surgical Pathology". Longmans, London.
Parkinson G.H.R. (ed) (1988) "An Encyclopaedia of Philosophy". Routledge, London.
Parrington J. and Coward K. (2003) The spark of life. Biologist (London) 50: 5–10.
Pascal R. (1954) "The German *Sturm und Drang*". Manchester University Press, Manchester, UK.
Pathak S. and Multani A.S. (2005) Aneuploidy, stem cells and cancer. In: "Cancer, Cell Structures Carcinogens and Genetic Instability". Ed. L.P. Bignold, (EXS vol. 96) Birkhäuser, Basel.
Patrides C.A. (ed) (1980) "The Cambridge Platonists". Cambridge University Press, Cambridge.
Paul D.B. (2003). Darwin, Social Darwinism and Eugenics. In: "The Cambridge Companion to Darwin". Eds J. Hodge, G. Radick. Cambridge University Press, Cambridge.
Paulsen F. (1895) "The German Universities, Their Character and Historical Development". Translated by E.A Perry. Introduction by N.M. Butler. Macmillan, New York.
Peel J.D.Y. (1971) "Herbert Spencer: the Evolution of a Sociologist". Heinemann Educational, London.
Pfitzner W. (1886) On the pathological anatomy of cell nuclei / *Zur pathologischen Anatomie des Zellkerns*. Virchow's Arch. 103: 275–300. (In German).
Pickering M. (1993) "Auguste Comte, an Intellectual Biography". Cambridge University Press, Cambridge.
Pinel P. (1813) "Philosophical Description and Methodical Classification of Disease, or the Analytical Method Applied to Medicine" / *Nosographie Philosophique, ou La Mèthode de l'Analyse appliquèe a la Mèdicine*. 5th edn. J. A. Brosson, Paris. (In French).
Pinkard T.P. (2002) "German philosophy 1760–1860: the Legacy of Idealism". Cambridge University Press, Cambridge.
Poggi P. and Maurizio B. (eds) (1994) "Romanticism in science: science in Europe, 1790–1840". With editorial assistance of Berendina van Straalen. Kluwer Academic, Dordrecht and Boston, MA.

Literature cited

Politzer G. (1934) "Pathology of Mitosis" / *Pathologie der Mitose.* Gebrüder Borntraeger, Berlin. (In German).
Porter R. (1997) "The Greatest Benefit to Mankind". Harper-Collins, London.
Rabl M. (ed) (1907) "Virchow's Letters to his Parents 1839–1864 / *Rudolf Virchow Briefe an Seine Eltern, 1839 bis 1864.* Originally Wilhelm Engelmann, Leipzig. Translated by L.J. Rather and published in 1990; Science History Publications, Canton, MA.
Raby P. (2001) "Alfred Russell Wallace. A Life". Princeton University Press, Princeton, NJ.
Rather L.J. (1962) Harvey, Virchow, Bernard, and the Methodology of Science. Introduction to "Disease, Life and Man (Translations of selected articles by R. Virchow)", Collier edition, New York, pp 13–38.
Rather L.J. (1971) The place of Virchow's "Celllular Pathology" in Medical Thought. (Introduction to Dover edition of Virchow's "Cellular Pathology" – see Virchow, 1858) pp v–xxvii.
Rather L.J. (1972) "Addison and the White Corpuscles. An Aspect of Nineteenth-Century Biology". Wellcome Institute of the History of Medicine, London.
Rather L.J. (1975) Langenbeck on the mechanism of tumour metastasis and the transmission of cancer from man to animal. Clio Med. 10:213–225.
Rather L.J. (1978) "The Genesis of Cancer. A Study in the History of Ideas". The Johns Hopkins University Press, Baltimore.
Rather L.J. (1990a) "A Commentary on the Medical Writings of Rudolph Virchow". Norman Publishing, San Francisco.
Rather L.J. (1990b) "Reading Wagner: a Study in the History of Ideas". Louisiana State University Press, Baton Rouge.
Rather L.J., Rather P. and Frerichs J.B. (1986) "Johannes Müller and the Nineteenth Century Origins of Tumor Cell Theory". Science History Publications, Canton, MA.
Reinhardt K.F. (1960) "Germany 2000 years". Frederick Ungar, New York.
Ribbert H. (1911) "The Cancers of Mankind" / *Das Karzinom des Menschen.* Friedrich Cohen. Bonn. (In German).
Richardson M.K. and Keuck G. (2002) Haeckel's ABC of evolution and development. Biol. Rev. 77: 495–528.
Corr E. and Richter W. (ND) "TH Aachen: a city and its High School" / *TH Aachen: eine Stadt und ihre Hochschule".* Verlag J. A. Mayer. No place. Undated but thought to be 1995 – 125th anniversary of opening of the Technical College (*Technische Hochschule*).
Robbins S.L. and Cotran R. (2004) "Pathologic Basis of Disease". 7th edn. Eds V. Kumar, A. Abbas and N. Fausto. Saunders, Philadelphia.
Ross R.J. (1998) "The Failure of Bismarck's *Kulturkampf*: Catholicism and State Power in Imperial Germany, 1871–1887". Catholic University of America Press, Washington DC.
Roux W. (1888) Contribution to the developmental mechanisms of embryos / *Beiträge zur Entwickelungsmechanik des Embryos.* Virchow's Arch 114:113–159. Partial translation by H. Laufer. In: "Foundations of Experimental Embryology". Eds B.H. Willier and J.M. Oppenheimer. Hafner Press, New York, 1974.
Rüegg W. (2004) Themes (chapter 1) In: "A History of the University in Europe". Ed. W Rüegg. vol. 3. Cambridge University Press, Cambridge, pp 3–32.
Russell B. (1958) "Introduction to Western Philosophy". Sheed and Ward, London.
Sachse A. (1927) "Friedrich Althoff and his Work" *Friedrich Althoff und sein Werk.* (In German).
Sandberg A.S. (1990) "The Chromosomes of Human Cancer and Leukemia". 2nd edn, Elsevier, New York, pp 2–10.
Sandler I. (1983) Pierre Louis Moreau de Maupertuis – a precursor of Mendel? J. Hist. Biol. 16: 101–136.
Schattenfroh S. (2002) "Charité Guide Book". Charité University Hospital, Berlin.
Schipperges H. (1994) "Rudolph Virchow" / *Rudolph Virchow.* Rowohlt, Hamburg. (In German).

Schmiedebach H.P. (1990) Robert Remak (1815–1865). A Jewish physician and researcher between recognition and rejection. Z. Arztl. Fortbild. (Jena) 84: 889–894.

Schopenhauer A. (1844) "The World as Will and Representation". Translated by E.F.J. Payne. 1966. Dover Publications, New York.

Schottländer J. (1888) On Nuclear and Cell Division Processes in the Endothelia of the Inflamed Cornea / *Über Kern- und Zelltheilungsvorgänge in den Endothelien der entzündeten Hornhaut*. Arch. f. Mikr. Anat. 31: 424–476. (In German).

Schubert-Soldern R. (1962) "Mechanism and vitalism: philosophical aspects of biology". Translated by C.E. Robin. Burns & Oates, London.

Schwaiger M. (1979) In memoriam Karl Heinrich Bauer. Dtsch. med. Wschr. 104: 441–443. (In German).

Schwalbe J. (1901) "Virchow Bibliography" / *Virchow – Bibliographie*. G. Reimer, Berlin. (In German).

Schwarz H. (1943) "Imperial Privy Council in the Seventeenth Century". With a supplement The social structure of the Imperial privy council, 1600–1674, by Henry F. Schwarz and John I. Codding. Harvard University Press, Cambridge MA.

Sherwin-White A.N. (ed) (1967) "Fifty Letters of Pliny". Oxford University Press, London.

Shimkin M.B. (1977) "Contrary to Nature". U.S. Dept Health, Education and Welfare, Publication No (NIH) 79–720, Washington DC.

Sigerist H.E. (1942) Review of "The Doctors Mayo". Amer. Hist. Rev. 47: 901–903.

Silverman M.E., Grove D. and Upshaw C.B. (2006) Why does the heart beat? The discovery of the electrical system of the heart. Circulation 113: 2775–2781.

Simon J. (1878) Some points of science and practice concerning cancer. Br. Med. J. i: 219–224.

Simpson A.J., Caballero O.L., Jungbluth A., Chen Y.T. and Old L.J. (2005) Cancer/testis antigens, gametogenesis and cancer. Nat. Rev. Cancer 5: 615–625.

Singer C. and Underwood E.A. (1962) "A Short History of Medicine". 2nd edn, Oxford University Press, Oxford, UK.

Spranger E. (1960) "Wilhlem von Humboldt and the Reform of the Education System" / *Wilhelm von Humboldt und die Reform des Bildungswesens*. M. Niemeyer, Tubingen. (In German).

Spencer H. (1875) "Foundations of Philosophy (System of Synthetic Philosophy, vol. 1)". Authorised German edition of the 4th English edition. Translated from English to German by B. Fetter, *Grundlagen der Philosophie (System der synthetischen Philosophie, I. Band). Autorisirte deutsche Ausgabe. Nach der vierten englischen Auflage übersetzt von B. Vetter*. Schweizerbart, Stuttgart. (In German).

Stern C. (1969) Richard Benedict Goldschmidt, April 12, 1878–April 24, 1958. Perspect. Biol. Med. 12: 179–203.

Sturtevant A.H. (1965) "History of Genetics". Harper and Row, New York.

Sweet P.R. (1978) "Wilhelm von Humboldt: a Biography". Ohio State University Press, Columbus, Ohio.

Taddey G. (ed) (1977) "Encyclopaedia of German History, Persons, Events, Institutions" / *Lexicon der Deutschen Geschichte, Personen, Ereignisse, Institutionen*. Alfred Kröner, Stuttgart. (In German).

Taylor A.J.P. (1951). "The Course of German History, a Survey of the Development of Germany since 1815". 2nd edn. Hamish Hamilton, London, p. 1.

Taylor R. (1997) "Berlin and its Culture: a Historical Portrait". Yale University Press, New Haven, CT.

Triolo V.A. (1964) Nineteenth century foundations of cancer research, origins of experimental research. Cancer Res. 24: 4–27.

Tubiana M., Dutrieux J. and Pierquin B. (1996) One century of radiotherapy in France. Int. J. Radiation Oncol. 35: 227–242.

Velpeau A. (1856) "A Treatise on the Diseases of the Breast and Mammary Region". Translated by M. Henry. Sydenham Society, London.

Literature cited

Vickers B. (ed) (1987) "English science, Bacon to Newton". Cambridge University Press, Cambridge and New York.
Virchow R. (1847) On the developmental history of cancer along with remarks on fat formation in the animal body and pathological resorption / *Zur Entwickelungsgeschichte des Krebses, nebst Bemerkungen ueber Fettbildung im thierschen Körper und pathologische Resorption.* Virchow's Arch. 1: 94–201. (In German).
Virchow R. (1854a) "Handbook of Special Pathology and Therapeutics" / *Handbuch der speciellen Pathologie und Therapie.* vol. 1. Verlag Ferdinand Enke, Erlangen, pp 328–9. (In German).
Virchow R. (1855) Cellular Pathology. Virchow's Arch. 8: 3–39. English translation in Rather L.J. (1962) pp 86–115.
Virchow R. (1858) "The Cellular Pathology Based on Physiological and Pathological Tissue Teaching" / *Die Cellularpathologie in ihrer Begründung auf physiologische und pathologische Gewebelehre.* 2nd edn. Translated by F. Chance, Dover Publishers, New York.
Virchow R. (1862–6) "The Disease-related Tumours" / *Die Krankhaften Geschwülste.* vol. 1 (1863), A. Hirschwald, Berlin. (In German).
Virchow R. (1870) "The Cellular Pathology" / *Die Cellular Pathologie*, 4th edn (of Virchow, 1858, above), A. Hirschwald, Berlin. (In German).
Virchow R. (1880) The Nature and Causes of Disease / *Krankheitswesen und Krankheitursachen.* Virchow's Arch. 79: 1–19; 185–228. (In German).
Virchow R. (1884) On Metaplasia / *Ueber Metaplasie.* Virchow's Arch. 97: 410–430. (In German).
Virchow R. (1886) Origin and Pathology / *Descendenz und Pathologie.* Virchow's Arch. 103: 1–14; 205–215; 413–436. (In German).
Virchow R. (1888) On the diagnosis and prognosis of carcinomas / *Zur Diagnose und Prognose des Carcinoms.* Virchow's Arch. 111: 1–24. (In German).
Virchow R. (1891) The state of cellular pathology / *Der Stand der Cellularpathologie.* Virchow's Arch. 126: 1–11. (In German).
Virchow R. (1892) Study and research. Smithsonian Ann. Rpts. for the year 1894: 653–666.
Virchow R. (1894) The founding of the Berlin University and the transition from the philosophic to the scientific age. Smithsonian Ann. Rpts for the year 1894: 681–696.
Virchow R. (1898) Recent Progress in Science and its influence on Medicine and Surgery. Lecture delivered at the opening of the Charing Cross Medical School, and published in Berl. klin. Wnschr, 35: 897– (In German).
Vogel J. (1847) "The Pathological Anatomy of the Human Body". Translated by G.F. Day. H Baillière, London.
Von Baer K. E. (1827) On the genesis of the ovum of mammals and man. Letter to the Imperial Academy of Sciences, St Petersburg, printed by Leopold Voss, Leipzig. Translated by C.D. O'Malley, with Introduction by B. Cohen. Isis 47: 117–153, 1956.
Von Haller A. (1757) "A Dissertation on the Motion of the Blood, and on the Effects of Bleeding, together with a Second Dissertation on the Motion of the Blood and Effects on Bleeding". Whiston and White, London. Reprinted by Classics of Medicine Library, Gryphon Editions, New York, 1998.
Von Hansemann David Paul. All works by this author are listed in Appendix E
Von Hansemann F.D. (1968) "The Ancestors and Descendants of David Justus Ludwig Hansemann and Fanny Hansemann, nee Fremery" / *Die Vorfahren und Nachkommen von David Justus Ludwig Hansemann (1790–1864) und Fanny Hansemann, geborene Fremery (1801–1876).* C.A. Starke, Limburg/Lahn. (In German).
Von Hansemann G. (1863) "The Economic conditions of the *Zollverein* with particular respect to the Linen, Cotton and Wool Industry" / *Die wirthschaftlichen Verhältnisse des Zollvereins; insbesondere in Beziehung auf die Leinen-, Baumwollen-, und Wollen-Industrie.* Berlin. (In German).

Von Hansemann G. (1871a) "Eduard von Hartmann's Philosophy of the Unconscious for the Consciousness of Wider Circles" / *Eduard von Hartmann's Philosophie des Unbewussten für das Bewusstsein weiterer Kreise.* Printed in Cöln und Leipzig. (In German).

Von Hansemann G. (1871b) "Atoms and their movements. An attempt to Generalise from the Krönig-Clausius Theory of Gases" / *Die Atome und ihre Bewegungen. Ein Versuch zur Verallgemeinerung der Krönig-Clausius'schen Theorie der Gase.* Printed in Cöln und Leipzig. (In German).

Von Leyden E. (1891) Clinical Experiences on the diagnostic significance of Koch's lymph / *Klinische Erfahrungen über die diagnostische Bedeutung der Koch'schen Lymphe.* Veröffentlichungen der Hufeland'schen Gesellschaft in Berlin. Vörträge, in 1891/92. A Hirschwald, Berlin, pp 33–64. (In German).

Von Leyden E. et al., (1902) "Report of the Committee for Cancer Research" / *Bericht über die vom Komitee für Krebsforschung am 15. Oktober 1900 erhobene Sammelforschung.* Gustav Fischer, Jena. (In German). (Full names of co-authors are not given in the original).

Wagner R.P. (1999) Rudolph Virchow and the genetic basis of somatic ecology. Genetics 151: 917–920.

Wallace A. (1889) "Darwinism". Macmillan, London.

Walshe W.H. (1846) "The Nature and Treatment of Cancer". Taylor and Walton, London.

Wedl C. (1855) "Rudiments of Pathological Histology". Translated by G. Busk. Sydenham Society, London.

Weiner D.B. (1968) "Raspail, Scientist and Reformer". Columbia University Press. New York.

Weismann A.G. (1891–2) "Essays upon Heredity and Kindred Biological Problems". Translated by E.B. Poulton, S. Schönland and A.E. Shipley. vol. 1 1891; vol. 2 1892. Oxford University Press, Oxford.

Weismann A.G. (1893) "Germ Plasm: A Theory of Heredity / *Das Keimplasma; eine Theorie der Vererbung.* Originally published by G. Fischer, Jena, 1892. Translated by W.N. Parker, and H. Rönnfeldt. Walter Scott Ltd, London.

Whitman R.C. (1919) Somatic mutation as a factor in the production of cancer; a critical review of v. Hansemann's theory of anaplasia in the light of modern knowledge of genetics. J. Cancer Res. 4: 181–202.

Whittaker T. (1901) "The neo-Platonists: a Study in the History of Hellenism". Cambridge University Press, Cambridge.

Williams C.J.B. (1856) "Principles of Medicine". John Churchill, London.

Williams E.A. (2002) "A Cultural History of Medical Vitalism in Enlightenment Montpellier". Ashgate, Aldershot, U.K.

Willis R.A. (1948) "Pathology of Tumours". Butterworth and Co, London.

Willis R.A. (1950) "Principles of Pathology". Butterworth and Co, London.

Willis R.A. (1934) "The Spread of Tumours in the Human Body". Butterworth and Co, London.

Willis R.A. (1958, 1962) "The Borderland of Embryology and Pathology". Butterworth and Co, London.

Willis R.A. (1962) "The Pathology of the Tumours of Children". Oliver and Boyd, Edinburgh.

Wilmut I., Schnieke A.E., McWhir J., Kind A.J. and Campbell K.H. (1997) Viable offspring derived from fetal and adult mammalian cells. Nature 385: 810–813.

Wilson E.B. (1924) "The Cell in Development and Heredity". 3rd edn. Macmillan, New York.

Witkowski J.A. (1983) Experimental pathology and the origins of tissue culture: Leo Loeb's contribution. Med. Hist. 27: 269–288.

Wohlrab F. and Henoch U. (1988) The life and work of Carl Weigert (1845–1904) in Leipzig 1878–1885. Zentralbl. Allg. Pathol. 134: 743–751. (In German).

Wolf J.H. (1999) "Medical Historical Aspects of the Internal Workings of the 125-year History of the Hospital in Berlin-Friedrichshain" / *Medizinhistorische Streiflichter auf die inwendigen Facetten der 125-jährigen Krankenhausgeschichte im Berliner Friedrichshain.* Published by the Hospital in Friedrichshain, Berlin. pp 21–107. (In German).

Literature cited

Wolff J. (1907) "The Science of Cancerous Disease from Earliest Times to the Present" / vol. 1 of *Die Lehre von der Krebskrankheit von den ältesten Zeiten bis zur Gegenwart*. Translated by B. Ayoub, and with an Introduction by P. Sarco. Science History Publishers, Sagamore Beach, MA, 1990.

Wolpert L. (1995) Evolution of the cell theory. Phil. Trans. R. Soc. Lond. B. Biol. Sci. 349:227–233.

Wright G.P. (1954) "An Introduction to Pathology". 2nd edn. Longmans Green and Co, London.

Yamagiwa K. and Ichikawa K. (1918) Experimental Study of the Pathogenesis of Carcinoma. J. Cancer Res. 3:1–29.

Zimmerman A. (2001) "Anthropology and Antihumanism in Imperial Germany". University of Chicago Press, Chicago.

Zimstein G. (2001) Thomas Henry Morgan. In: "Darwin and Co / A History of Biology in Portraits" / *Darwin & Co. Eine Geschichte der Biologie in Portraits*. vol. II. Eds I. Jahn and M. Schmitt. CH Beck, Munich, pp 28–43. (In German).

Index

Aachen and Munich Fire Insurance Society 3
Aachen 4
Abbe 43
abstractionism 89
abstractionism and inwardness 36
achromatic connecting threads 152, 202
achromatic figure 197, 257
achromatic lenses 43
achromatic spindle 149, 205
achromatic threads 131
acromegaly 99
Adami, John George 105, 118, 119
Adamkiewicz 257
adaptation 52, 94
adenoma 298
adenoma malignum 298
adrenal glands 225
aetiology 170, 243, 281, 296, 308, 309
aetiology of tumours 95
Agaziz 115
ageing 232
ageing and cancer 301
alkylating agents 83, 90, 111
alloplasia 92, 94
Althoff, Friedrich Theodor 15
Altmann 161
altruism 32, 33, 86, 89, 99, 112, 136, 221, 225, 250, 259, 299, 305
altruistic growth 99
Amann Jr. 239
American Type Culture Collection 80, 90
amplification 86
anaplasia 47, 108, 139, 142, 251, 253, 286, 300, 301
anaplasia, degree of 168, 260
anaplasia, expressed as deviation from normal tissue 303
anaplasia, manifest by increasing deviation from the mother tissue 246
anaplasia, philosophically 89
anaplasia, possible underlying genomic disturbance 110
anaplastic change 142, 168, 283
anatomical pathologists 114

ancestral heredity 48
aneuploidy 83, 107, 110
aniline dyes 111
anisotropia 215, 220
anti-Aristotelianism 35
anti-Darwinism 115
anti-Ultramontane movement 10
aplastic change 73
apoachromatic lenses 43
archiblast 240
Aristotle 25, 26, 46, 52, 57
Aristotle's "Four Causes" 35
Aristotle's theories of Categorisation 51
Arnold, Julius 42, 67ff (article summarised), 124, 153, 159, 288
arsenic 111
Aselli 58
asymmetric cell division 135, 256
asymmetric cell division, fate of smaller daughter cell 258
asymmetric mitotic division 76, 84, 129, 141, 150, 163, 174
asymmetric mitosis as cause of tissue changes 255
Auerwald 4
Austro-Prussian War 4
auxiliary plasmata 51
Avicenna 57
axolotl larva 134

bacteria as not producing specific toxins 160
bacteriology 281, 282
Baer, Karl Ernst von 46, 47, 51, 55
"balances", as a philosophical concept 26
balances of chromosomes 80
Bard 46, 47, 187, 213, 214, 218, 221
Barry, Martin 47
Barthez 26
Basedow's disease 308
Bashford 104, 296
Bauer, Karl Heinrich 107, 119
Baumgarten 153, 164, 212
Beattie 105
Behring, von 159, 282
Benda 316

Beneden, van   63
Beneke, Rudolph   101, 117, 286, 291
Berenblum   108
Bergmann, von   15
Berlin Medical School   7
Bernard, Claude   41
Bichat, Xavier   44, 54
Bildung   6, 11
Billroth   34, 35, 211, 251
Biogenic Law   31
biological theory   93
"biologistic sociology"   32, 33, 112
Bismarck   11, 13, 33, 38
Bizzozero   51, 161, 195
Bland-Sutton   105 (quotes), 118
blastema   44, 45, 59
blastoderm   135
blastomatosis   95
blastomeres   101
blastula   50, 53, 216
blood, Grawitz's concept of   301, 306
blood-borne nature of metastasis   62
blood group antigens   110
blood transfusions   249
Blumenthal   295, 297
Boerhaave   73, 293
Bose, Countess   184
Böhmer's haematoxylin   146, 192
Boll   255
Borelli   58
Borst, Maximilian   94f (translations), 104, 107, 115, 117
Boveri, Theodor   63, 117, 118, 133, 150, 161, 223, 235, 238
Boveri, ideas similar to Hansemann's   101-104
Boveri's theory mentioned by Hansemann   316
Bridges, C.B.   106
Brücke   12
Bücher   159
Buchner   160
Büngner, von   165
Burdette   108
Burschenschaft   13
Bütschli   214

cacoplasia   58, 90
cacoplastic change   73
cadherins   110
Cambridge (Neo-) Platonists   57

Camphausen   4
Canada balsam   193
cancer à deux   294
cancer therapies   315
cancroid   87, 171, 298
cantharides   315
capacity for independent existence   53, 62, 76, 299
capacity for independent existence, increased   78, 110, 297
carcinogens   110
carcinomata   84
carcinomata of the epidermis   168
carcinomata versus sarcomata   153, 175, 243
Carlsbad Decrees   280
Carmalt   248
cataplasia, see kataplasia
cell death, physiological   278
cell division   151
cell division, delay of   206
cell division, multipartite   102, 163
cell divisions, specificity of   280, 288
cell embolisms   249
cell rests   61
"Cell State"   31
cell theory   44, 110
cells, hyperchromatic   132, 148
cells, hypochromatic   132, 147, 152
cells, lineage fidelity of   76
cells, specificity of   46, 89, 212-214, 220, 250, 254, 259, 306
cells with normal chromatin content (normochromatic)   132, 147
cell-type specificity of mitotic appearances   82, 280
cell-type specific location   173
cellular adaptation   46
cellular altruism   32
cellular pathology   159, 307
"Cellular Pathology" (Virchow)   29, 45
centrosomes   197, 199, 201, 203
Charité Hospital   14
Charrin   159
"chemical" mechanisms in tumour formation   316
chemotherapy, experimental   304, 305
chorio-carcinoma   281, 286
chromatic connecting threads (in mitoses)   151
chromatin   133
chromatin content of nuclei   149

chromatin deficiency 125
chromatin increases in resting cells 234
chromatin-poor mitoses 128
chromosomes, see also mitoses
chromosomal instability 84
chromosomes, number of 148, 204
chromosomes, perishing of individual 256
chronic irritation 60, 294
clastogenesis 83
cleavage of the egg 135
cleavage spheres 215
cloudy swelling 311
coagulation, in relation to fixation 203
coagulating lymph 58
coal tar 111
Coën 176, 195
Cohnheim, Julius Friedrich 6, 12, 30, 61, 186
compensatory hypertrophy (of the kidney) 228
Comte, Auguste 32, 38, 86, 89
conceptuality, excessive, in philosophy 26
Congress of Vienna 3
connective tissue 60
connective tissues, unity of 214
Cornil 69
Cowdry 108
Cruikshank, William 58, 72
curability 283
cure 283
Curie, Marie 111
curriculum vitae, Hansemann's 5, 317
cytopathology 283
cytoplasm, constriction of 154

Danish War 4
Darwin, Charles 26, 30, 32, 37, 49, 52, 233
Darwin, Erasmus 30, 37
"Darwin's bulldog", see Huxley, Thomas Henry
"Darwinian variations" 300
Darwinism 115
de Bovis 294
de Vries, Hugo 135, 217, 218, 252
death 232
de-differentiation 53, 106, 223, 251, 258, 287, 291, 293, 299, 303
delay in appearance of tumour 110
Descartes, René 26, 35, 57, 71, 113
Descartes, mechanistic theory of tissue formation 35
destined progressions of cell types 114

developmentalist theory 46, 55
diagnosis of malignant tumours 86, 282, 283
diagnostic cytology 86
diaster phase of mitosis 206
Dickson 105
differentia (Aristotle) 51
differential utilization of the genome 109
"differentiated out" (completion of embryonic differentiation) 142
differentiation 33, 39, 46, 48, 51, 52, 77, 78, 86, 110, 137, 140, 142, 216, 217, 301
differentiation by division of labour 214
diphtheria 282
Discount Bank 4
dispermic eggs 101
dispirem 203
Disse 173, 244
divisions, of nuclei, reduction 238, 288
dogmas, origins in medicine 280
Dolly, the sheep 62, 82, 90
Donné 43
dormant cells 279
Dr habil. 9, 15
Drasch 210
Dubois-Reymond 311
Duelling Corps 13
"dysanaplasia" 90
dyscrasia 307
"dysde-differentiation" 90

Eberth 161
egg 47, 78, 133, 136, 138, 142, 169, 214, 215, 220, 222, 251
eggs, primordial 252
eggs, shaken dispermic 101, see also Boveri
Ehrlich-Altmann granules 189
embryological reversion 62, 283
embryonal cells 299, 300
embryonal epithelial cells 142
embryonal theory 61
embryonic tissues 86
endocrine mechanisms and organs 110
endometrium 78
endothelioma 286
eosin 42
epidermis 50, 164, 196, 278
epithelial character of cells 172ff, 240ff
epithelio-mesenchymal interactions 92
epithelium, squamous 213
euplasia 58
euplastic tissues 73

"Evo-Devo"   114
evolution   52
Ewing, James   105, 115, 118
exhaustion   231

Farmer, Moore and Walker   104, 288, 290
    (reply to Hansemann's letter in Lancet)
fatty conditions   311
fertilisation   78, 126, 236, 297
fertilisation by leukocytes   126
Fibiger   103, 313, 314
fibro-plasia   59
fibrous degeneration   198
Fichte, Johann Gottlieb   27, 36
field theory   292, 297
Fischer   176
fixation   42, 127, 130, 133, 145, 201, 311
Flemming, Walter   7, 63, 65ff (article summarised), 125, 126, 146, 150-153, 161, 162, 164, 165, 171, 174, 184, 188, 190, 200, 210, 211, 235, 257, 288
forces, see plasias
forces, plastic   26, 57-59, 71
Fortschrittspartei, see Progress Party
Foulds, L.   109
Franco-Prussian War   4
Fredrick the Great   31
Friedrich III (Emperor)   70
Freiherr   10
Freud, Sigmund   12
Friedländer   15, 153
Friedrich Wilhelm IV   4
Friedrich-Wilhelms *Gymnasium*   6
Friedrichshain Hospital   9, 15
Friorep   13, 14
Froschauer, Justinian von   250
functions, division of   137
functions, dual, of organs   231
functions, negative   226
functions of cancer cells   291
functions, positive   226, 228
Fütterer   153

Galen   25
galls (crown) of plants   107, 221
Garré   165
gastrula   216, 217
gastrulation   47
Gaub   59
Gaylord   296
Geheimrat   10

gemmules   49, 55
generational stages   135-6, 138-9, 169, 217, 221-225, 233, 250, 255
genetic instability   106, 110
geotropism   296
germ layers   47
German Customs Union   3
German medical schools   6
German philosophy   27
German Romantic movement   37
German Universities   11
germinal centres   211
germinal cells   48
giant cells   152, 163
Goethe, Johann Wolfgang von   37, 46, 55, 280
Goldschmidt, Richard Benedict   114, 119, 120
Goodsir, John   44, 50, 54, 86
graininess (in photograms)   194
granulation tissue   212
Grawitz   171, 186, 248, 279
growth direction   217
growth direction change   255
growth energy   136, 139
growth, excessive, of tumour cells   85, 95
growth factor   110
growth factor genes   86
gymnasia   11

habilitation doctorate   9, 15
Häcker   216
Haeckel, Ernst   31, 32, 38, 59, 86
haematoxylin   42, 133, 146
Hahn, E.   295
Haller, Albrecht von   27
Hanau   141, 248, 295
Hansemann Platz   4
Hansemann, Adolph   4
Hansemann, David Justus   3, 17
Hansemann, Gustav   5, 18
harmonies, philosophical concept of   26
Harvey   25
Hatschek   218
Hauptplasmen   51, 85, 103, 108
Hauptplasmen, ejection of   259
Hauser   104, 147, 148, 170, 236, 259, 288
Hegel, Georg Wilhelm Friedrich   XVII, 27, 36, 37
Heidenhain   161
Helmholtz   12, 183

Index

Henle 12, 45
Herder, Johann Gottfried 37
Heredity, theories of 294
Hertwig, O. 50, 126, 140, 159, 161, 214, 215, 217, 219, 237
heteroplasia 58
heteroplastic tumours 60, 239
Hewson, William 58, 72
Hippocrates 25
His 6, 12, 13, 211, 214, 218
histogenesis 99, 243
histological accommodation 188, 212-216, 218, 248
histological adaptation 187
histological methods 311
histological substitution 46, 52
Hofmann, Friedrich 58, 71
Hoffmann, Ludwig 15
Home, Everard 72, 73
homeoplasia 58
homeoplastic tumours, Virchow on 60
homograft 110
homunculus 55
Hooke, Robert 182
Hume, David 310
humoural pathology 160, 281
Hunter, John 58, 72
Hunter, William 72
Huxley, Thomas Henry 31, 38
hybridizing of plants 30
hyperplasia 59
hypertrophy 58

idioplasmas 138, 217
ids 49
ignoramus et ignorabimus 311
illiberalism 34
immune sera 315
immuno-identity 110
incubation period 165, 209
infection theory 294
infective agents 111
Innerlichkeit 36
integrins 110
interphase 208, 209
interstitial cells of the testis 281
ionizing radiations 111
irradiated cells 83
irritation theory 296
isotropia 215, 220

Israel, Oskar 8, 14, 43, 96-100 (article in full), 287

Jensen 295
Johns Hopkins Hospital 6
Junkertum 33

Kaiserin-Friedrich-Stiftung 9, 15
Kaiserin Viktoria (Empress Victoria) 74
Kant, Immanuel XVII, 27, 36
Karg 177, 241, 244, 259
kataplasia 98, 101, 286, 291
keratinisation 168
kidney 227
kidney anlage 218
kidney, mixed tumour of 287
Kiel Medical School 7
Klebs, Edwin 30, 42, 69, 73, 125, 126, 134, 141, 146, 147, 152, 153, 155, 187, 241, 253
Koch 30, 281
Koch's Postulates 282
Koch's preparation ("Tuberculin") 277
Koller 108
Kölliker 12, 45, 47, 173
Kowalevski 47
Kowalewsky 136
Kraft 165
Kulturkampf 13, 31, 38
Kusserow, Ottilie von 5

lacteals 58
Laennec 58
Lamarck, Jean Baptiste 55
Lanceraux 59, 227
Landerer 160
Lang, Albert 222
Langenbeck 53, 62 (extract from Rather's translation)
Langerhans Islets 307
Le Dran 58
Le Dran-Hunterian model 60
Leber 159
Lebert 42, 59
Leeuwenhoek 43
Leipzig Medical School 6
Lessing, Gotthold Ephraim 27, 37
Levine 107
Leyden, von 277, 295
Lieberkühn's crypts 164
lineage fidelity 46
liver 165

Lobstein, Jean 58, 59, 73, 90
Lockhart-Mummery, John Percy 108, 119
Loeb 223
Lubarsch, Otto 8, 83, 92-94 (translations of excerpts), 117, 316, 324
Lücke 248
Ludford 107
Ludwig, Carl 7, 13, 27
lymph 58
lymph cells 196
lymph glands 164
lymph nodes 198
lymphocytes 206

Mach 308
main plasmata, see *Hauptplasmen*
malignant mixed tumour of the kidney 287
Malpighi 43, 58
Malpighian body 140
Mann, Thomas 34
Martin, W.A. 68ff (article summarised), 124, 125, 153f
Martinotti 189
Maupertuis, Pierre-Louis de 49, 55
Mayo Clinic 6
Mayzel 161
"Medical Reform" 13, 28
Mendelian genetics 114
mercuric chloride , see sublimate
metabolic products 160
metaplasia 46, 53, 59, 85, 94, 186, 212, 213, 296, 306
metastases 60, 246, 260
metastases, histological appearances compared to primary tumour 171
Metchnikoff, Elie 8, 15, 159, 250
Michaelis, L. 295
microscopy 42
microscopy, three-dimensional, see three-dimensional microscopical study
militarism 33, 34
mitoses, abortive forms 149, 154, 163
mitoses, asymmetrical, see asymmetric mitotic division
mitoses, hyperchromatic 94, 128, 150, 253
mitoses, incomprehensible 149
mitoses, in metastases compared to primary tumours 171
mitoses, multipolar 153, 237
mitoses, number of 163, 304
mitoses, quadripartite 134

mitoses, tripartite 147, 281
mitotic catastrophe 84
mixed tumours 87
modifier genes 86
monaster phase 204
monism 38
Moore 104, 288, 290
Morgagni 44
Morgan 86, 101, 106
Morpugo 164
motility of tumour cells 248
mounting media 42
mouse tumours 304, 305
mucous membranes 164
Müller, H.F. 190, 205
Müller, Johannes 12, 14, 44, 50, 59, 123, 171, 279
multinucleate cells 206
multipolar cell 149
multipolar mitosis 102
museums, of anthropology, pathology etc 14
mutation, somatic, see somatic mutation
Muybridge 190
Mystic philosophers 36

Nägeli 49, 183, 217
Naturphilosophie 28, 37
Nebenplasmen 51, 85, 103, 108
Neelsen 177
negative function 226
neohumoralism 45
neoplasia 59
neotenic forms 301
Newton 36
Nicholson, Gilbert de Pouton 108, 119
nitrosamines 111
Noeggerath 170, 259
nuclear fusion 63
nuclear migration 209
nutritive foci 44

Oberling 108
Oken 46
omnes metabolica per cellulae 44
omnes rera pathologica per cellulae locis 46
omnis cellula e cellula 29, 44, 45, 48, 54, 60
omnis cellula e cellula ejusdem generis 46, 213
oncogenes 110, 112
ontogenesis 301
ontogenetic development 135

Index

oogenesis 78
oogenic de-differentiation 112
Orth 298, 313, 316
osteomalacia 311
over-philosophising 113
oxygen 208, 209

Paley, William 37
pancreas 307
pancreas, role in diabetes 227
Pander 46
Pangenesis 233
panmerism 134
parablast 240
paracrine 110
paraffin, cause of tumours 111
paraffin embedding 42
parasites as causes of tumours 279, 280, 294
parenchyma of organs 242
parthenogenesis 78, 90
Pasteur, Louis 41
pathological mitoses 83, 145
pathology, philosophy of 28
Perl 245
Petit 58
Pfitzner 69 (article summarised), 125
philosophy of pathology 28
photomicrographs 172, 193
phylogenesis 301
Pius IX, Pope 38
plasias 57
plasmata 49, 85, 138
plastic forces 26, 57-59, 71
Plato 26, 57
Pliny the Younger 26, 35
Plotinus 57, 71
pluricentricity, of tumours 292
pluri-polar mitoses, see multipolar mitoses
Poa nemoralis 139, 221
Podwyssozki 176, 195
poisons 164
polar bodies 47, 76, 78, 127, 139, 151, 169, 202, 235, 258
polar bodies, expulsion of 133
Politzer 108
Polyploidy, see aneuploidy
positive functions 226, 228
precancerous conditions 313
predispositions to cancer 313
preformationist theories 46, 55
pre-tumourous anaplasia 94

Probius 14
Progress Party 13
proliferation capability 293
prosoplasia 108, 139, 141, 171, 252, 287, 299
protoplasmic poisons 280
Prussia 33
Prussian Bank 4

quadripolar mitosis 104
Quincke 214

Rabl 299
radionecrosis 314
radiotherapy 314, 315
radium 314
Raspail, François-Vincent 42, 54
ray treatment 314
Realschule 10
Recklinghausen, von 187, 212
re-differentiation 53, 94, 106
reduction division 238, 288
regeneration 52, 163, 165, 196, 197, 219, 223
regeneration, permanent 161
Reinhardt 13
Reinke 210
Remak 46, 214
rest pause, see interphase
retinoblastoma 86
Retzius 174
"revolt against morphology" 114
1848 revolution 9, 34
Rhenish Provincial Assembly 4
Ribbert, Moritz 83, 91, 117, 145, 169, 172-175, 212, 241, 259, 291, 299, 316
Richtungskörperchen, see polar bodies
rickets 311
Rodolphi 12
Roger 159
Rokitansky 45
Rosa 300
Rous, Peyton 111, 314
Roux, Wilhelm xvii, 47, 135, 137, 234, 308
Royer-Collard 61
Rudolph Virchow Hospital 9, 15

Salamandra maculata 190
Salix purpura 139
sarcomata 84, 150, 152, 177, 239, 240, 242, 256
Schelling, Friedrich Wilhelm Joseph von 28, 37

369

Schimmelbusch 194
Schleiden 44
Schmidt, Herman 161, 186, 212
Schneider 161, 190
Schopenhauer, Arthur 27, 36
Schottländer 64ff (article summarised), 125, 134, 150, 154, 174, 257
Schütz 155, 165, 167, 210
Schwann 12, 44
Schwarz 205
sclerosis of the skin 164
Scott 300
secretion 161, 162, 296
secretion, internal 306
sectioning 42
selenium 315
seminum morbii 59, 279
Society for the Encouragement of Industriousness 4
somatic mutation 107, 109
specialisation 77
specificity of cells, see cells, specificity of
specificity of cells, lineage fidelity, see cells, lineage fidelity
specificity of cell divisions, see cell divisions, specificity of
Spencer, Herbert 33, 39, 86, 89, 305
sperm 47, 78
spindles 152, 202
spindles, bent 202
Stahl 26, 58
staining *en bloc* 133
staining of histological sections 42, 192
starvation 164
Sticker 305
Strassburger 63, 161, 183
Streitkultur 27, 45
Ströbe 169, 170, 175, 176, 210, 259
stroma 242
Sturm und Drang movement 37
Sublimate (mercuric chloride) 42, 145, 191, 192
survival of the fittest 33
Swammerdam 43

tar 111
therapeutics 281
Thiersch 6, 13, 242, 255
Thiroloix 227
Thomasius, Christian 27, 36
three-dimensional microscopical study 175

thyroid gland 225
thyroid secretion 308
tissue changes in carcinomas as effects of anaplasia 255
toxins 280
transition images 185, 188, 212
transplantation experiments 76, 138, 221
transplanted tissue 249
traumatic theory 294
traumatic theory as envisaged by Virchow 60
tripartite divisions of nuclei 281
tuberculin 277
tuberculin test 278
tumour cells, see also anaplasia
tumour cells, intra-tumoural morphological heterogeneity 87
tumour cells, motility of 248
tumour fragments in urine 177
tumour progression 84
tumour suppressor genes 86, 110
tumours, transplantable in mice 304, 305

Ultramontane movement 16
unequal egg cleavage 215, 218, 235
unicentricity of tumours 292
University of Berlin, medical faculty 12

van Beneden 161
variation in plants and animals under domestication 26, 32
Vasale 161, 195
Verborn 308
Vierordt 228
Virchow, Rudolph 7, 8, 13, 14, 20, 25, 32, 34, 38, 41, 45, 46, 50, 52, 53, 55, 63, 73, 85-87, 89, 94, 113-115, 123, 126, 138, 141, 159, 160, 165, 177, 182, 185, 187, 215, 233, 238, 248, 279-281, 283, 293, 296, 299, 300, 306, 311 (see also Table of Contents for major discussions)
Virchow, interest in anthropology 13
Virchow, personality 8
Virchow, his thinking 28
Virchow's Archives 13
Virchowism 295
vitalism 26
Vorländer, Daniel 5
Vorländer, Mathilde 5

Wagner, E.L. 6

Index

Wagner, Richard   27, 37
Waldeyer   63, 190, 236, 248, 281
Walker   104, 288, 290
Wallace, Alfred Russell   31, 38
Weigert, Carl   6, 7, 12
Weismann, August   49, 50, 79, 139, 169
Whitman, R.C.   106 (extracts of article), 119
Wilberforce, Samuel   38
Willis, Rupert Allan   108, 119
Wolff, Caspar   27, 36, 46, 71, 101
World War I   10
Wright   108

Wundt, Wilhelm   12

Xenophanes   30
X-ray examinations   311
X-ray therapy, fractionation of dosage   315

Zeiss   43
Ziegler   187, 241
Zollverein, see German Customs Union
"Zoonomia"   30, 37
zygote   78